Dermatology
at a Glance

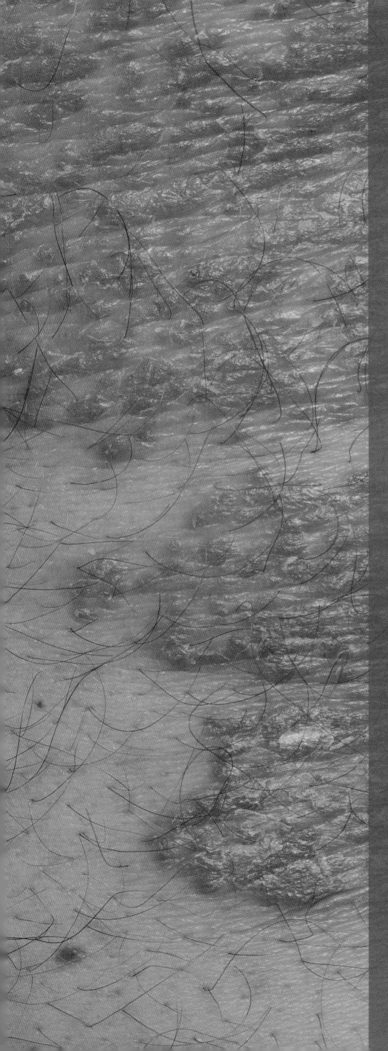

Dermatology at a Glance

Second Edition

Mahbub M.U. Chowdhury
MBChB, FRCP, FAcadMEd
Consultant Dermatologist and Honorary Senior Lecturer
The Welsh Institute of Dermatology
University Hospital of Wales
Cardiff, UK

Ruwani P. Katugampola
BM, FRCP, MD (Cardiff)
Consultant Dermatologist
The Welsh Institute of Dermatology
University Hospital of Wales
Cardiff, UK

Andrew Y. Finlay
CBE, MBBS, FRCP (London), FRCP (Glasgow)
Professor of Dermatology
Division of Infection and Immunity
Cardiff University School of Medicine
Cardiff, UK

WILEY Blackwell

Registered Offices
John Wiley & Sons, Inc., 111 River Street, Hoboken, NJ 07030, USA
John Wiley & Sons Ltd, The Atrium, Southern Gate, Chichester, West Sussex, PO19 8SQ, UK

Editorial Office
9600 Garsington Road, Oxford, OX4 2DQ, UK

For details of our global editorial offices, customer services, and more information about Wiley products visit us at www.wiley.com.

Wiley also publishes its books in a variety of electronic formats and by print-on-demand. Some content that appears in standard print versions of this book may not be available in other formats.

Library of Congress Cataloging-in-Publication Data
Names: Chowdhury, Mahbub M. U., author. | Katugampola, Ruwani P., author. |
    Finlay, Andrew Y., author.
Title: Dermatology at a glance / Mahbub M.U. Chowdhury, Ruwani P.
    Katugampola, Andrew Y. Finlay.
Description: Second edition. | Hoboken, NJ : Wiley, [2020] | Series: At a glance series | Includes
    bibliographical references and index. | Identifiers: LCCN 2019014351 (print) |
    LCCN 2019015534 (ebook) | ISBN 9781119392651 (Adobe PDF) |
    ISBN 9781119392729 (ePub) | ISBN 9781119392613 (pbk.)
Subjects: | MESH: Skin Diseases | Dermatology–methods | Handbook
Classification: LCC RL71 (ebook) | LCC RL71 (print) | NLM WR 39 | DDC 616.5–dc23
LC record available at https://lccn.loc.gov/2019014351

Cover Design: Wiley
Cover Image: Courtesy of Cardiff and Vale NHS Trust

Set in 9.5/11.5pt Minion Pro by SPi Global, Pondicherry, India
Printed and bound in Singapore by Markono Print Media Pte Ltd

10 9 8 7 6 5 4 3 2 1

Contents

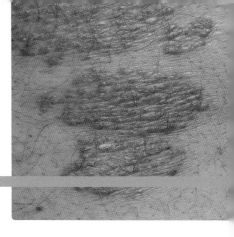

Preface to the Second Edition

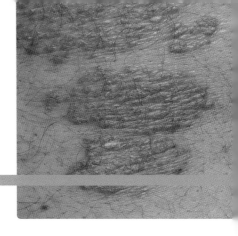

The first edition of *Dermatology at a Glance* was highly commended at the BMA Book Awards. We received excellent feedback from a wide readership including medical students, nurses, general practitioners, and postgraduate doctors, and so we decided to keep to the similar overall structure of the book for the second edition. We have included readers' suggestions such as more basic science and therapeutics, expansion of the clinical picture quiz section both online and in the book, and all diagrams, many photos and tables have been revised and enlarged for clarity where possible.

Dermatology is currently expanding at an exciting pace with new research findings and powerful new treatments such as the biologics. So we have updated all the chapters and expanded some, such as the chapters on topical drugs, psoriasis, blistering skin diseases, skin infestations, nail and hair diseases, and hereditary skin diseases. New diagrams and photos have been added where needed.

Extra chapters on dermoscopy (Dr Ausama Atwan), hidradenitis suppurativa (Dr John Ingram), cosmetic dermatology (Dr Maria Gonzalez), diagnostic pathways, systemic therapies, drug reactions, and pruritus have been added to further aid the reader in diagnosing and managing skin conditions and to stay up-to-date with new developments. The three new invited chapter authors are all working now or recently in the academic dermatology department in Cardiff. They are all recognised experts in their subject areas and have been a fantastic addition to the team.

We hope you enjoy this second edition!

Mahbub M.U. Chowdhury
Ruwani P. Katugampola
Andrew Y. Finlay
Cardiff
April 2019

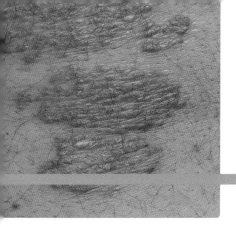

Preface to the First Edition

This book is especially designed for medical students, general practitioners, and nurses with a special interest in dermatology. You will find all the facts to help you pass dermatology undergraduate exams. It is also a great starting point when studying for higher exams such as the MRCP or MRCGP. It gives you the basics in clear, understandable language and then builds on them.

All you need to know about each topic is presented on one open spread. This attractive double page layout is an ideal format for studying and revising. This book uses all the experience that has made the 'At a Glance' series highly successful. Clear original diagrams and tables make complex subjects simple and there are over 300 clinical photographs. We have highlighted any key points and specific clinical warnings across the book. There is a Best of the Web section to guide your online dermatology searches.

Dermatology at a Glance is written by three experts in clinical dermatology, who have special expertise in skin allergy, paediatric dermatology, medical dermatology, and quality of life. They are all based in the Cardiff Dermatology Department, which is known internationally as a world leader in dermatology education (www. dermatology.org.uk).

Clinical dermatology is a fascinating subject. We hope that reading this book will help you become as enthusiastic as we are about the largest organ in the body, the skin, and its clinical challenges.

Mahbub M.U. Chowdhury
Ruwani P. Katugampola
Andrew Y. Finlay
Cardiff
January 2013

About the Authors

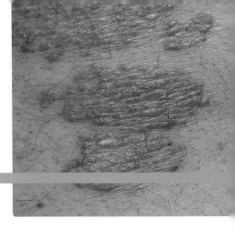

Mahbub M.U. Chowdhury MBChB, FRCP, FAcadMEd

Dr Chowdhury was Academic Vice President of the British Association of Dermatologists and Chair of the Education Subcommittee from July 2017 to 2019 and has led UK Dermatology education, research, and training policy. Since 2016, he has been Chair of the RCP Dermatology Specialty Exam Board and has played a key role in setting standards for this international exam since the inaugural exam board in 2009.

As Committee Member of the British Society for Cutaneous Allergy, he has written the postgraduate cutaneous allergy curriculum and supervised the first UK fellowship in cutaneous allergy. He is an international expert in skin allergy and has over 100 published articles and book chapters and has co-edited two other textbooks.

He has over 20 years of experience in dermatology teaching for medical and postgraduate students and was the Chairman for dermatology registrar training in Wales. His research interests include latex allergy, occupational dermatology, contact dermatitis, and medical education and training for all grades of healthcare professionals including nurses and physician associates. In recognition of his teaching and research contributions, he was appointed as Honorary Senior Lecturer at Cardiff University in 2019.

Ruwani P. Katugampola BM, MD (Cardiff), FRCP

Dr Katugampola has a special interest in paediatric dermatology and vulval dermatoses. She has over 20 published articles and book chapters. She is involved in dermatology education by teaching and examining medical students and postgraduate doctors. Her research interests include rare congenital cutaneous porphyrias.

Andrew Y. Finlay CBE, MBBS, FRCP (London and Glasgow)

Professor Andrew Finlay was Head of the Academic Dermatology Department at Cardiff University. He has been involved in dermatology education for over 40 years and created the highly successful distance-learning international Diploma in Practical Dermatology for GPs. He has led research on developing ways to measure the impact that skin disease has on people's lives and on their families: questionnaires developed by his team, such as the DLQI, are used routinely across the world. Previously President of the British Association of Dermatologists and author of 400 articles, he was awarded the British Society for Investigative Dermatology Medal for contributions to dermatology research.

Contributing Authors

Dr Ausama Atwan MD, MSc, EBDV, FAcadMEd
Specialty Doctor in Dermatology
Royal Gwent Hospital
Newport, UK
Chapter 11 Dermoscopy

Dr John R. Ingram MA, MSc, DM (Oxon), FRCP (Derm), FAcadMEd
Senior Lecturer and Honorary Consultant Dermatologist
Division of Infection and Immunity
Cardiff University
Cardiff, UK
Chapter 18 Hidradenitis Suppurativa

Dr Maria L.R. Gonzalez MBBS, DDSc, MSc (Medical Education)
Consultant Dermatologist
Specialist Skin Clinic
Cardiff, UK
Chapter 51 Cosmetic Dermatology

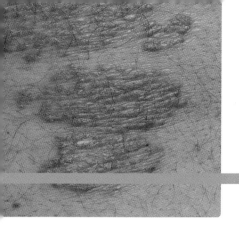

Foreword

When I was a medical student, I craved for short textbooks that would quickly give me an overview of the important things to learn in a topic such as dermatology, so that I could see the wood for the trees and get a sense of the whole rather than the details. And if that book also had lots of summary tables, key points and illustrations, I was in heaven. Thankfully, the medical students of today, and also others such as general practitioners and nurses who want a succinct overview of the important bits of dermatology, are blessed with this second edition of *Dermatology at a Glance* by Chowdhury, Katugampola and Finlay. Writing succinctly is not easy, and trying to capture each topic on a double-paged spread like the other *At a Glance* series is challenging, yet the authors have succeeded in getting the right balance of detail, evidence and patient perspectives into this practical and useful book. It is also fun to read, especially with the quiz at the end. The authors have put a lot of thought into the book structure, and as well as the traditional topic-based layout including areas such as melanoma, skin cancer, fungal infections and systemic disease, they have included sections such as 'the red face' or 'the elderly skin', or a 'child with a rash', because that is how people present in the real world. Written by a very experienced team who have delivered dermatology teaching for many years, the book is a masterpiece for entry level reading in dermatology. I commend it to all who are interested in finding out more about the skin in health and disease.

Hywel C. Williams DSc, FMedSci
Professor of Dermato-Epidemiology and Co-Director of the
Centre of Evidence-Based Dermatology, University of
Nottingham and Nottingham University Hospitals NHS Trust,
Queen's Medical Centre, Nottingham, UK

Acknowledgements

We wish to thank and acknowledge the following for their input during the preparation of both editions of this book: our patients for having given signed permission for their clinical images to be published and our consultant colleagues for the use of clinical images of their patients including Dr Mazin Alfaham, Dr Rim Al-Samsam, Professor Alex Anstey, Dr Phil Atkins, Dr J. Davies, Dr Maria Gonzalez, Professor Keith Harding, Dr Peter Holt, Dr Manju Kalavala, Professor Mike Lewis, Dr Colin Long, Dr Andrew Morris, Dr Catherine Roberts, Dr Rachel Abbott, Dr Richard Motley, Dr Julian Nash, Dr Girish Patel, Professor Vincent Piguet, Dr Hamsaraj Shetty, Dr Graham Shortland, Dr David Tuthill, and Mr Patrick Watts. We would like to thank Dr Kenneth May for preparing the histology illustrations and Miss Fiona Ruge for the direct immunofluorescence images. We would like to thank all recent surgical fellows and specialist registrars, Sister Beverly Gambles, Sister Sue Parkes, and Dr Dev Shah for their help with obtaining specific photographs.

We would especially like to thank the clinical photographers of the Media Resources Centre, University Hospital of Wales, Cardiff, for taking all of the clinical images and the Cardiff and Vale University Local Health Board, the copyright owner of all of the clinical images in this book, for permission to reproduce these images. We wish to thank the British Association of Dermatologists for permission to reproduce the photograph of Dr John Pringle. We also thank Mosby Elsevier for permission to reproduce figures from Chapter 7, Systemic therapy (Dr R.E.A. Williams) and Chapter 12, Surgical Techniques (Dr P.J.A. Holt) In: Finlay and Chowdhury (2007: 118, 221, 224, 234, 240). We thank Wounds UK for permission to reproduce the table published in: Newton (2011).

We would also like to thank our dedicated nursing staff in the Dermatology Day Treatment Unit, University Hospital of Wales, Cardiff, for organising photographs of practical treatments and phototherapy.

Karen Moore provided excellent editorial support throughout the preparation of the first edition of the book and we would like to thank her colleagues and the artists for the superb artwork. For the second edition, we would like to thank James Watson, Yoga Mohanakrishnan, Fionnguala Sherry-Brennan, and Monisha Swaminathan for their support and guidance.

We would like to thank all of our UK and international visiting medical students who have inspired us to write this book for future generations of doctors.

Last, but not least, we wish to thank our families for their unfailing long-term patience and support during the preparation of this book and this new edition.

Conflict of Interests

Andrew Y. Finlay is joint copyright owner of the DLQI, CDLQI, FDLQI, FROM-16 and other quality of life measures: Cardiff University and Andrew Y. Finlay receive royalties from their use. Andrew Y. Finlay has been a paid consultant on advisory boards to pharmaceutical companies who market biologics for psoriasis, including Novartis, Eli Lilly, and Sanofi. Mahbub M. Chowdhury has been a paid consultant on advisory boards for pharmaceutical companies marketing hand eczema and psoriasis treatments including Basilea and Leo. Mahbub M. Chowdhury is paid as Associate Editor for Essential Evidence Plus website updating 80 dermatology modules annually. Ruwani Katugampola has no conflicts of interest.

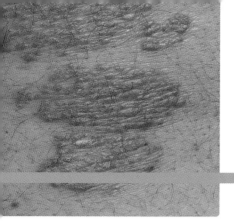

List of Abbreviations

Ab	antibody
ABPI	ankle brachial pressure index
ACD	allergic contact dermatitis
ACE	angiotensin converting enzyme
AD	atopic dermatitis
AGEP	acute generalized exanthematous pustulosis
AIDS	acquired immunodeficiency syndrome
AIP	acute intermittent porphyria
AJCC	American Joint Committee on Cancer
ANA	antinuclear antibody
ANCA	anti-neutrophil cytoplasmic antibody
AP	actinic prurigo
APC	antigen presenting cell
AR	autosomal recessive
ART	active retroviral therapy
BAD	British Association of Dermatologists
BCC	basal cell carcinoma
BJD	British Journal of Dermatology
BM	basement membrane
CAD	chronic actinic dermatitis
CDC	Centers for Disease Control and Prevention
CDLQI	children's dermatology life quality index
CEP	congenital erythropoietic porphyria
CMV	cytomegalovirus
CRP	C-reactive protein
CT	computed tomography
CTCL	cutaneous T cell lymphoma
CXR	chest x-ray
CYA	ciclosporin A
DHFR	dihydrofolate reductase
DLE	discoid lupus erythematosus
DLQI	dermatology life quality index
DNA	deoxyribonucleic acid
DRESS	drug reaction with eosinophilia and systemic symptoms
DVT	deep vein thrombosis
EASI	eczema area and severity index
EB	epidermolysis bullosa
ECG	electrocardiogram
EPP	erythropoietic protoporphyria
ESR	erythrocyte sedimentation rate
FBC	full blood count
FP	Fitzpatrick
FROM-16	family reported outcome measure
FTU	finger tip unit
5-FU	5-fluorouracil
GC	glucocorticoid
GCS	glucocorticosteroids
GI	gastro-intestinal
GvHD	graft versus host disease

HAART	highly active anti-retroviral treatment
HGPRT	hypoxanthine phosphoribosyl transferase
HHV	human herpes virus
HIV	human immunodeficiency virus
HPV	human papilloma virus
HS	hidradenitis suppurativa
HSV	herpes simplex virus
ICD	irritant contact dermatitis
Ig	immunoglobulin
IL	interleukin
IMF	immunofluorescence
IP	incontinentia pigmenti
IRIS	immune reconstitution inflammatory syndrome
IU	international units
KA	keratoacanthoma
KS	Kaposi's sarcoma
LASER	light amplification by stimulated emission of radiation
LP	lichen planus
LPP	lichen planopilaris
LS	lichen sclerosus
MAPK	mitogen activated protein kinase
MCC	Merkel cell carcinoma
MCP	mercaptopurine
MCV	mean corpuscular volume
MDT	multidisciplinary team
MED	minimal erythema dose
MHC	major histocompatibility complex
MI	methylisothiazolinone
MM	malignant melanoma
MMR	measles, mumps, and rubella
MRI	magnetic resonance imaging
MTX	methotrexate
NF	neurofibromatosis
NICE	National Institute for Health and Care Excellence
NMSC	non-melanoma skin cancer
NSAID	non-steroidal anti-inflammatory drug
OCD	obsessive–compulsive disorder
PASI	psoriasis area and severity index
PCP	pneumocystis carinii pneumonia
PCR	polymerase chain reaction
PCT	porphyria cutanea tarda
PD	programmed death
PDE	phosphodiesterase
PDT	photodynamic therapy
PEST	psoriasis epidemiology screening tool
PIH	post-inflammatory hyperpigmentation
PLE	polymorphic light eruption
PUPPP	pruritic urticated papules and plaques of pregnancy
PUVA	psoralen and ultraviolet A

PVL	Panton–Valentine leucocidin	STI	sexually transmitted infection
PWS	port wine stain	TB	tuberculosis
QALY	quality adjusted life year	TEN	toxic epidermal necrolysis
RAR	retinoid A receptor	TGN	thioguanine nucleotide
RAST	radioallergosorbent test	TNF	tumour necrosis factor
RNA	ribonucleic acid	TPMT	thiopurine methyltransferase
RXR	retinoid X receptor	TS	tuberous sclerosis
SC	subcutaneous	UP	urticaria pigmentosa
SCC	squamous cell carcinoma	UV	ultraviolet
SCORAD	SCORing Atopic Dermatitis	UVA	ultraviolet A
SCORTEN	SCORe of Toxic Epidermal Necrosis	UVB	ultraviolet B
SIGN	Scottish Intercollegiate Guidelines Network	UVR	ultraviolet radiation
SJS	Stevens–Johnson syndrome	VP	variegate porphyria
SLE	systemic lupus erythematosus	WCC	white cell count
SMO	smoothened receptor	XLD	X-linked dominant
SPF	sun protection factor	XLR	X-linked recessive
SSMM	superficial spreading malignant melanoma	XO	xanthine oxidase
SSSS	staphylococcal scalded skin syndrome	XP	xeroderma pigmentosa

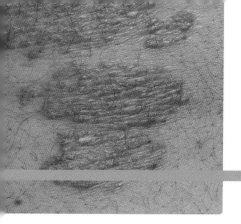

About the Companion Website

This book is accompanied by a companion website:

www.wiley.com/go/chowdhury/dermatology

Scan this QR code to visit the companion website:

The website features clinical picture quizzes and an image bank to help prepare for dermatology examinations.

Principles
of Dermatology

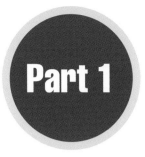

Part 1

Chapters

1 Evidence-Based Dermatology

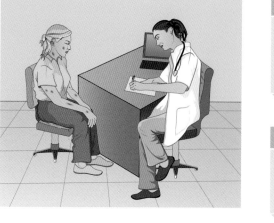

Figure 1.1 Influences on Clinical Decision-Taking.

Patient-Related Influences

- Adherence
- Worries
- Quality of life
- Age
- Family and friends
- Financial status
- Ethnicity
- Attitude and behaviour
- Education and intelligence

Disease-Related Influences

- Disease severity
- Causes and treatment
- Guidelines

Physician-Related Influences

- Influence of colleagues
- Time constraints
- Influence of pharmaceutical companies
- Experience

Practice-Related Influences

- Cost
- Practice setting
- Treatment availability
- Bureaucracy in prescribing

Influences on Clinical Decision-Taking

Drug prescription statistics across Europe show that there are vast differences in drug usage in dermatology from country to country. The diseases and the science of medicine are the same, but prescribing practice is hugely influenced by local custom and experience, habit and prejudices. There must be something wrong.

Clinical decision-taking is very complex and a wide range of issues influence the clinician (Figure 1.1). But the foundation of high-quality decision-taking should be evidence-based scientific information about the disease and its possible treatment. This information should then be tailored to the individual patient's needs, preferences, and values.

Much of the management advice given in this book is not evidence based. Some may later be shown to be incorrect. Although the authors have tried to give evidence-based information, this book gives their current opinions and some of their biases. So how could this be improved? How can clinical practice become based more on evidence and less on opinion?

Guidelines

It is helpful to have the well thought out views of others available in an easily digested form to guide you over therapy. Until recently, guidelines in dermatology and across the rest of medicine were usually written by a small group of self-appointed 'experts' who reached a consensus in discussion, based on their current practice. The likelihood of bias or missing the results of recent research was obvious. However, there has been a revolution in guideline writing. The processes are now designed to be structured and open. There is a formal literature review and guidelines are based on all the available evidence. When published, the strength of evidence

backing up each recommendation is given. There is an open process of wide consultation before final acceptance and publication, and a date for review is set, usually after three or four years.

If you read any guidelines, make sure that their production was rigorous and evidence based, such as the British Association of Dermatologists' (BAD) guidelines (www.bad.org.uk/healthcare-professionals/clinical-standards/clinical-guidelines) or the European Dermatology Forum guidelines (www.euroderm.org).

Systematic Reviews

A systematic review is a very detailed structured literature review that aims to answer a specific research or therapy question. By having clear criteria for papers that will or will not be included and by searching very widely for all possible papers, it is possible to be confident in the results of such reviews. The study results may be combined by a process of meta-analysis. The Cochrane Group, named after the Cardiff chest physician and epidemiologist, coordinates and publishes these reviews: the Cochrane Skin Group reviews are at http://skin.cochrane.org.

UK Clinical Trials Network

If a drug works really well, the number of patients needed to prove effectiveness is very small. Only a handful of patients were needed to demonstrate that isotretinoin works in severe acne. But most advances in treatment are of smaller additional benefit and large double-blind trials are essential.

The problem is that there are over 2000 different skin diseases: a dermatologist may only see some of these once every few years. It is impossible in a single centre to carry out prospective double-blind trials on such uncommon conditions.

Dermatology at a Glance, Second Edition. Mahbub M.U. Chowdhury, Ruwani P. Katugampola, and Andrew Y. Finlay.
© 2020 John Wiley & Sons Ltd. Published 2020 by John Wiley & Sons Ltd.
Companion website: www.wiley.com/go/chowdhury/dermatology

It is also very costly. Many important clinical questions therefore remain unanswered.

So what can be done? The UK Dermatology Clinical Trials Network is based at the Centre of Evidence Based Dermatology at Nottingham University, led by Professor Hywel Williams. The network allows large numbers of dermatologists across the UK to contribute to high quality clinical studies. Key clinical questions can now be answered about rare conditions or about common conditions that no pharmaceutical company is interested in funding.

Key Points

- Clinical decisions should ideally be based on evidence.
- Systematic reviews identify current evidence and knowledge gaps.

Dermatology: The Best on the Web

Free Open Access Journals

Acta Dermato-Venereologica: http://www.medicaljournals.se/acta
BMC Dermatology: http://www.biomedcentral.com/bmcdermatol
Dermatology Online Journal: http://dermatology.cdlib.org
Many others at Directory of Open Access Journals: www.doaj.org
and at: http://www.openaccessjournals.com/dermatology-journals.html

Detailed Information About Skin Diseases

American Academy of Dermatology: http://www.aad.org
New Zealand Dermatological Society (DermNet NZ): http://dermnetnz.org
eMedicine on Dermatology: http://emedicine.medscape.com

Dermatology Images

DermIS: Universities of Heidelberg and Erlangen: www.dermis.net
Global Skin Atlas: www.globalskinatlas.com
Interactive Medical Media (US company): www.dermnet.com

Clinical Guidelines

British Association of Dermatologists. Evidence-based guidelines, more than 25 topics: www.bad.org.uk/healthcare-professionals/clinical-standards/clinical-guidelines
European Guidelines: European Dermatology Forum, more than 45 topics: http://www.euroderm.org

Quality of Life Questionnaires, including DLQI

Division of Infection and Immunity, Cardiff University: https://www.cardiff.ac.uk/medicine/resources/dermatology-questionnaires

Evidence-Based Dermatology

Centre of Evidence Based Dermatology, Nottingham University: www.nottingham.ac.uk/research/groups/cebd/index.aspx
Cochrane Skin Group: evidence-based dermatology reviews: http://skin.cochrane.org
UK Dermatology Clinical Trials Network: www.ukdctn.org

Patient Support Groups

British Association of Dermatologists list, more than 60 UK groups: www.bad.org.uk/for-the-public/patient-support-groups
Changing Faces: www.changingfaces.org.uk
National Eczema Society: www.eczema.org
Psoriasis Association: http://www.psoriasis-association.org.uk
Vitiligo Society: www.vitiligosociety.org.uk

Patient Information Leaflets

British Association of Dermatologists, more than 170 leaflets: www.bad.org.uk/for-the-public/patient-information-leaflets

Resources for Medical Students

British Association of Dermatologists: excellent online resources and information aimed at medical students: www.bad.org.uk/healthcare-professionals/education/medical-students
BAD undergraduate essay prize, and BAD Undergraduate dermatology project/elective grants: www.bad.org.uk/healthcare-professionals/education/medical-students/undergraduate-awards
Chiang, N. and Verbov, J. (2014). *Dermatology: A Handbook for Medical Students and Junior Doctors*. British Association of Dermatologists (BAD). A 72-page free book online aimed at UK medical students. www.bad.org.uk/healthcare-professionals/education/medical-students
DermSchool: annual national dermatology meeting for medical students: www.bad.org.uk/healthcare-professionals/education/medical-students/dermschool-event
DermSoc. How to set up a medical student dermatology society in your medical school: www.bad.org.uk/healthcare-professionals/education/medical-students/dermsoc
DOIT: European e-learning platform for medical students (medical schools need to register): http://www.cyberderm.net/en/home/start.html
Intranet lectures for medical students: www.bad.org.uk/healthcare-professionals/education/medical-students/intranet-lectures-for-medical-students
Rees, J. Skin Cancer 909: A Textbook of Skin Cancer for Medical Students. Free book online aimed at medical students. http://skincancer909.com

Dermatology News and Reference

Medscape: US-based news and reference: http://emedicine.medscape.com/dermatology

e-Learning Sample Sessions

Department of Health and BAD project: five open access sessions: http://www.e-lfh.org.uk/programmes/dermatology/sample-sessions

Free iPhone Apps

British Association of Dermatologists' free learning tool for medical students: https://itunes.apple.com/gb/app/dermatology-medical-student/id670207116?mt=8
My Psoriasis (MyPso). For patients to track their psoriasis activity. (Funder Leo.)
Psoriasis 360. PASI and DLQI calculator by Janssen EMEA (Cardiff University app).
PsoriasisTx. Advancing psoriasis and psoriatic arthritis management. (Curatio CME Institute.)
References On Tap (previously PubMed On Tap).
SCORAD Index Linkwave. Measures eczema (calculator in English).
Skin and Allergy News: The latest dermatology news.
Virtual Dermatoscope (Cardiff University app).

Dermatology at a Glance, Second Edition. Mahbub M.U. Chowdhury, Ruwani P. Katugampola, and Andrew Y. Finlay.
© 2020 John Wiley & Sons Ltd. Published 2020 by John Wiley & Sons Ltd.
Companion website: www.wiley.com/go/chowdhury/dermatology

Free Android Apps

Dermatology Glossary
    Fitzpatrick's Dermatology Flashcards
    Dermatology In-Review
    Practical Dermatology

Subscription Services

Essential Evidence Plus: evidence-based clinical support system www.essentialevidenceplus.com

Dermatology Postgraduate Distance Learning Course

MSc, PgDip in Practical Dermatology (distance learning), Cardiff University
    MSc in Clinical Dermatology (full-time), Cardiff University: https://www.cardiff.ac.uk/medicine/courses/postgraduate-taught

3 Dermatology: Then and Now

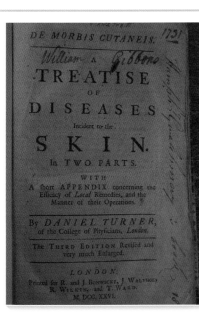

Figure 3.1 Frontispiece of the first dermatology textbook in English, 1726 edition, by Daniel Turner.

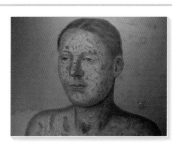

Figure 3.2 Pemphigus foliaceus, from *Atlas of Skin Diseases*, Sydenham Society, late nineteenth century.

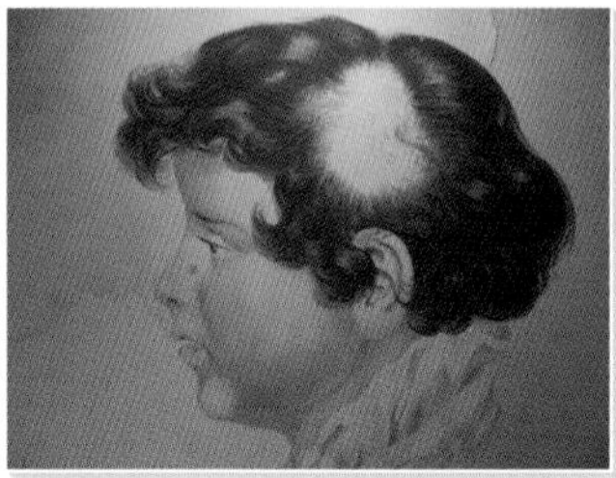

Figure 3.3 Alopecia areata, from *Atlas of Skin Diseases*, Sydenham Society, late nineteenth century.

Figure 3.4 'Cleopatra's Needle'. The plaque commemorates the dermatologist Sir Erasmus Wilson, who transported this 3450-year-old Luxor obelisk to the Embankment, London, in 1877.

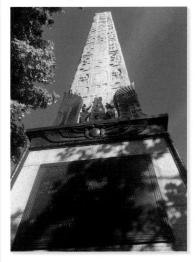

Figure 3.5 Dr John Pringle (1855–1923), who described adenoma sebaceum, 'Pringle's disease'.

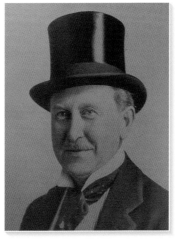

Figure 3.6 Moulage of lupus vulgaris and cutaneous horn, from John Pringle's 1903 translation of *Jacobi's Portfolio of Dermochromes*.

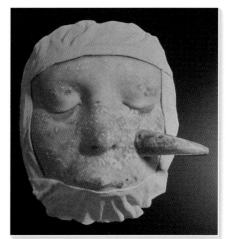

Table 3.1 Key figures of twentieth-century dermatology.

Sir Archibald Grey (1880–1967) – founded the British Association of Dermatologists in 1921.

Dr Geoffrey Dowling (1891–1976) – an exceptional clinician and clear thinker who influenced a generation of British dermatologists.

Dr Frederic Mohs (1910–2002) – first used histologically controlled removal of skin cancer in 1936 in Wisconsin. The technique was named after him and is described in Chapter 10.

Dr Albert Kligman (1916–2010) – US dermatologist whose career spanned the introduction of topical steroids to the recognition of topical retinoids being effective in photodamage, a word he invented. Controversial because of his use of prisoners in clinical testing in the 1950s and 1960s

Dr Arthur Rook (1918–1991) – a consultant first in Cardiff then in Cambridge, founded the *Textbook of Dermatology*, now the massive four volume standard textbook used by dermatologists worldwide.

Dermatology at a Glance, Second Edition. Mahbub M.U. Chowdhury, Ruwani P. Katugampola, and Andrew Y. Finlay.
© 2020 John Wiley & Sons Ltd. Published 2020 by John Wiley & Sons Ltd.
Companion website: www.wiley.com/go/chowdhury/dermatology

Historical Highlights

- *1572* – The first printed book on dermatology, *De Morbis Cutaneis*, was published by Geronimo Mercuriali. He later presided over a disastrous medical response to the plague in Venice in 1576.
- *Eighteenth century: Dermatology emerges as a specialty* – Skin diseases were usually dealt with by general physicians. Daniel Turner (1667–1740) trained as a surgeon, and in 1712 published the first skin disease book in English, *A Treatise of Diseases Incident to the Skin*, with detailed treatment recipes (Figure 3.1).
- *Eighteenth and nineteenth centuries: Classification war* – Across science there was a huge drive to classify, in dermatology led by Joseph Plenck (1735–1807) from Vienna. Rival French and English classifications of skin disease were published; Robert Willan's (1757–1812) system (inspired by Plenck's) eventually won. Many of the disease names are still in use, including their mistakes (e.g. mycosis fungoides meaning 'fungus fungus', now known to be a T-cell lymphoma). Willan first described erythema nodosum.

  Thomas Bateman (1778–1821) described molluscum contagiosum, alopecia areata, and senile purpura. Clinical illustrations from the *Sydenham Society Atlas* (Figures 3.2 and 3.3) are still accurate.
- *Nineteenth century: German, Austrian, and French dominance* – Many skin diseases are named after the French or German dermatologists who first described them. Austrian physician von Hebra (1816–1880) founded the influential Vienna Dermatology School and discovered the cause of scabies. In London, Erasmus Wilson (1809–1884), founded the *Journal of Cutaneous Medicine*, named lichen planus, and brought Cleopatra's Needle from Egypt to London (Figure 3.4). John Pringle described adenoma sebaceum (Figures 3.5 and 3.6).
- *The golden age of skin hospitals* – There were huge numbers of dermatology beds: L'Hôpital St Louis in Paris had 1100, of which 700 were reserved for scabies. Often ineffective topical treatment was used for psoriasis, fungal disease, syphilis, and tuberculosis.

Twentieth Century

Key figures of twentieth-century dermatology (Table 3.1).

1903: Neils Finsen was awarded the Nobel Prize for UVB treatment of lupus vulgaris (skin tuberculosis).

1920s: X-rays used for fungal skin infections and skin cancer.

1930–1950: Antibiotics conquer fatal cellulitis and tuberculosis. Goeckerman (tar + UVB) and Ingram regimes (dithranol + UVB) widely used for psoriasis.

1940s: 'Dermatology and Venereology' grew as a single specialty as the skin and mucosal problems of syphilis and gonorrhoea were so common. But in the Second World War specialists treated sexually transmitted disease in the troops and the speciality of genitourinary medicine developed from this. In Europe, only the UK, Eire, and Malta have dermatology and venereology as separate specialities.

1950s: Topical steroids: the biggest ever advance for eczema.

1960s: Griseofulvin for fungal infection.

1970: PUVA for psoriasis, and topical azoles for fungal infection.

1980s: Isotretinoin cures severe acne and ichthyoses alleviated with etretinate or acitretin. Aciclovir introduced for herpes simplex.

AIDS: explosion of HIV induced skin disease, e.g. Kaposi's sarcoma, until retrovirals introduced.

1990s: Terbinafine and itraconazole finally cure fungal infections. Ciclosporin for psoriasis, developed when psoriasis improvement was noticed after transplantation. New insight into psoriasis immunopathogenesis.

Twenty-First Century

- Biologics for psoriasis revolutionise treatment of severe psoriasis, drastically reducing need for dermatology beds. Next biologic revolution starting for eczema, hidradenitis suppurativa.
- Development of daycare treatment centres across the UK.
- Dermatology cancer therapy becomes major part of speciality.
- New subspecialities develop: cancer surgery, cutaneous allergy, photodermatology, paediatric dermatology, genital dermatology, post-transplant dermatology.
- Dermoscopy introduced as clinical diagnostic technique.
- Cosmetic dermatology grows rapidly in response to consumer/patient demand and new procedures (e.g. laser treatment).

The Spreading of Knowledge

- *Moulages* – Incredibly realistic wax 3D models of skin diseases for teaching (Figure 3.6), created from 1867 by Jules Barreta, Hôpital St Louis, Paris. Worth seeing there or at Gordon Museum, London.
- *British Journal of Dermatology (BJD)* – Founded in 1888 by Malcolm Morris and Henry Brooke, the *BJD* is one of the top dermatology journals worldwide. In 1921 Sir Archibald Grey and the *BJD* team founded the British Association of Dermatologists.
- *Journal of Investigative Dermatology* – The highest impact scientific dermatology journal, official journal of the main European, American, and Japanese scientific dermatology societies.
- *World Congress of Dermatology* – Held every five years since the first in Paris in 1889; held in London in 1896 and 1952. Now four-yearly: Vancouver 2015, Milan 2019, Singapore 2023.

Skin Disease: Cultural Aspects

- *Films* – Turner's housekeeper/lover in *Mr Turner* has a scabby skin condition. www.skinema.com describes:
  - Actors with skin conditions (e.g. Tom Cruise and acne).
  - Villains with skin conditions (e.g. Al Pacino in *Scarface*).
  - Realistic roles of ordinary people with skin disease.
- *Television* – The TV series *The Singing Detective*, a musical drama by Dennis Potter, was a focused portrayal of the anguish of severe psoriasis; Potter had psoriatic arthropathy. There were 240 references to dermatology in the 180 episodes of the comedy series *Seinfeld*, many depicting skin disease in a negative way.
- *Literature* – Psoriasis in literature is reviewed by Frans Meulenberg (1997). John Updike had psoriasis, as did the main characters of *From the Journal of a Leper* and the novel *The Centaur*. Vladimir Nabokov (author of *Lolita*) had psoriasis but mostly ignored it in his writings. In *The Unconsoled* Kazuo Ishiguro describes a man with severe skin disease.
- *Art* – Paul Klee (1879–1940), modern artist, had scleroderma, altering the way he used a paintbrush. There appears to be a basal cell carcinoma beneath Michelangelo's (1475–1564) eye in one of his self-portraits. In the *Mona Lisa* (1503) by Leonardo da Vinci, the yellow spot at the medial aspect of the left upper eyelid may be a xanthelasma: have a close look next time you are in Paris.
- *Politics* – The Canadian finance minister Jim Flaherty resigned in 2014 because of pemphigoid. The President of Ukraine, Viktor Yushchenko, was poisoned by dioxin in 2004. His face became disfigured by chloracne, with cysts and hyperpigmentation. Hidradenitis suppurativa had a major psychological effect on Karl Marx (1818–1883). Jean-Paul Marat (1743–1793) was murdered in the bath he was taking to relieve his (possible) dermatitis herpetiformis.

4 How the Skin Works

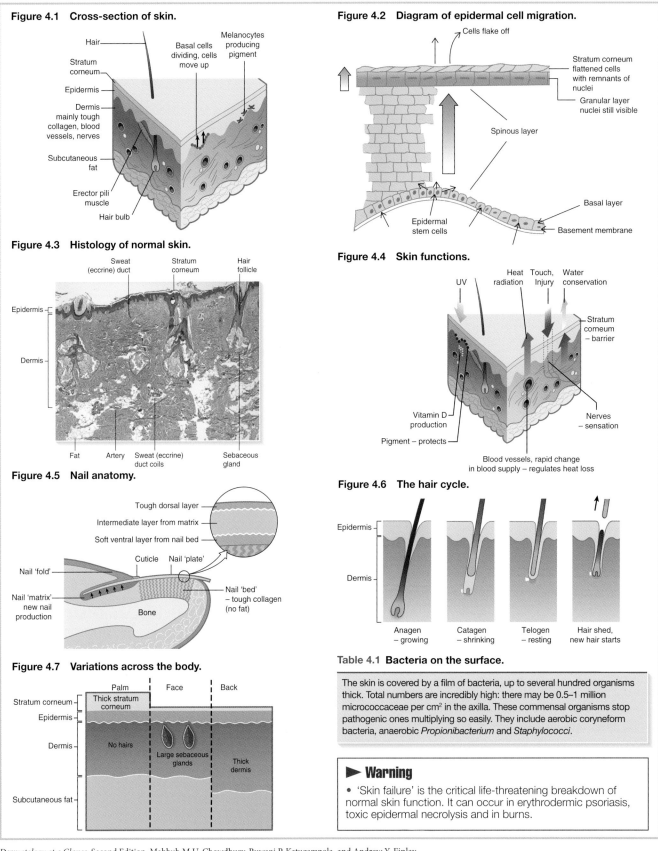

Figure 4.1 Cross-section of skin.

Figure 4.2 Diagram of epidermal cell migration.

Figure 4.3 Histology of normal skin.

Figure 4.4 Skin functions.

Figure 4.5 Nail anatomy.

Figure 4.6 The hair cycle.

Figure 4.7 Variations across the body.

Table 4.1 Bacteria on the surface.

The skin is covered by a film of bacteria, up to several hundred organisms thick. Total numbers are incredibly high: there may be 0.5–1 million micrococcaceae per cm^2 in the axilla. These commensal organisms stop pathogenic ones multiplying so easily. They include aerobic coryneform bacteria, anaerobic *Propionibacterium* and *Staphylococci*.

► **Warning**
• 'Skin failure' is the critical life-threatening breakdown of normal skin function. It can occur in erythrodermic psoriasis, toxic epidermal necrolysis and in burns.

Dermatology at a Glance, Second Edition. Mahbub M.U. Chowdhury, Ruwani P. Katugampola, and Andrew Y. Finlay.
© 2020 John Wiley & Sons Ltd. Published 2020 by John Wiley & Sons Ltd.
Companion website: www.wiley.com/go/chowdhury/dermatology

Critical Role of Evolution

Without the stratum corneum, a highly effective waterproof layer, the body would rapidly dry out and die. But the skin, at the surface between inside and out, is maximally vulnerable to trauma.

Evolution's brilliant solution is to constantly replace the stratum corneum, with a feedback mechanism so that if there is any damage, replacement rate is rapidly stepped up. Various cell 'layers' are described in the epidermis, but in reality the epidermis is dynamic. There is a constant flow of new cells produced above the dermo-epidermal junction that flatten to form the stratum corneum when they reach the top, making a new stratum corneum every month (Figure 4.2).

Ultraviolet Protection

Ultraviolet (UV) radiation from the sun can cause dermal damage and promote skin cancer. Melanocytes, positioned above the dermoepidermal junction, produce melanin in response to UV, resulting in temporary darkening, a tan. The high concentration of melanin in the deeply black skin of many African peoples provides very effective protection, whereas white skin in Northern climes allows meagre sun exposure to be sufficient for vitamin D production.

Heat Regulation

The blood flow through the dermis can be rapidly altered by valves regulating blood flow through capillaries in the upper dermis or by short-circuiting blood through dermal arterio-venous anastomoses.

If the core body temperature goes up, say during strenuous exercise, the amount of blood near the surface is massively increased, so heat radiates away from the body. The skin looks redder (flushed) because there is so much blood near the surface. If the core temperature remains too high, the sweat glands are turned on and the latent heat of evaporation results in some cooling.

If the core body temperature drops, blood supply to the skin surface is shut off. So the skin looks pale and feels cool. If this skin response is not sufficient to increase the core temperature, shivering starts and erector pili muscles contract ('goose pimples'), in a prehistoric but ineffective effort to increase the insulation.

Sensory

The range of different skin sensations includes touch, soreness, pain, itch, tickle, heat, cold, and pressure. There is an obvious protective function, for example, immediate withdrawal of a hand after feeling a dangerously hot area. These skin sensors provide critical interfaces between the body and the external world. Confirmation of limb positioning, intimate caressing, and fine finger activities such as typing on your smartphone all depend on correctly functioning skin sensations.

Vitamin D Production

Vitamin D is essential for calcium and phosphate regulation (Chapter 43). Lack of vitamin D causes rickets, poorly formed bone, typically with curved tibia, or osteomalacia. Vitamin D is in the diet, mainly in milk and eggs, or is generated in the skin by ultraviolet B (UVB) from the sun acting on 7-dehydrocholesterol. This only happens outdoors, as UVB does not go through window glass. People with dark skin who live in the north and cover up their skin risk developing rickets.

Immunological Functions

Langerhans cells in the epidermis are constantly on the alert for any unusual chemical touching the skin. New foreign chemicals are learnt by Langerhans cells, and information passed via the lymph nodes to circulating T-cells. If the chemical is encountered again, a brisk inflammatory response is triggered, 'delayed hypersensitivity', attacking the unwanted antigen (Chapter 35).

Sebaceous Glands

The sebaceous glands are active from about 15 weeks *in utero*, but quickly become smaller at birth. They do not function again until puberty. Every hair follicle has a sebaceous gland attached to it. The glandular cells fall apart in the middle of the gland to produce the sebum (i.e. holocrine secretion). The sebum then lubricates the hair shaft and the surrounding skin. Sebum may have a protective function against bacteria and fungi.

Nails

- Fingernails are evolutionary remnants of our ancestors' claws.
- Nails are still important for fine manipulations such as untying knots or starting to peel an adhesive label.
- Most societies decorate nails and diseased nails can be a handicap in those jobs where normal looking hands are important.
- Nail is produced by the nail matrix (Figure 4.5). This consists of rapidly dividing, specialised epidermal cells situated densely at the proximal end of each nail, protected by the overlying nail fold and cuticle.
- The epidermis under the nail contributes only minimally to new nail plate.
- Fingernails grow about 4 cm/year.

Regional Variation and Clinical Relevance (Figure 4.7)

- Facial skin contains very large sebaceous glands: acne, a disease of sebaceous glands, is most prominent on the face.
- Palmar and plantar skin has very thick stratum corneum with different keratin components. Genetic conditions such as tylosis (palmoplantar hyperkeratosis) can be confined to these sites.
- Where two skin surfaces come together in the body folds (flexures), the stratum corneum becomes moist and so a less efficient barrier. Superficial infections (e.g. intertrigo) occur and creams are absorbed more easily.
- The skin on the back is subject to extensive stress and has a thick dermis. Injury or surgery causes more obvious scarring.

Skin and Hair Colour

There is wide racial variation in the amount and type of pigment that is produced by melanocytes and then transferred to keratinocytes in the epidermis. The main dark pigments are eumelanins and the red–yellow pigments are phaeomelanins (seen in blond or pale-skinned individuals). Red hair also contains intensely coloured trichochromes. Red and blonde-haired people have a much higher lifetime risk of developing skin cancer.

Key Points
- Skin has several critical functions essential to life.
- Severe disease results in skin failure, high morbidity, or even death.

5 The Burden of Skin Disease

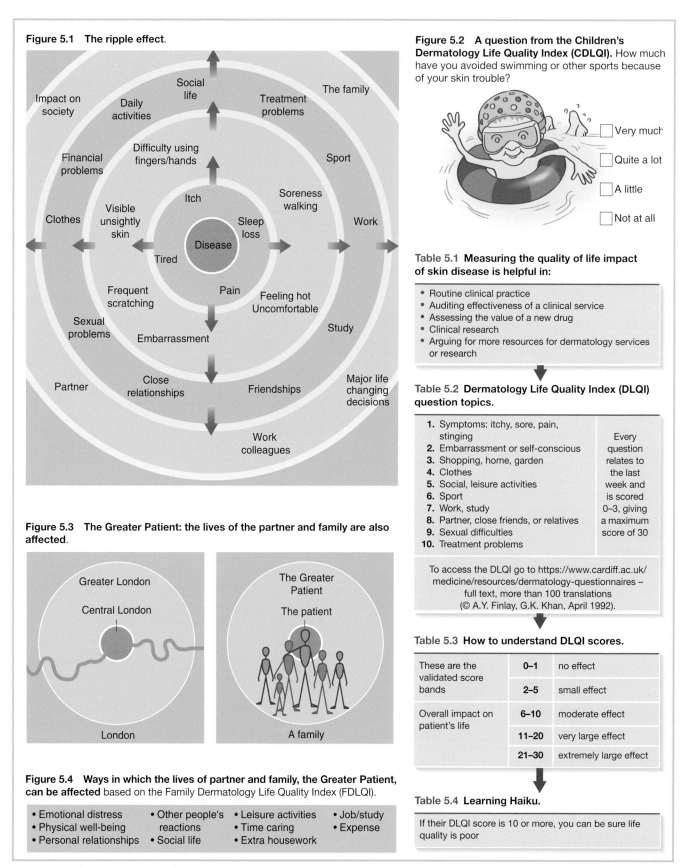

Figure 5.1 The ripple effect.

Figure 5.2 A question from the Children's Dermatology Life Quality Index (CDLQI). How much have you avoided swimming or other sports because of your skin trouble?

- Very much
- Quite a lot
- A little
- Not at all

Table 5.1 Measuring the quality of life impact of skin disease is helpful in:

- Routine clinical practice
- Auditing effectiveness of a clinical service
- Assessing the value of a new drug
- Clinical research
- Arguing for more resources for dermatology services or research

Table 5.2 Dermatology Life Quality Index (DLQI) question topics.

Question topics	
1. Symptoms: itchy, sore, pain, stinging 2. Embarrassment or self-conscious 3. Shopping, home, garden 4. Clothes 5. Social, leisure activities 6. Sport 7. Work, study 8. Partner, close friends, or relatives 9. Sexual difficulties 10. Treatment problems	Every question relates to the last week and is scored 0–3, giving a maximum score of 30

To access the DLQI go to https://www.cardiff.ac.uk/medicine/resources/dermatology-questionnaires – full text, more than 100 translations (© A.Y. Finlay, G.K. Khan, April 1992).

Figure 5.3 The Greater Patient: the lives of the partner and family are also affected.

Table 5.3 How to understand DLQI scores.

These are the validated score bands	0–1	no effect
	2–5	small effect
Overall impact on patient's life	6–10	moderate effect
	11–20	very large effect
	21–30	extremely large effect

Figure 5.4 Ways in which the lives of partner and family, the Greater Patient, can be affected based on the Family Dermatology Life Quality Index (FDLQI).

- Emotional distress
- Physical well-being
- Personal relationships
- Other people's reactions
- Social life
- Leisure activities
- Time caring
- Extra housework
- Job/study
- Expense

Table 5.4 Learning Haiku.

If their DLQI score is 10 or more, you can be sure life quality is poor

Dermatology at a Glance, Second Edition. Mahbub M.U. Chowdhury, Ruwani P. Katugampola, and Andrew Y. Finlay.
© 2020 John Wiley & Sons Ltd. Published 2020 by John Wiley & Sons Ltd.
Companion website: www.wiley.com/go/chowdhury/dermatology

How Skin Disease Affects Peoples' Lives

Many patients with skin disease experience a major impact on their quality of life, although some continue their lives as normal (Figure 5.1). Chronic inflammatory skin diseases such as severe psoriasis, eczema, acne, and hidradenitis suppurativa cause the greatest life quality impairment and disfiguring diseases such as vitiligo and alopecia areata also cause major problems. Virtually all aspects of patients' lives can be affected, including home care, shopping, choice of clothes, social activities, sport, study, work, and personal and sexual relationships. Patients experience itchiness and embarrassment, and the treatment itself, especially if topical, can add to the burden.

Understanding Patient's Quality of Life Impact Helps Clinical Practice

One of the main reasons that people seek help for their skin disease is that it is disrupting their lives. When taking clinical decisions in dermatology, clinicians are influenced by how severely they think the patient's life is affected. If you understand this impact accurately, your clinical decisions will be more appropriate. Simply ask 'How is your skin disease affecting your life at the moment?' Formal measurement with a quality of life questionnaire may be helpful (e.g. when considering prescribing a systemic therapy). If you identify psychological problems, such as depression, or the need for counselling, refer the patient for additional expertise and support.

How to Measure the Impact of Skin Disease on Life Quality

There are dermatology-specific questionnaires such as the Dermatology Life Quality Index (DLQI) or Skindex, disease-specific questionnaires, such as the Psoriasis or Acne Disability Indices, and generic measures that can be used across all diseases (Table 5.1).

Comparison with Non-skin Diseases

It is important to be able to compare the impact on quality of life of a skin disease with a non-skin disease (e.g. diabetes or ulcerative colitis), so that the burden of skin disease is understood when decisions are being taken about health care resource allocation. Generic quality of life questionnaires such as the SF-36, EuroQol, or WHO-BREV are used. Questions cover all the ways that diseases, across the whole of medicine, can affect people's lives. Severe psoriasis causes as much life quality impairment as diabetes or heart failure, using the SF-36.

Dermatology Life Quality Index

The DLQI (Tables 5.2 and 5.3) is used in many clinical research studies as a patient reported outcome measure to find out how effective treatments are, from the patient's point of view. This information complements the traditional measures of extent of disease or number of lesions, as the degree of impact experienced by a patient may not be predictable by examining the skin, but is strongly influenced by the patient's personality and attitudes, current circumstances, and their experiences of the reaction of others to their skin problem.

Rule of Tens: Using Quality of Life Scores to Help Define Disease Severity

The Rule of Tens states that if a patient with psoriasis has:
- Body surface area affected >10% (one hand surface area is equivalent to 1% body surface area, see Chapter 12) *or*
- PASI (psoriasis area and severity index score) >10 *or*
- DLQI (dermatology life quality index score) >10

then consider that the patient has severe psoriasis.

This indicates the need to consider aggressive therapy, possibly systemic. The Rule of Tens is used to guide the clinical decision whether biological therapies should be used in psoriasis.

Major Life-Changing Decisions

Skin disease not only affects patients now, but may have a profound influence on major life-changing decisions, such as what career to follow, whether to have children, or whether to move to another city or country. Having a skin disease may therefore have long-term repercussions on whole life development.

Children

Children's lives can also be severely disturbed by skin disease. School work, play, holiday activities, and choice of clothes can all be affected. The simple 10-question CDLQI, available as a text or cartoon version, measures these effects (Figure 5.2).

The Greater Patient

If a patient has a skin disease, the lives of the patient's partner and family members may also be affected (Figure 5.3). The patient (at the centre) impacts on the Greater Patient (the partner and/or affected family members). Parents of a child with severe atopic dermatitis have disturbed sleep and family activities have to be curtailed; the partner of a man with severe psoriasis finds that her social and sexual life is affected. This secondary effect on the Greater Patient can be measured using the FDLQI (Figure 5.4) or the Family Reported Outcome Measure (FROM-16).

Utility Measures

This is a way of 'converting' life impairment experienced by a patient into hypothetical cash, time, or lifespan equivalents.

Example – 88% of people with acne attending a hospital clinic would rather have a cure for their acne than be given £500.

Quality adjusted life years (QALY) are used as a method of calculating the benefit of a treatment, so that the benefit can be compared with the benefit from other interventions and also with its cost.

Key Points
- Try to understand both the patient's and the relative's experience and think of ways to improve their situation.
- Remember to use the routine question 'How much is your skin disease affecting your life at the moment?'
- Measurement of skin disease impact may help improve decisions.

▶ **Warning**
- Don't rely on guesswork to understand how your patient's life is affected by the skin disease – ask!

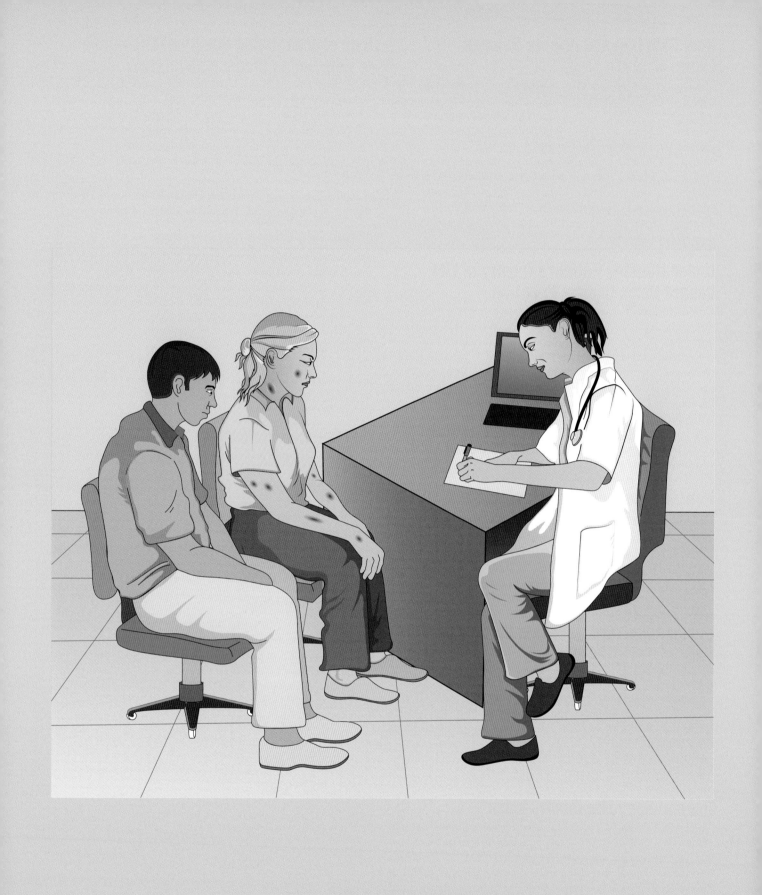

The Patient Consultation

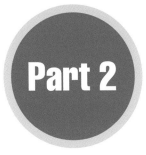

Part 2

14

Part 2 The Patient Consultation

6 Taking the History

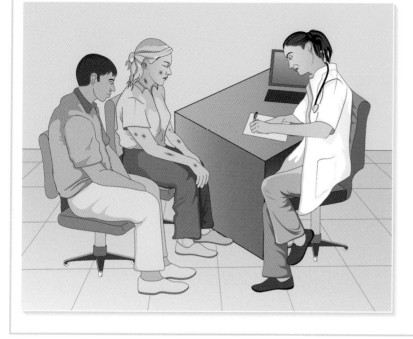

Figure 6.1 For the next few minutes, my only concern is the patient in this room. I won't let anything distract me, and I will focus and attend to this patient, making sure they feel cared for and respected (Feldman, 2010).

Table 6.1 Key questions when discharging an outpatient.

Are arrangements in place in case further support needed?
Is the patient happy to be discharged?
Has the patient been taught to self-manage?
Has the GP been fully informed?

Why Taking a History is Important

Skin disease is very visible. Most doctors (despite protesting ignorance) can instantly diagnose several common skin diseases. There are several hundred rarer skin conditions that dermatologists rapidly recognise: this is one of the attractions and satisfactions of clinical dermatology. So why bother with a history?

- Taking an accurate history is at the heart of good medicine.
- If you don't take an accurate history you will miss vital information.
- You need to know about the previous history of the skin condition and its response to treatment to be able to judge what therapy should be suggested.
- You can't tell how much the patient's life is being affected by just examining the skin.
- You need to know what drugs the patient is taking because they may have caused or be making the skin condition worse. The drugs you plan to prescribe for the patient's skin disease may be contraindicated or interact with their current medication.
- You need to know the family history in case there is a genetic aspect to the condition or in case the condition is infectious.
- You need to know about the impact of the patient's work on the skin condition and the influence of the skin condition on the patient's ability to work.
- You need to know about associated conditions such as atopic diseases or diabetes.
- You need to be able to assess the psychological impact of the disease. Is the patient depressed because of the skin problem? Are they particularly worried about the medication you are planning to prescribe to them, or about a procedure you plan to perform on them?

- You need to know about the family to assess how much support is available for the treatment you may suggest.

Patients are eager to show you their skin problem straight away ('the rolled up trouser leg syndrome'). If so, look briefly but carefully and explain that you want to ask a few questions before you examine them fully.

Structured History Taking

Introduction
- Use general open question (e.g. 'What is the problem?')

Current Complaint
- When started?
- Course of disease (steady, intermittent)?
- Main symptoms?
- Which areas are affected?
- What makes it better or worse?

Past Medical History
- Details of previous skin disease
- Ask about common skin diseases (e.g. eczema, psoriasis, acne).
- Ask about common systemic diseases with skin manifestations (e.g. diabetes, TB, immunosuppression, and/or HIV).

Drugs and Allergies
- Current topical and systemic drugs.
- Other topical and systemic drugs used in the past for skin disease and their benefit.

Dermatology at a Glance, Second Edition. Mahbub M.U. Chowdhury, Ruwani P. Katugampola, and Andrew Y. Finlay.
© 2020 John Wiley & Sons Ltd. Published 2020 by John Wiley & Sons Ltd.
Companion website: www.wiley.com/go/chowdhury/dermatology

- History suggesting contact allergy (e.g. nickel, perfume).
- History of allergy to systemic drugs.
- History of immediate allergy (e.g. latex).

Social History
- Current impact of skin disease on life and work?
- Impact of work on skin disease?
- Alcohol? (alcoholism is a risk factor in worsening of psoriasis).
- Smoker? (smoking is strongly associated with palmoplantar pustulosis and hidradenitis suppurativa).
- History of high sun exposure or sunbed use?

Family History
- Eczema, asthma, hay fever?
- Psoriasis?
- Genetic disease?
- Skin cancer?

Key Points to a Successful Consultation
- Greet the patient by name and introduce yourself.
- Address the patient appropriately and respectfully. Do not assume that using the patient's first name will always make them feel at ease, it may be perceived as over-familiar.
- Initially let the patient talk uninterrupted. Patients will talk only for a few minutes on average. This saves time later and the patient feels happy to have told you what is important to them.
- Listen to the patient.
- Repeat your understanding of the key information the patient has given you.
- Sit at the same height as the patient, at an angle, not divided by desk or computer.
- Have lots of eye contact with the patient.
- Check that the patient understands what you are saying to them.
- Seek permission from the patient for students to be present.

Special Circumstances

Children
Although the main history comes from the parent, involve the child. Does the child really want treatment for that wart, or is it just the parent?

Elderly
The elderly usually need more time. Accept it. You may need to speak more slowly and clearly. The elderly may have their own ideas about what is best for them. Listen, they are often right.

Language and Translations
If a person needs a translator, look around the clinic staff and students for someone fluent. You may need to rebook the appointment when a translator can be there to ensure that you can communicate. When speaking through a translator still speak directly to the patient and also use sign 'language' to give your meaning directly to the patient.

Adolescents
- Try to empathise.
- Try to imagine what it is like for them, even though they might appear to be rude or difficult.
- Speak to them, not to the parent.
- Indicate subtly that you are listening to them and taking their side when a disagreement breaks out with a parent.
- Be aggressive with treatment, show that you want them to get results.
- Be aware of potential major adherence problems.

History Taking with Experience
Experience will allow 'homing in' on critical relevant information. However, do not be over-confident: you still need to have a structure to ensure you do not miss relevant information.

Why Recording the History is Important
Clinical Reasons
- To avoid repetitive history taking.
- Quality control that you have covered all key aspects of history.
- Clear record of current drugs and dosages.
- Comparative purposes for future consultations.

Medico-Legal Reasons
- Evidence that a careful history was taken.
- Evidence that particular information was given.

Multi-Tasking in the Clinic
Apart from the core business of history taking, patient examination, and clinical decision-taking, there are many demands on time in the clinic. You need to learn to address these but always place the patient at the centre of them.
- Seek permission for teaching, do not assume it.
- If you need to discuss matters with a colleague, explain to the patient why this may help them.
- You may need to answer a phone to silence it ringing, but explain to the caller that you will phone them back after the consultation.
- If you must take the call, ask the patient and explain why.
- The patient will approve of you seeking more information online or from books if you give a running commentary.
- Dictating letters about a patient in front of them, and copying the letter to the patient, can be very helpful to a consultation: the patient knows that the letter has definitely been written. This also gives the patient the opportunity to flag up any mistakes.
- Manage clinic issues between patients, not during consultations.

How to Take Clinical Decisions: The Art of Medicine
To take a clinical decision you need accurate information from a detailed history and examination. Decisions should be informed by scientific evidence. Local and national guidelines seek to provide evidence-based guidelines based on the most reliable relevant science (Chapter 1).

But there are many non-scientific influences on decision-taking: some influences are good, others bad. Non-clinical influences are patient, clinician, and practice related. Examples include where a patient lives, intelligence, age, personality, family members' influence, clinician time constraints, relationships with colleagues, and prescribing bureaucracy. You need to be aware of these influences to ensure that your decision is best for that patient.

One of the commonest decisions that a dermatologist takes is whether or not to discharge an outpatient from the clinic. To ensure that this decision is taken appropriately, the clinician should consider some key points (Table 6.1).

Processing patient information, scientific knowledge, and the other influences constitutes the art of medicine: clinical medicine is complex, challenging, and rewarding.

Key Point
- A structured history is essential for diagnosis and management.

▶ Warning
- Don't skimp on the history just because the disease is visible.

7 How to Examine the Skin

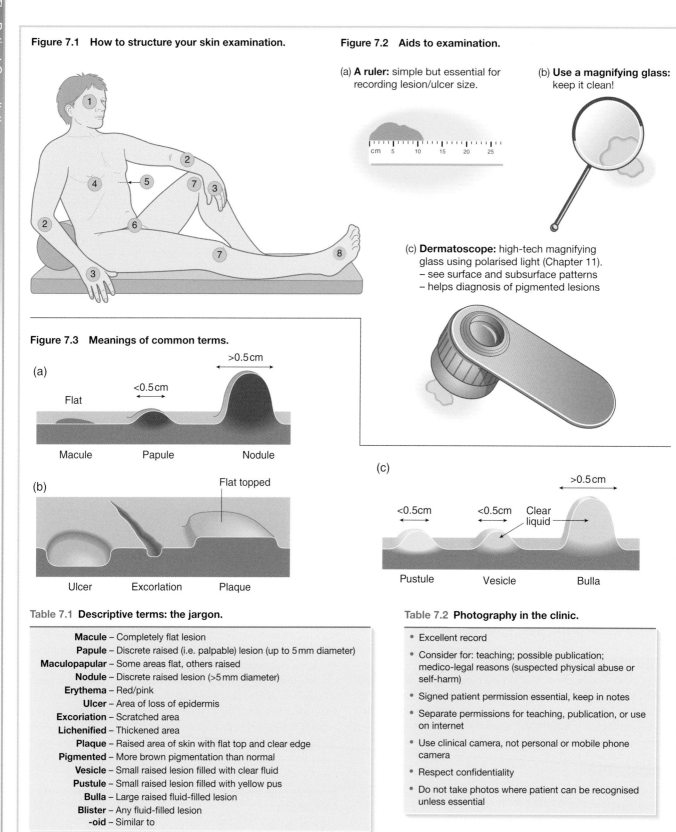

Figure 7.1   How to structure your skin examination.

Figure 7.2   Aids to examination.

(a) **A ruler:** simple but essential for recording lesion/ulcer size.

(b) **Use a magnifying glass:** keep it clean!

cm 5 10 15 20 25

(c) **Dermatoscope:** high-tech magnifying glass using polarised light (Chapter 11).
– see surface and subsurface patterns
– helps diagnosis of pigmented lesions

Figure 7.3   Meanings of common terms.

(a)

>0.5cm

<0.5cm

Flat

Macule   Papule   Nodule

(b)

Flat topped

Ulcer   Excorlation   Plaque

(c)

<0.5cm   <0.5cm   Clear liquid   >0.5cm

Pustule   Vesicle   Bulla

Table 7.1 Descriptive terms: the jargon.

Macule – Completely flat lesion
Papule – Discrete raised (i.e. palpable) lesion (up to 5 mm diameter)
Maculopapular – Some areas flat, others raised
Nodule – Discrete raised lesion (>5 mm diameter)
Erythema – Red/pink
Ulcer – Area of loss of epidermis
Excoriation – Scratched area
Lichenified – Thickened area
Plaque – Raised area of skin with flat top and clear edge
Pigmented – More brown pigmentation than normal
Vesicle – Small raised lesion filled with clear fluid
Pustule – Small raised lesion filled with yellow pus
Bulla – Large raised fluid-filled lesion
Blister – Any fluid-filled lesion
-oid – Similar to

Table 7.2 Photography in the clinic.

- Excellent record
- Consider for: teaching; possible publication; medico-legal reasons (suspected physical abuse or self-harm)
- Signed patient permission essential, keep in notes
- Separate permissions for teaching, publication, or use on internet
- Use clinical camera, not personal or mobile phone camera
- Respect confidentiality
- Do not take photos where patient can be recognised unless essential

Dermatology at a Glance, Second Edition. Mahbub M.U. Chowdhury, Ruwani P. Katugampola, and Andrew Y. Finlay.
© 2020 John Wiley & Sons Ltd. Published 2020 by John Wiley & Sons Ltd.
Companion website: www.wiley.com/go/chowdhury/dermatology

Examination Optimal Conditions

First you need to get the patient in the best position to be examined:
- Privacy
- Chaperone
- Patient undressed
- On a couch
- Bright light

Essential

- Willingness to examine the patient properly
- Thinking seeing (not just looking)
- Ruler handy (Figure 7.2)
- Magnifying glass and dermatoscope available (Figure 7.2)

Simple Structure

You need a simple structure to make sure that you have seen all the skin. 'Start at the top and work your way down' (Figure 7.1).

Scalp

- Think about the scalp and the hair separately
- Feel the scalp as the hair may be too thick to see much
- Part the hair to see the scalp
- Pick up hair at the edge of the scalp to see the edge of the rash (e.g. psoriasis)
- Any baldness? If yes, any alopecia areata 'exclamation mark' hairs (Chapter 30)?
- Any scarring (flat, shiny, bald areas free of follicle openings)?
- Any unusual hair thickness or twistiness?

Ears

External Pinnae

- Signs of solar damage especially at the edge
- Scaliness suggesting seborrhoeic dermatitis
- Discrete tender area on prominent ridge suggesting chondro-dermatitis

External Auditory Meatus

- Psoriasis
- Eczema

Face

- Examine areas of maximum sun damage: forehead, upper cheeks, and nose. Any sign of skin cancer?
- Hair growth normal (also eyelashes, eyebrows)?
- Eyes: mucosal surfaces
- Lips, mouth: check tongue, gums, and buccal mucosal surface inside cheeks (e.g. white net-like pattern of lichen planus)

Neck, Axillae, and Arms

Flexures

- Axillae: erythrasma, hidradenitis suppurativa, fungal infection, flexural psoriasis, seborrhoeic dermatitis?
- Antecubital fossae: atopic eczema?

Extensors

- Elbows: psoriasis?

Hands

- Wrists: scabies?
- Finger webs: irritant contact dermatitis, scabies?
- Nails: fungal infection, psoriasis?

Trunk: Back, Chest, Abdomen, and Buttocks

- Upper trunk: acne?
- Flexures: intertrigo?
- Nipples: atopic eczema, contact dermatitis, Paget's disease?
- Umbilicus: psoriasis?

Genitalia, Perineum, Groins, and Perianal Skin

- Contact dermatitis
- Fungal infection
- Intertrigo
- Genital warts or discharge

Legs

- Flexures: atopic eczema?
- Knees: psoriasis?
- Lower legs: varicose veins?
- Ankles: venous eczema?

Feet

- Soles: pustular psoriasis?
- Toe webs: fungal infection?
- Toenails: fungal infection, onychogryphosis?

General Points: All Areas

- Hair growth pattern normal?
- Hair pigmentation normal?
- Skin pigmentation normal?
- Condition symmetrical?
- Sun damage pattern (differences covered–uncovered areas)?

Individual Lesions

- Where?
- Size: diameter?
- Colour? Variable pigment?
- Raised or flat?
- Edge: smooth or irregular? (Figure 7.3)

Recording Examination Findings

- Essential for later comparison and for medico-legal reasons
- Write down immediately main positive and negative findings
- Record lesion measurements immediately

Special Situations

- Patient shy or refuses examination
- Chaperone essential
- Try to understand patient's concern: religious, cultural, personality?
- Explain why examination is essential to provide best advice
- Sometimes patients allow examination of only one or more limited areas
- If permission refused, record this but still try to provide advice, with caveats

Key Points

- Remember to 'start at the top and work your way down'.
- Keep clear records of history and examination.

► Warning

- It's tempting to only look at the skin areas mentioned by the patient.
- If you don't examine the skin fully, you may make the wrong diagnosis or prescribe the wrong treatment.

Diagnostic Clues

Figure 8.1 Differential diagnosis of rashes based on affected body site(s).

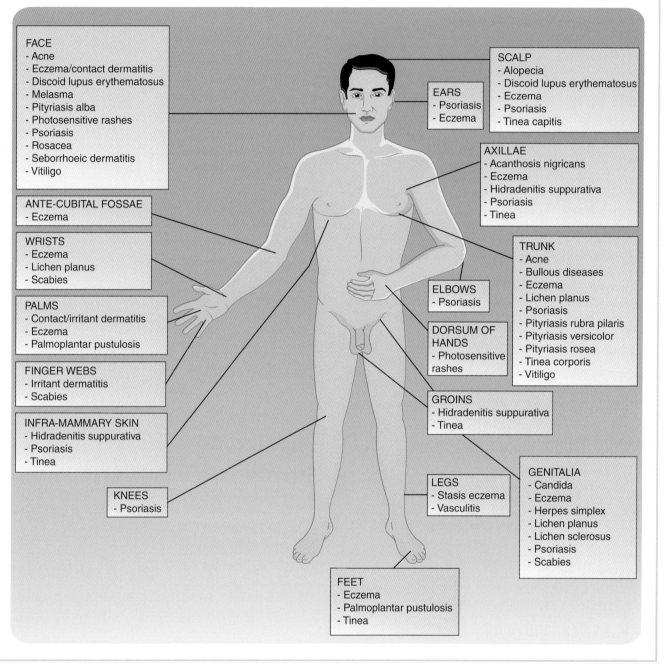

FACE
- Acne
- Eczema/contact dermatitis
- Discoid lupus erythematosus
- Melasma
- Pityriasis alba
- Photosensitive rashes
- Psoriasis
- Rosacea
- Seborrhoeic dermatitis
- Vitiligo

ANTE-CUBITAL FOSSAE
- Eczema

WRISTS
- Eczema
- Lichen planus
- Scabies

PALMS
- Contact/irritant dermatitis
- Eczema
- Palmoplantar pustulosis

FINGER WEBS
- Irritant dermatitis
- Scabies

INFRA-MAMMARY SKIN
- Hidradenitis suppurativa
- Psoriasis
- Tinea

KNEES
- Psoriasis

SCALP
- Alopecia
- Discoid lupus erythematosus
- Eczema
- Psoriasis
- Tinea capitis

EARS
- Psoriasis
- Eczema

AXILLAE
- Acanthosis nigricans
- Eczema
- Hidradenitis suppurativa
- Psoriasis
- Tinea

TRUNK
- Acne
- Bullous diseases
- Eczema
- Lichen planus
- Psoriasis
- Pityriasis rubra pilaris
- Pityriasis versicolor
- Pityriasis rosea
- Tinea corporis
- Vitiligo

ELBOWS
- Psoriasis

DORSUM OF HANDS
- Photosensitive rashes

GROINS
- Hidradenitis suppurativa
- Tinea

GENITALIA
- Candida
- Eczema
- Herpes simplex
- Lichen planus
- Lichen sclerosus
- Psoriasis
- Scabies

LEGS
- Stasis eczema
- Vasculitis

FEET
- Eczema
- Palmoplantar pustulosis
- Tinea

Dermatology at a Glance, Second Edition. Mahbub M.U. Chowdhury, Ruwani P. Katugampola, and Andrew Y. Finlay.
© 2020 John Wiley & Sons Ltd. Published 2020 by John Wiley & Sons Ltd.
Companion website: www.wiley.com/go/chowdhury/dermatology

The aim of this chapter is to help with the diagnosis of rashes and lesions based on their symptoms or characteristic features and distribution based on body site (Figure 8.1).

Itchy Rashes

Individual lesions (wheals) lasting less than 24 hours – Urticaria

Dry/scaly rash – Eczema, lichen planus, psoriasis, tinea infection, early mycosis fungoides

Burrows, papules, track marks – Scabies

Blistering rash – Bullous pemphigoid, dermatitis herpetiformis, insect bites

Skin Rashes Based on Shape of Individual Lesions

Discoid (coin shaped) – Discoid eczema, psoriasis, mycosis fungoides, discoid lupus erythematosus, tinea infection

Annular (ring-like with central clearing) – Granuloma annulare, tinea incognito

Arcuate (half-moon shaped) – Subacute cutaneous lupus erythematosus

Serpiginous (serpent-like or wavy) – Cutaneous larva migrans, elastosis perforans serpiginosa

Targetoid (resembles archer's target) – Erythema multiforme

Linear – Phytophotodermatitis

Skin Lesion Based on Colour

Skin coloured
- Soft – skin tag (fibroepithelial polyp), neurofibroma
- Warty – Seborrhoeic keratosis, viral wart
- Firm – benign intradermal naevus, dermatofibroma, keloid or hypertrophic scar, molluscum contagiosum, basal cell carcinoma

Yellow/orange – Sebaceous gland hyperplasia, xanthalasma, xanthogranuloma, pilomatrixoma

Dark brown/black – Seborrhoeic keratosis, benign melanocytic naevus, giant comedone, solar lentigo, naevus of Reed, lentigo maligna, malignant melanoma

Blue – Blue naevus, venous lake

Red – Spider naevus, pyogenic granuloma, haemangioma, Spitz naevus

Skin Lesion Based on Surface Appearance

Central dimple (umbilication) – Molluscum contagiosum

Punctum – Epidermoid cyst, pilar cyst

Dimpling – Dermatofibroma

Warty – Seborrhoeic keratosis, viral wart

Hyperkeratotic – Cutaneous horn, hyperkeratotic actinic keratosis, keratoacanthoma, squamous cell carcinoma

Ulcerated – Basal cell carcinoma, squamous cell carcinoma, pyogenic granuloma

Completely flat – freckles, vitiligo, lentigo maligna, malignant melanoma

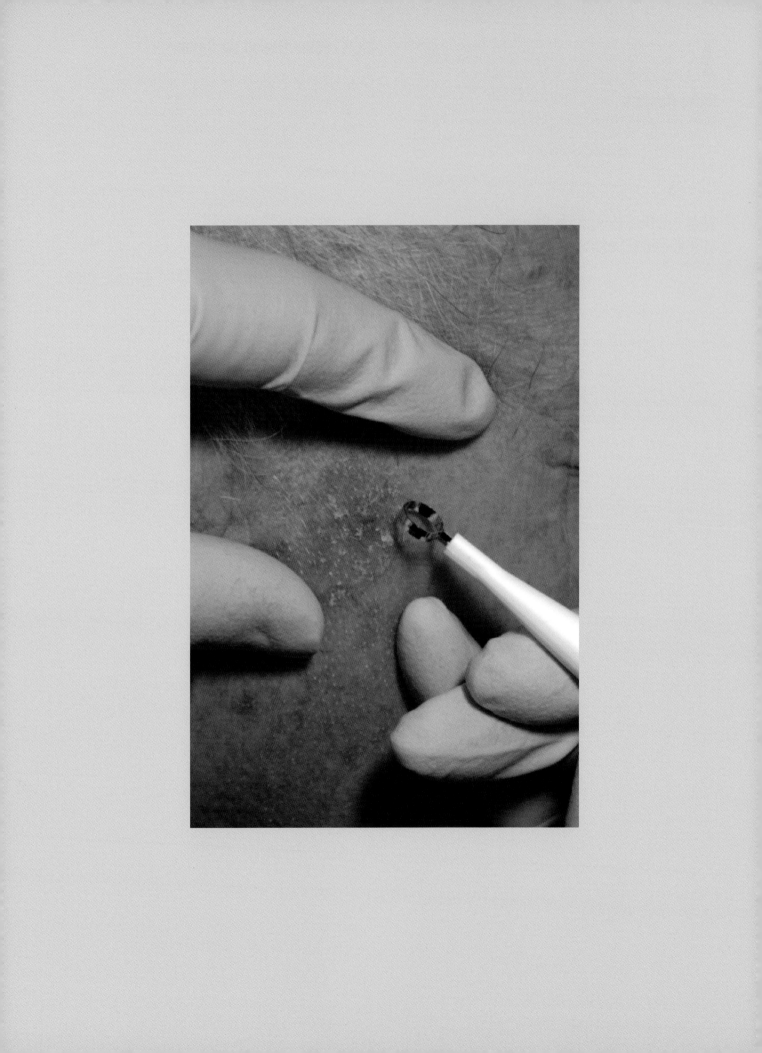

Basic Procedures

Chapters

9 Surgical Basics

Table 9.1 Pre-surgical counselling.

- Obtain informed consent, either formal verbal or written
- Explain risks, e.g. infection, bleeding, nerve damage, pigment change, recurrence of lesion
- Warn regarding type of scar and risk of keloid, e.g. on chest, shoulder
- Warn regarding limitation of use of limbs and/or time off work

Table 9.2 Surgery procedures used in dermatology.

- Shave biopsy
- Punch biopsy
- Curettage
- Incisional biopsy
- Excision

Figure 9.1 Anatomy of the face to show location of branches of the facial nerve in relation to the fascia and parotid gland, and the overlying facial and superficial temporal arteries.

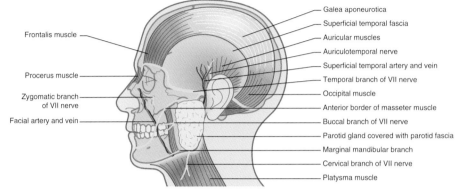

Frontalis muscle
Procerus muscle
Zygomatic branch of VII nerve
Facial artery and vein

Galea aponeurotica
Superficial temporal fascia
Auricular muscles
Auriculotemporal nerve
Superficial temporal artery and vein
Temporal branch of VII nerve
Occipital muscle
Anterior border of masseter muscle
Buccal branch of VII nerve
Parotid gland covered with parotid fascia
Marginal mandibular branch
Cervical branch of VII nerve
Platysma muscle

Figures 9.1, 9.4, 9.6 reproduced with permission from Finlay and Chowdhury (2007).

Figure 9.2 Benign mole removed by shave excision with half blade and haemostatic applied with cotton bud leaving a circular defect.

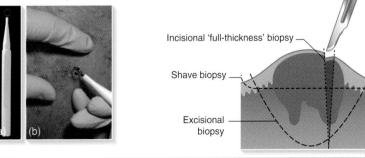

Figure 9.3 (a) **4 mm punch biopsy.** (b) **Punch biopsy on cheek.**

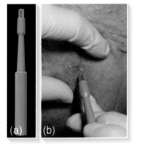

Figure 9.4 Punch biopsy: stretch the skin (a), at right angles to the intended direction of the scar (b), remove the biopsy by cutting (c), do not crush the specimen. The defect (d) is then sutured (e).

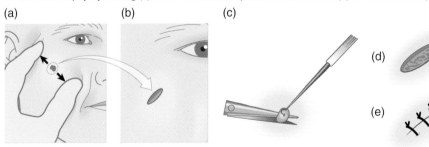

(a) (b) (c) (d) (e)

Figure 9.5 (a) **Curette.** (b) **Curette with sharp margin used on cheek.**

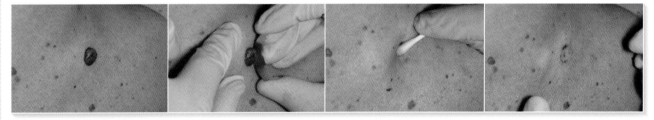

Figure 9.6 Types of skin biopsies.

Incisional 'full-thickness' biopsy
Shave biopsy
Excisional biopsy

Figure 9.7 Skin tumour marked with 5 mm margin and ready for full ellipse excision.

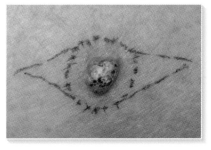

Dermatology at a Glance, Second Edition. Mahbub M.U. Chowdhury, Ruwani P. Katugampola, and Andrew Y. Finlay.
© 2020 John Wiley & Sons Ltd. Published 2020 by John Wiley & Sons Ltd.
Companion website: www.wiley.com/go/chowdhury/dermatology

The ability to perform some basic skin surgery is an essential part of a dermatologist's skills and many GPs now also undertake simple procedures. Up to 60% of referrals to dermatology may need some surgical intervention.

Preparation Prior to Surgery

Full counselling is essential prior to any surgical procedure to explain why the procedure is necessary, what will be done and possible complications (Table 9.1). This avoids any conflict and potential complaints afterwards.

Preoperative history should include past medical history and drug history including anti-coagulants (warfarin, apixaban, rivaroxaban) and anti-platelets (e.g. clopidogrel, aspirin) which may need to be stopped prior to surgery.

Basic understanding of anatomy is essential to perform surgery safely, particularly on the face and neck (e.g. branches of the facial nerve and superficial temporal arteries need to be avoided; Figure 9.1).

Local Anaesthesia

Local anaesthesia with 1 or 2% lidocaine is used with adrenaline (1 : 80 000 or 1 : 200 000) or without adrenaline. A person weighing 70 kg can have a maximum of 50 ml 1% lidocaine with 1 : 200 000 adrenaline. Adrenaline causes vasoconstriction to reduce bleeding and also increases the duration of the anaesthesia.

Use lidocaine with caution in patients taking non-selective beta-blockers as this can lead to hypertension and reflex bradycardia.

Nerve blocks use less volume and can give effective anaesthesia (e.g. supra/infraorbital). Digital ring blocks for finger anaesthesia usually use plain lidocaine without adrenaline to reduce the risk of ischaemia.

The pain of local anaesthetic injections can be reduced (e.g. in children) with the use of tetracaine gel (Ametop®) used 30 minutes preoperatively. Other tricks include using 0.5% plain lidocaine without preservative with a small gauge (30 g) needle followed by 1% lidocaine with 1 : 200 000 adrenaline.

Always check the anaesthetic has been effective before starting the procedure!

Side effects of local anaesthetic include accidental insertion and injection into blood vessels and resulting toxicity, pain, and temporary weakness of muscles (e.g. difficulty raising the eyebrows or closing the eyes after injecting the temple area).

Haemostasis

Solutions such as 20% aluminium chloride and 20% isopropyl alcohol or silver nitrate are used to stop bleeding in simple procedures (e.g. shave biopsy). Other options include electrocautery (current passing through high resistance metal), which produces heat with the cautery tip applied lightly to the wound surface. Avoid alcohol-based antiseptics when using this method because of the risk of fire.

Diathermy also generates heat by resistance to current which passes through the tissues. The use of the diathermy may include deliberate sparking with superficial damage to the skin and light scarring. If direct contact is made with the skin using the diathermy tip then the heat is produced at a deeper level and is more likely to cause scarring.

Deeper wounds can have firm pressure around the edge of the wound to stop bleeding and then be sealed with diathermy, or an absorbable suture is tied around the vessel. Electrocoagulation (bipolar AC current) can be used for deeper wounds with the current applied with forceps to the tissue and through to the vessel causing necrosis. Care must be taken with electrosurgery instruments because of possible interference with pacemakers and implantable cardioverter defibrillators. This may need to be discussed in advance with the cardiologist.

Surgical Procedures (Table 9.2)

Shave biopsy – Local anaesthetic is injected subcutaneously under the lesion without elevation. The skin is stretched firmly. A razor blade or surgical blade is then moved to and fro under the lesion to remove it, leaving a flat surface (Figure 9.2).

Punch biopsy – The skin is infiltrated with local anaesthetic around the area of biopsy. The skin is stretched at right angles to the preferred alignment of the scar (Figures 9.3 and 9.4). A 3–6 mm punch is rotated into the skin releasing the area of skin still attached to the base. This skin is lifted gently and cut beneath with sharp scissors. Suturing is with 6-0 polyamide (Ethilon®) on the face or 4-0 on the limbs. Sutures can be removed after 5–7 days for the face and 7–10 days for the trunk and limbs.

Curettage – Disposable ring curettes that have a sharp and blunt side are used (Figure 9.5). The curette's sharp side is used to separate (scrape) tumour from the underlying skin with a gentle regular sideways action under local anaesthetic.

Incisional biopsy – This is used to diagnose inflammatory skin conditions, infiltrative disorders, and skin cancers (e.g. panniculitis, vasculitis, or squamous cell carcinoma). This technique allows histological examination of the dermis and dermal–fat interface. The skin is removed as a narrow but deep wedge and sutured as in punch biopsy (Figure 9.6).

Full excision – This technique is used for full removal of skin tumours such as basal cell carcinoma, squamous cell carcinoma, and melanoma. Awareness of skin tension lines allows prediction of the best surgical scar. The skin must be marked with a sterile pen prior to local anaesthetic use. Antiseptics such as chlorhexidine 0.05% aqueous or iodine solutions can be used.

Ellipse excision ideally has a length : breadth ratio of 3 : 1 (Figure 9.7). Sutures should enter and exit the wound perpendicular to the surface and surface sutures should have minimum tension. Subcutaneous sutures include vicryl (Ethicon®) and polydioxanone (PDS®). These retain 50% of their strength at three to six weeks postoperatively. Surface sutures include Ethilon® or Prolene® from 3-0 to 6-0 (finer suture).

A dressing such as iodine (Inadine®) overlying antibiotic ointment (Polyfax®) can be used. This is followed with application of white soft paraffin (Vaseline®) daily for 7–10 days once the dressing is removed to prevent the wound from drying and crusting which tends to leave a worse scar.

Key Points
- Simple surgical procedures are now commonly undertaken for diagnosis and management.
- No surgery should be considered 'minor'.
- Give full explanation prior to the procedure.
- Warn all patients regarding possible complications such as bleeding, infection, and scarring.

▶ Warning
- Do not start the procedure unless the patient is 100% sure he or she wishes to proceed.

10 Key Procedures

Table 10.1 Some procedures used in dermatology.

- Cryotherapy
- Laser
- Botulinum toxin injections
- Iontophoresis (Chapter 13)
- Trichloroacetic acid treatment
- Mohs' micrographic surgery
- Full thickness skin graft/flap repair
- Nail surgery

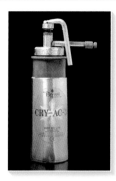

Figure 10.1 Cryogun.

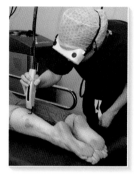

Figure 10.2 Pulse dye laser to treat vascular lesion on leg.

Figure 10.3a and b Axillary hyperhidrosis treated with multiple botulinum toxin injections.

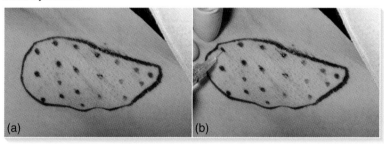

(a) (b)

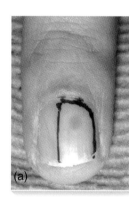

Figure 10.4a Glomus tumour under nail plate marked prior to surgery.

(a)

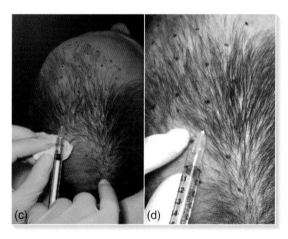

(c) (d)

Figure 10.3c and d Botulinum toxin for scalp hyperhidrosis.

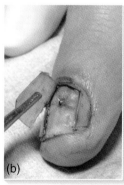

Figure 10.4b Nail reflected under ring block and biopsy taken of tumour.

(b)

Figure 10.5 Mohs' surgery. The tumour is debulked with curettage. A thin plate encompassing the entire margin and wound bed is excised. The tissue is then divided into quadrants and the cut edges marked with dye. The surgical margin is sectioned horizontally to include the epidermis and deep margins and examined under the microscope. Any tumour seen has breached the surgical margin and can be located to the exact location in the wound (quadrant b in this case). Further tissue can be removed until the surgical margins are tumour free. (Reproduced with permission from Finlay and Chowdhury 2007.)

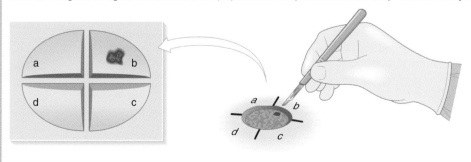

Dermatology at a Glance, Second Edition. Mahbub M.U. Chowdhury, Ruwani P. Katugampola, and Andrew Y. Finlay.
© 2020 John Wiley & Sons Ltd. Published 2020 by John Wiley & Sons Ltd.
Companion website: www.wiley.com/go/chowdhury/dermatology

This chapter describes other key procedures that are used in dermatology as listed in Table 10.1.

Cryotherapy

Liquid nitrogen cryosurgery is the most common form of cryotherapy used, with temperatures reaching down to −30°C. This achieves destruction of the tissue.

The spray technique with a cryogun is easiest to use (Figure 10.1). The aim is to achieve an ice field quickly with the spray tip held up to 1 cm away from the skin surface. Freeze times vary, with 5–10 seconds used for viral warts, solar keratoses and seborrhoeic warts. Bowen's disease, superficial basal cell carcinomas (BCC) and small squamous cell carcinomas (SCC) can be treated with 30–60 seconds and a second refreeze after thawing.

Certain tumours are not suitable for treatment with cryotherapy (e.g. morphoeic BCC, large tumours >2 cm in diameter, and ill-defined tumours).

Cryosurgery is painful and so young children less than 12 years of age may not tolerate it. Local anaesthetic can be used prior and two cycles of freezing may be needed in larger areas.

Side effects include pain, large blisters, and swelling. If plantar warts are treated they may limit walking for a few days. Hyper and hypopigmentation can occur in patients with darker skin and hence may need to be avoided in this group.

Laser (Light Amplification by Stimulated Emission of Radiation)

This has been used for many years in dermatology to treat vascular and pigmented lesions, scars, tattoos, and increased hair growth. Laser treatments are frequently requested by patients so a basic understanding is useful (Chapter 51).

Lasers currently used include CO_2, pulse dye (Figure 10.2) and erbium:YAG. The components of the laser include laser medium, optical cavity, and pumping system. Atoms in the laser medium are excited by an external source of energy into an unstable state and electrons then returning to their resting state emit energy. This energy is emitted as light which travels as photons. These photons are reflected by mirrors allowing a portion of the light to travel out of the optical cavity as a laser light delivered along fibreoptic cables. When the laser is used on the skin the light must be absorbed by the tissue for clinical effect. Chromophores (e.g. water, melanin, haemoglobin, or tattoo ink) are specifically targeted by laser light of certain wavelengths causing photothermal damage.

Vascular lesions can be treated with pulse dye laser (595 nm wavelength), KTP laser (585–595 nm), and Nd:YAG (long pulse 1320 nm). Pigmented lesions such as benign epidermal and dermal pigmented lesions can be treated where the chromophore is melanin (e.g. Nd:YAG 532–1064 nm). Tattoos can also be removed with various lasers to remove colours including black, blue, green, and red pigments. Laser resurfacing has become more popular with pulsed CO_2 and erbium:YAG lasers for photodamaged facial skin and scars.

Potential problems with lasers include discomfort, pigmentation, scarring, and infections for the patient (e.g. herpes simplex virus) and operator (e.g. human papilloma virus and HIV).

Xanthelasma Treatment

Xanthelasma can be painted with 95% trichloroacetic acid. There is a risk of this acid entering the eye and so it is applied with a cotton bud or orange stick to ensure only the area involved is treated. Repeated treatments are often necessary.

Other options for xanthelasma treatment include curettage and cautery under local anaesthetic.

Botulinum Toxin

This is used commonly for hyperhidrosis particularly in the axillary area. This can be a painful treatment but if high amounts of sweat are being produced it can be very effective. Multiple injections are required around the site affected (e.g. axilla, scalp) (Figure 10.3).

Nail Surgery

Nail surgery may be required to take biopsies of pigmented lesions and other tumours of the nail matrix and nail bed. This requires prior ring block and haemostasis is important. Special nail instruments are required to elevate the nail and to expose the nail matrix and nail bed. The centre of the lesion should be biopsied and a punch or small incisional biopsy may be sufficient for histological diagnosis (Figure 10.4).

Mohs' Micrographic Surgery

This is a method invented by Mohs in the United States to completely remove invasive BCC under histological control. The initial bulk of the tumour is removed by curettage creating a saucer-like defect. A further margin of skin is removed from the side and base of the wound and a horizontal section is taken of the surgical margin. The entire surgical margin can be examined histologically and then correlated to the area that may need further skin margins removed (Figure 10.5).

Mohs' surgery is useful for excision of BCC and SCC on the face where skin preservation is important (e.g. eyelids and nose). This is the treatment of choice for undefined margins or morphoeic BCC. It is time-consuming and expensive and requires great surgical expertise to ensure good results.

Closure may require full thickness skin grafts, skin flap repairs, or secondary intention healing.

Key Points
- Laser treatments are widely available; however, the appropriate laser needs to be determined by the type of lesion to be treated.
- Mohs' surgery is a very specialised technique used to remove ill-defined tumours at critical sites.

▶ **Warning**
- Liquid nitrogen cryotherapy is quick and easy to use but can leave disfiguring pigmentary changes and scarring.

11 Dermoscopy

Ausama Atwan

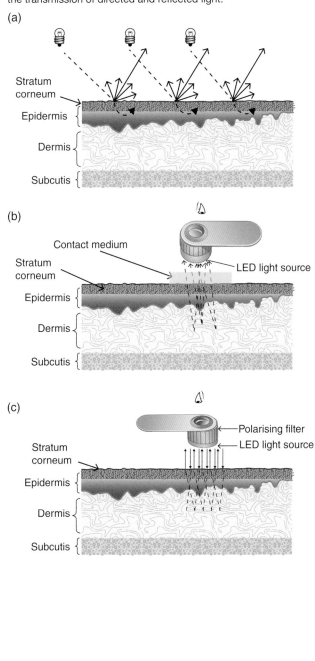

Figure 11.1   How Dermoscopy works. (a) Normally, most light rays falling on the skin's surface will be deflected and scattered by the stratum corneum. Only a fraction can penetrate the epidermis. (b) Applying a contact medium (e.g. medical gel) on the skin's surface increases light penetration, allowing better visualisation of deeper structures. (c) Cross-polarised dermatoscopes enhance the transmission of directed and reflected light.

(a)

(b)

(c)

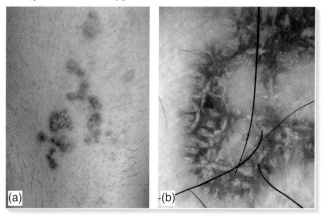

Figure 11.2a and b   Wickham's striae in lichen planus seen clearly with dermoscopy as short white lines.

(a)   (b)

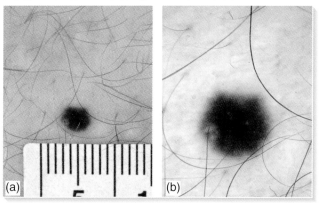

Figure 11.3a and b   The lines and holes forming the network are symmetrical in this benign reticular naevus.

(a)   (b)

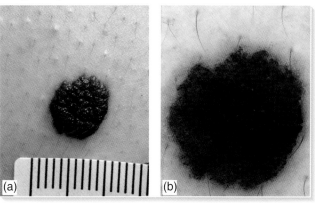

Figure 11.4a and b   Globules (clods) seen throughout this benign compound naevus.

(a)   (b)

Dermatology at a Glance, Second Edition. Mahbub M.U. Chowdhury, Ruwani P. Katugampola, and Andrew Y. Finlay.
© 2020 John Wiley & Sons Ltd. Published 2020 by John Wiley & Sons Ltd.
Companion website: www.wiley.com/go/chowdhury/dermatology

Figure 11.5a and b The peripheral globules (and the asymmetrical network) make this naevus suspicious.

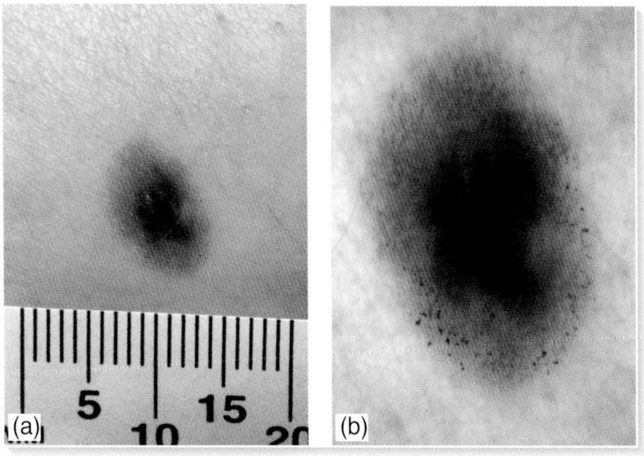

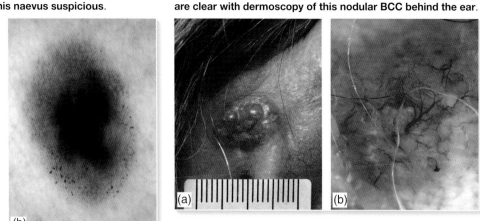

Figure 11.8a and b Focused branching (arborizing) vessels are clear with dermoscopy of this nodular BCC behind the ear.

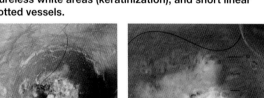

Figure 11.6a and b Short lines emerging from a structureless black blotch is classical for starburst pattern.

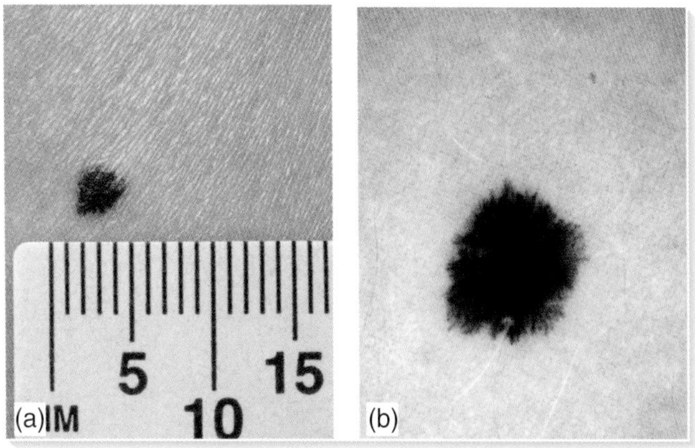

Figure 11.9a and b Dermoscopy of this SCC shows structureless white areas (keratinization), and short linear and dotted vessels.

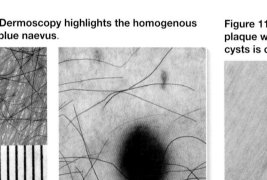

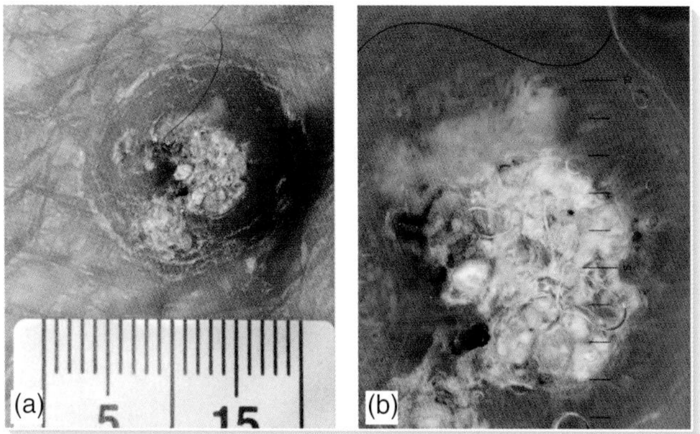

Figure 11.7a and b Dermoscopy highlights the homogenous blue pigment in this blue naevus.

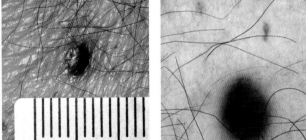

Figure 11.10a and b A sharply demarcated pigmented plaque with comedo-like openings and shiny, white, milia-like cysts is classical for seborrhoeic keratosis.

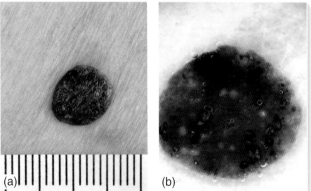

Figure 11.11a and b Numerous dotted vessels and white scales are nicely seen in this Bowen's disease.

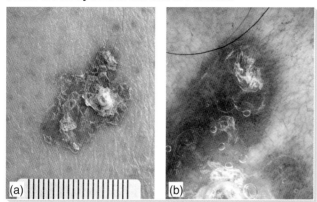

Figure 11.12a and b With dermoscopy of this facial actinic keratosis, the scales are seen more clearly and the erythema is interrupted by multiple white holes giving this 'strawberry' appearance.

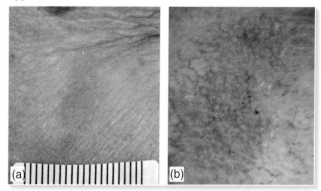

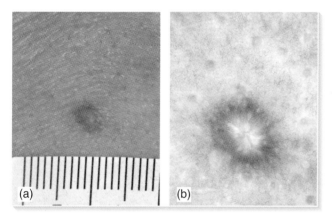

Figure 11.13a and b This lesion clinically has many differentials but dermoscopy highlights the structureless scar-like area centrally and the delicate peripheral network seen in dermatofibroma.

Dermoscopy, also known as dermatoscopy, is the use of a hand-held, non-invasive, diagnostic tool, the dermatoscope. It allows better visualisation of skin structures that cannot be seen by the naked eye, to enhance clinical diagnostic accuracy. Dermoscopy must be used in conjunction with, not instead of, a full clinical history and examination.

How Does it Work?

Normally the majority of light falling on the skin surface is deflected and scattered, so only the very superficial skin can be seen by the naked eye (Figure 11.1a). However, applying an oil or medical gel between the dermatoscope and the skin surface alters the light reflectance of the stratum corneum, enhancing light penetration and visualisation of deeper skin structures (this technique uses a 'contact dermatoscope') (Figure 11.1b). Alternatively, cross-polarised filters within the dermatoscope can enhance the transmission of directed and reflected light, allowing better visibility of skin structures (so called 'polarised dermatoscopes') (Figure 11.1c). 'Hybrid dermatoscopes' have both contact and polarised modes.

Value of Dermoscopy in Clinical Practice

Dermoscopy is commonly used to aid the diagnosis of skin lesions, mainly in the early detection of melanoma. Dermoscopy-trained clinicians have a greater ability, with increased diagnostic sensitivity, to accurately diagnose early melanoma compared to peers who rely on naked eye examination. Dermoscopy is also valuable in differentiating benign skin lesions from cancerous ones that can look clinically similar. The use of dermoscopy can therefore increase diagnostic specificity and reduce unnecessary excisions of benign lesions. Moreover, dermoscopy has been shown to be helpful in diagnosing some inflammatory skin conditions (such as lichen planus [Figure 11.2a and b], eczema, psoriasis, rosacea, pityriasis rosea), scalp disorders (alopecia areata, lichen planopilaris, tinea capitis), and nail disease. The dermatoscope is therefore sometimes called 'the dermatologists' stethoscope'.

Dermoscopy in Melanocytic Lesions

When examining a skin lesion with the dermatoscope, the first step is to recognise if the lesion is melanocytic (i.e. whether it is arising from melanocytes). Benign and atypical naevi, Spitz naevus, blue naevus, and melanomas all arise from melanocytes. It is important to note that not every pigmented lesion is melanocytic. For instance, seborrhoeic keratosis and dermatofibroma can be pigmented, but these do not develop from melanocytes. For melanocytic lesions, four dermoscopic patterns can be observed:

- **Reticular (network) pattern**

In benign naevi, the network lines are symmetrical and fade away at the periphery (Figure 11.3a and b).

- **Globular (clods) pattern**

Monomorphic globules are normally seen in naevi in children and in benign compound naevi (Figure 11.4a and b). However, asymmetry in globules sizes and distribution within a naevus may indicate growth and malignant transformation (Figure 11.5a and b).

- **Starburst pattern**

Radial eccentric lines emerging from a dark blotch (Figure 11.6a and b). This is typical for Spitz naevi or Spitz-like melanomas.

- **Homogeneous blue pattern**

Structureless homogenous blue area (Figure 11.7a and b). If blue naevi are longstanding with no change they are usually benign whereas recent and changing blue naevi may suggest melanoma.

In some cases, more than one pattern can be seen in the same lesion. The patient's age and clinical history are important in these (as in any) cases to guide the diagnosis.

Dermoscopy in Non-Melanocytic Lesions

- **Basal cell carcinoma (BCC)**

Occasionally BCC can be difficult to distinguish from benign conditions such as intradermal naevi and sebaceous hyperplasia. In such cases dermoscopy can be very helpful to show the classical branching (arborizing) vessels seen in nodular BCC (Figure 11.8a and b). It also helps to distinguish superficial BCC from other mimicking lesions (actinic keratosis and Bowen's disease).

- **Squamous cell carcinoma (SCC)**

This skin cancer arises from epidermal keratinocytes. Excess keratin produced by cancerous keratinocytes is typically seen under the dermatoscope as white areas. In addition, as SCCs are growing lesions that need a blood supply, dermoscopy reveals irregular linear vessels (Figure 11.9a and b).

- **Seborrhoeic keratosis**

These benign lesions can look suspicious, especially when inflamed. Using dermoscopy, however, helps by showing a sharply demarcated plaque with holes (comedo-like openings) and occasionally shiny white dots (milia-like cysts) (Figure 11.10a and b).

- **Bowen's disease (squamous cell carcinoma in situ)**

Dermoscopy can facilitate the diagnosis of this by showing clusters of small, dotted vessels and white scales which result from keratin production (Figure 11.11a and b).

- **Actinic (solar) keratosis**

These are commonly seen on sun-exposed areas and can have various degrees of keratinization. The dermatoscope shows an erythematous patch with scaling. When seen on the face, the erythema can be interrupted with white circles (representing keratinization in follicular openings), giving the appearance of the surface of a strawberry (Figure 11.12a and b).

- **Dermatofibroma (histiocytoma)**

There are various subtypes of dermatofibroma and it is not always straightforward to diagnose. However, dermoscopy typically shows a structureless, scar-like area centrally with a delicate network in the periphery (Figure 11.13a and b). Palpation of the lesion during examination can often be helpful to differentiate this from reticular melanocytic naevi.

Limitations of Dermoscopy

Dermoscopy has become an indispensable tool in dermatology practice, especially in countries where skin cancers are commonly seen. However, skin conditions can have various presentations and in some clinical scenarios dermoscopic features are not specific. For instance, some melanomas lack pigment (amelanotic) or are only minimally pigmented (hypopigmented), so none of the usual melanocytic features can be seen. Clinical judgement has to be balanced based on the patients' age, risk factors, and full history of lesion duration, evolution, and symptoms. Dermoscopy is helpful to aid the diagnosis in conjunction with all of these factors.

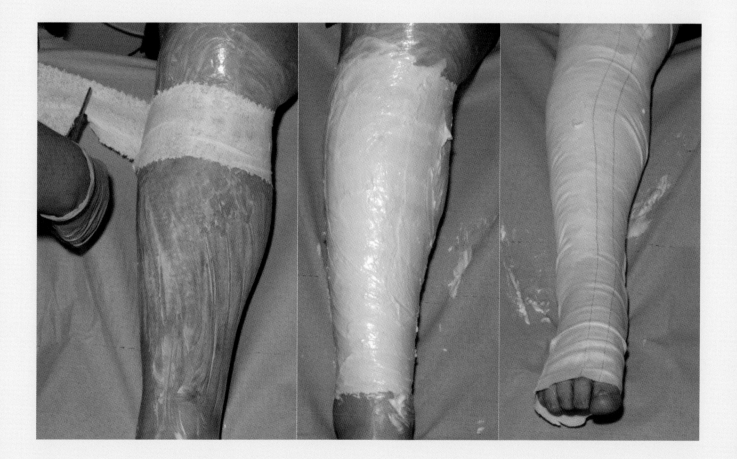

Treatments

Part 4

Chapters

12 Topical Therapy

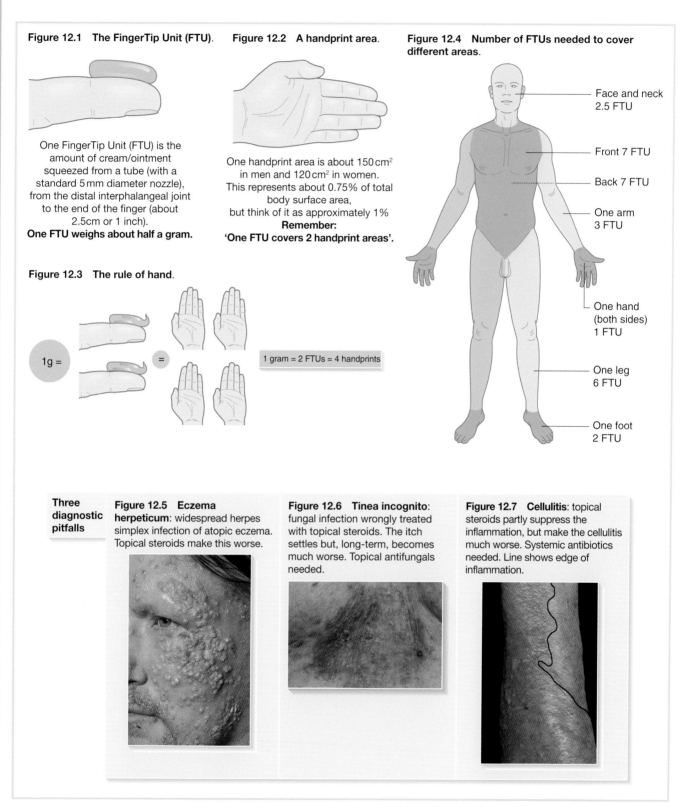

Figure 12.1   The FingerTip Unit (FTU).

One FingerTip Unit (FTU) is the amount of cream/ointment squeezed from a tube (with a standard 5 mm diameter nozzle), from the distal interphalangeal joint to the end of the finger (about 2.5cm or 1 inch).
One FTU weighs about half a gram.

Figure 12.2   A handprint area.

One handprint area is about 150 cm² in men and 120 cm² in women. This represents about 0.75% of total body surface area, but think of it as approximately 1%
Remember:
'One FTU covers 2 handprint areas'.

Figure 12.3   The rule of hand.

1g =   =

1 gram = 2 FTUs = 4 handprints

Figure 12.4   Number of FTUs needed to cover different areas.

Face and neck 2.5 FTU

Front 7 FTU

Back 7 FTU

One arm 3 FTU

One hand (both sides) 1 FTU

One leg 6 FTU

One foot 2 FTU

Three diagnostic pitfalls

Figure 12.5   Eczema herpeticum: widespread herpes simplex infection of atopic eczema. Topical steroids make this worse.

Figure 12.6   Tinea incognito: fungal infection wrongly treated with topical steroids. The itch settles but, long-term, becomes much worse. Topical antifungals needed.

Figure 12.7   Cellulitis: topical steroids partly suppress the inflammation, but make the cellulitis much worse. Systemic antibiotics needed. Line shows edge of inflammation.

Dermatology at a Glance, Second Edition. Mahbub M.U. Chowdhury, Ruwani P. Katugampola, and Andrew Y. Finlay.
© 2020 John Wiley & Sons Ltd. Published 2020 by John Wiley & Sons Ltd.
Companion website: www.wiley.com/go/chowdhury/dermatology

Figure 12.8 Sea of nonadherence.

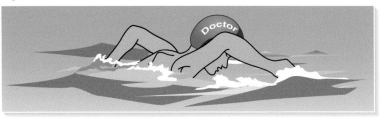

Table 12.1 Adherence.

Most topical preparations prescribed are only put on a few times or never even picked up from the pharmacy. To increase adherence:
- Be aware that patients do not use treatments as prescribed
- Explain/demonstrate to the patient how to use it
- Make it simple! Preferably only one topical application and only once a day
- Prescribe enough
- Provide a written treatment plan

Table 12.2 Don't undertreat.
- Do use high potency steroids in acute disease, for a few days
- Don't use high potency for long periods unless specialist supervision
- Do a risk/benefit analysis!

Table 12.3 The Yesterday Use question.

'What ointments/creams did you put on your skin yesterday?'
- If accurate, believable description: adherence may be good
- If admits none – good opening to discuss how to improve adherence

Topical skin treatment has a huge advantage over systemic therapy. The drug can go direct to the part of the skin that is diseased so high concentrations can be used with minimal risk. Cardiac drugs can harm the skin, but topical skin drugs do not harm the heart!

What Influences Absorption?
- Body site: the palm has very thick stratum corneum so absorbs little. The scrotum has thin stratum corneum so absorbs a great deal.
- Stratum corneum function: if the stratum corneum is moist (e.g. in body folds) much more will be absorbed than in dry exposed areas.
- Influence of the disease: if the stratum corneum is lost or diseased absorption is easier. So in treating psoriasis the drug gets in more easily at the diseased sites than the surrounding normal skin.
- Size of what is being absorbed: if the molecule is too large, very little will get in. Penetration enhancers such as propylene glycol may be added to topical drugs to increase drug absorption.
- When a topical drug is applied, most ends up on clothes.
- All topical drugs that get into the skin are eventually absorbed into the circulation, but the quantity is usually very small.

What is a Cream?
A cream is a semi-solid mixture of water and lipids. Creams usually look opaque white (like fresh cream). Water and lipids do not blend, but can form an 'emulsion' in which small droplets of one are suspended in the other: either droplets of lipids in water or droplets of water in lipids. If the cream is 'lipids in water' (e.g. aqueous cream), it will evaporate and so is cooling, and the cream will mix with water so it can be washed off. If the cream is 'water in lipids' (e.g. oily cream), it is more difficult to wash off. Because creams contain water, they can spread easily over moist areas of diseased skin whereas ointments slip off.

What is in a Cream?
- Active drug
- Base (the mixture of water and lipids)
- Emulsifying agents (which help to stabilise the emulsion)
- Antibacterials
- Perfumes (sometimes)

There may be a risk of developing allergic contact dermatitis to these different components, even though the active drug is not allergenic.

What is an Ointment?
Ointments are semi-solid mixtures of lipids (no water). They feel greasy and look transparent and grey. Drugs such as corticosteroids may be added to both cream and ointment bases.

Ointments stick well to dry diseased skin.

'If it's dry, use an ointment, if it's wet, use a cream.'

What is a Lotion?
A lotion is a liquid, usually water or sometimes alcohol, containing a medication. The liquid evaporates, leaving the medication spread over the surface.

What is an Emollient?
An emollient (or 'moisturiser') is something that moisturises and softens the skin surface. Both creams and ointments can be emollients. Commonly used emollient lotions in the UK include: E45®, QV© and Cetraben® lotion. Commonly used emollient creams in the UK include: Oilatum®, Ultrabase®, E45® and Epimax®. There is no good evidence that one emollient is better than another. In atopic eczema, emollients may prolong time to flare, reduce numbers of flares, and reduce corticosteroid use.

How Often Should Drugs be Applied?
The pharmacokinetics of many commonly used topical drugs are not well worked out. Traditionally, topical drugs have been used two to three times per day, often with no real evidence for that frequency. There may sometimes be a patient-perceived benefit from the emollient action of some drugs, encouraging more frequent use than is pharmacologically necessary. Potent topical steroids would probably be equally effective used only once daily. Adherence is greater for once daily than for twice daily.

Topical Steroids
Topical steroids revolutionised treatment of inflammatory skin disease in the 1950s. They are still the first choice for most inflammatory skin conditions.

The myths – 'Topical steroids are dangerous'. 'They should only ever be used very sparingly'.

The facts – Topical steroids have a range of potencies (strengths):
- *Mild potency* – minimal risk of side effects. Least effective. e.g. hydrocortisone 0.5, 1.0, 2.5%.
- *Moderate potency* – minimal risk of side effects. Mildly effective, e.g. clobetasone butyrate (Eumovate®).
- *Strong potency* – side effects only if used daily for more than two to three weeks. Safe to use for few days in acute situations. Very effective, e.g. betamethasone valerate (Betnovate®).
- *Very strong potency* – high risk of side effects. Extremely effective, e.g. clobetasol propionate (Dermovate®). Needed for resistant conditions (e.g. discoid lupus erythematosus), poor absorption sites (e.g. palms). There is a probable association between use of high potency topical steroids in pregnancy and low birth weight.

Side Effects of Potent Topical Steroids if used Widely in the Long-Term

Skin
- Thinning of dermis: 'atrophy'
- Telangiectasia
- Fragility of skin, easy bruising and tearing
- Striae
- Rosacea, acne, perioral dermatitis
- Hirsutism
- Contact allergy (Chapter 35).

Systemic Absorption (Inflamed Skin Absorbs Drugs More Easily)
- Cushing's syndrome
- Glaucoma
- Growth retardation in children

Topical Tacrolimus and Pimecrolimus
- Anti-inflammatory but not corticosteroids
- No skin thinning
- Local immunosuppressants
- Initial use may cause burning sensation
- Concern about long-term potential (so far unproven) for increasing skin cancer on treated skin exposed to the sun

Antibiotics

Topical antibiotics are the treatment of choice for bacterial infections such as impetigo, infected eczema, and erythrasma (fusidic acid 20 mg/g cream, neomycin, tetracycline). They are commonly used in the treatment of acne (erythromycin), but this widespread use encourages higher prevalence of antibiotic resistance and so is no longer recommended.

Antifungals

Topical antifungal agents such as terbinafine are very effective against dermatophyte infections. Terbinafine works by inhibiting ergosterol synthesis in fungal cell membranes. This changes the permeability of the membrane causing cell lysis. Human cells are not affected. As terbinafine is fungicidal, only a few applications are required to cure.

Yeast infections such as candida or seborrhoeic dermatitis are treated with topical azoles such as clotrimazole, ketoconazole, and imidazole. Azoles also work by altering the permeability of fungal cell walls, by inhibiting the enzyme cytochrome P450 and hence interfering with ergosterol biosynthesis.

Antivirals

Topical aciclovir is very effective in treating herpes simplex and herpes zoster. The mode of action of aciclovir is very clever; it is converted by viral enzymes to aciclovir triphosphate, which then inhibits HSV specific DNA polymerases. It is therefore harmless to normal human cells. Despite 40 years of use, resistance is very low and the drug remains very safe. Gertrude Elion was awarded the 1988 Nobel Prize partly for her work in developing aciclovir.

Infestation Therapies

The aim of any therapy for infestation is to use a drug that kills the insect or mite but does not affect human cells. Topical permethrin 5% is effective in scabies and head lice. Permethrin works as a neurotoxin and is more toxic to cold-blooded animals such as insects or fish.

Ivermectin is used to treat scabies, body and head lice, and tropical diseases including filariasis, onchocerciasis, and loa loa. Ivermectin interferes with glutamate-gated chloride channels in invertebrate nerves and muscles, paralysing and killing the insect or mite. Ivermectin can be taken systemically, although it may cause neurotoxicity, or used as a lotion (0.5%). A cream is available for rosacea, as *Demodex* may contribute to its pathogenesis. William Campbell and Satoshi Ōmura were awarded the 2015 Nobel Prize for discovering ivermectin. Since 1988 the pharmaceutical company Merck and Co have given the drug free for the treatment of onchocerciasis, an outstanding benefit to the human race.

Topical Retinoids

Topical retinoids are used in acne and to reverse photodamage. Retinoids are related to vitamin A and include tretinoin, adapalene, and tazarotene. They are widely used in acne; however, they are not as effective as the systemic retinoid isotretinoin which also dramatically reduces sebum formation.

Topicals for Psoriasis

Coal tar and tar derivatives were widely used for psoriasis in the twentieth century: they may still be useful for their soothing antipruritic affect. Topical dithranol (anthralin), although effective in chronic plaque psoriasis, is now seldom used because it stains skin and clothes and may cause irritation. However, both of these therapies may be useful in special circumstances where other treatments are contraindicated or not wanted by the patient (Chapter 15).

Vitamin D analogues (e.g. topical calcipotriol) are easy to use and are available in many formulations including for the scalp. Calcipotriol may work by binding to vitamin D receptors and altering cell differentiation. It is also marketed as a combination with the potent topical steroid betamethasone dipropionate.

Sunscreens

Sunscreens (Chapter 43) may work by partially blocking or reflecting sunlight or by chemically absorbing specific wavelengths. Inert blockers such as micronised titanium dioxide or zinc oxide are the most effective but are visible. Commonly used chemical ingredients include phenylbenzimidazole sulphonic acid (UVB), oxybenzone (UVB and UVA), homosalate (UVB), octyl methoxycinnamate (UVB), and avobenzone (UVA).

Topical Drugs for Pre-Malignancy or Malignancy

Treatment of actinic keratoses, BCC, and Bowen's disease may include 5-fluorouracil (5-FU). Synthesis of thymidine, which is required for DNA replication, is blocked by 5-FU as it inhibits thymidylate synthase. More rapidly dividing cancerous cells are affected more than normal cells. Topical use may cause inflammation and local discomfort.

Topical imiquimod 5% was originally licensed to treat genital viral warts, but is now also used to treat actinic keratoses, Bowen's disease, and superficial BCC. It modulates the innate immune response to recognise the abnormal cells and induces cytokines to get rid of them. Application usually causes some redness and soreness.

Drug Combinations and Formulations

The main reason that topical drugs are not effective is that they are not applied. The fewer drugs and the less the frequency of application, the more likely they will be applied. The best approach is therefore to ask a patient to use only one topical drug, only once a day. Combining drugs therefore makes sense.

Combination examples include calcipotriol/corticosteroid for psoriasis, antibiotic/corticosteroid for infected eczema, and adapalene/benzoyl peroxide for acne. Since the earliest times, pharmacists and doctors have created mixtures for topical application: unfortunately, most mixtures are made with no knowledge of the impact of the combination process on absorption or effectiveness.

Topical drugs need to be formulated to be as easy as possible to 'live with'. If they stain, sting, or feel uncomfortable, they simply won't be used.

Most topically applied drug ends up on clothes, sheets, or around the house rather than being absorbed. There is really no need to apply topical drugs 'thickly'.

Pharmacokinetics of Topical Applications

The published 'advised' frequency of application of topical drugs is seldom based on any evidence of pharmacokinetic data or effectiveness. In eczema the 'tradition' of applying topical corticosteroids twice daily may be partly based on the perceived emollient (rather than active) effect, even though once daily application may have a similar anti-inflammatory effect.

As topical applications are absorbed through the stratum corneum, a reservoir of drug is created in the stratum corneum from which more drug is gradually absorbed. This partly explains why once daily application may be almost as effective as more frequent application.

Compliance/Adherence

Clinicians (and medical students) need to be aware of the invisible "sea of nonadherence" in which we are all swimming (Figure 12.8). About 95% of dermatology patients underdose new topical therapies and 30% don't even collect their outpatient prescription drugs from the pharmacy. Awareness of nonadherence matters because lack of use means lack of effectiveness, longer time to cure, and wasted appointments. Also doctors get a distorted idea of the lack of effectiveness of therapies.

Patients may not use treatment because the treatments are messy and difficult, they take time, and it may be impossible to apply a regular topical therapy with many other pressures in people's lives. Patients need encouragement, teaching, and help with treatment: the simpler the regimen the better. It may be helpful to involve the patient's relatives as part of the caring team.

Key Points
- Very inflamed skin is disabling and uncomfortable.
- Potent steroids have minimal risks used in the short-term.
- A FTU weighs 0.5g and spreads over two handprints.

▶ Warning
- Treatment often fails because of poor adherence.
- Emollients accumulating in clothes or dressings may cause a fire hazard.

13 Practical Special Management

Table 13.1 **Examples of dermatology day care services.**

- Patient education on application of topical treatments, e.g. eczema
- Intensive topical treatments, e.g. for psoriasis, eczema
- Regular review and monitoring of patients with 'unstable' inflammatory skin diseases, e.g. eczema
- Phototherapy (Chapter 44)
- Management of leg ulcers (Chapter 52)
- Postoperative wound care following skin surgery, e.g. following skin graft, suture removal
- Infusion and monitoring of patients on biological therapy for severe psoriasis
- Iontophoresis for palmar plantar hyperhidrosis

Table 13.2 **Skin conditions treated with radiotherapy.**

Benign lesions	Malignant lesions
• Keloid scars	• Basal cell carcinoma • Squamous cell carcinoma • Cutaneous lymphomas (T and B cell subtypes) • Kaposi's sarcoma • Angiosarcoma • Merkel cell carcinoma

Table 13.3 **Potential complications of radiotherapy.**

Acute complications	Long-term complications
• Redness (erythema) • Peeling (desquamation) of the skin on treated area • Mild bleeding	• Skin atrophy with telangiectasia • Fibrosis of skin • Hyper or hypopigmentation of the skin • Alopecia of treated site (e.g. scalp) • Skin malignancies at site of radiotherapy (e.g. squamous cell carcinoma) • Lymphoedema

Figure 13.5   Infliximab infusion for severe psoriasis.

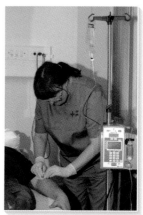

Figure 13.1   Application of moisturisers.

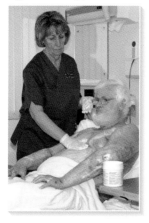

Figure 13.2   Application of coal tar.

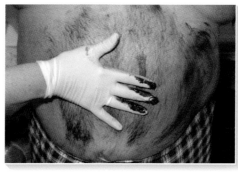

Figure 13.6   Iontophoresis of the (a) hands and (b) feet.

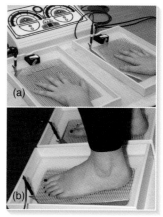

(a)

(b)

Figure 13.3   (a) Dithranol. (b) Application of dithranol.

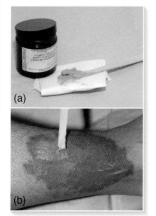

(a)

(b)

Figure 13.4   Zinc impregnated bandaging. (a) Either moisturisers or topical corticosteroids applied to the skin, (b) followed by the zinc impregnated bandages, (c) followed by cotton bandages (e.g. Tubifast®) to hold things in place.

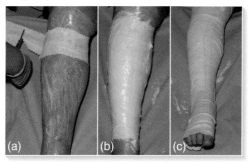

(a)   (b)   (c)

Figure 13.7   Application of topical cantharidin to a viral wart.

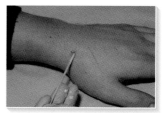

Dermatology at a Glance, Second Edition. Mahbub M.U. Chowdhury, Ruwani P. Katugampola, and Andrew Y. Finlay.
© 2020 John Wiley & Sons Ltd. Published 2020 by John Wiley & Sons Ltd.
Companion website: www.wiley.com/go/chowdhury/dermatology

Dermatology Day Care Services

Dermatology care in the UK is primarily an outpatient service. In addition to the outpatient consultations, many patients benefit from dermatology day care services that are mainly nurse-led (Table 13.1). The following are examples of the services provided by a dermatology day care unit.

Patient Education

Treatment of chronic inflammatory skin diseases such as eczema and psoriasis requires the use of several topical treatments including moisturisers and active treatments such as topical corticosteroids or calcineurin inhibitors.

Educating patients and parents of affected children regarding the appropriate application of the topical treatments, including quantities, and when and how to use them, helps to improve treatment compliance. Patients also require education about self-administration by injection of biological therapies for severe psoriasis.

Intensive Topical Treatment

Reasons for receiving topical treatment in a dermatology day care unit include the following:
- Severe extensive skin disease (e.g. eczema, psoriasis)
- Elderly individuals unable to reach body sites to apply treatment
- Co-morbidities that limit ability to use topical treatment (e.g. arthritis, impaired vision)
- Too messy to use at home (e.g. crude coal tar for psoriasis)
- Need careful application, as contact with unaffected skin may cause severe skin irritation (e.g. dithranol for large plaque psoriasis)

Moisturisers come in a variety of consistencies from lotions and creams to greasy emollients which can be used for any dry skin condition (e.g. eczema; Figure 13.1).

Coal tar, ranging in strength (1–20%), has been used for many years in the treatment of psoriasis and, less commonly, eczema (Figure 13.2). It is a relatively cheap, non-toxic treatment. Its exact mechanism of action is not known, but is thought to have antipruritic, antimicrobial, and anti-inflammatory properties. Because of its thick black consistency and smell, treatment in patients' own homes is not practical or acceptable, and therefore requires day treatment. Coal tar is applied to the affected skin, then covered with light cotton bandages and washed away after two hours. Treatment is repeated on a daily basis, with increasing strength of coal tar, until disease clearance.

Dithranol (anthralin), ranging in strength (0.1–10%), has also been used for many years as a successful treatment for plaque psoriasis (Figure 13.3a and b). Its exact mechanism of action is not known. It stains and irritates unaffected skin. Dithranol is carefully applied only to the psoriatic plaques, the areas covered with light cotton bandages and left for 30–60 minutes (short contact therapy). It is then removed with cotton wool and the skin washed. Treatment is repeated daily, with increasing strength of dithranol, until disease clearance.

Bandaging is used in the treatment of inflammatory skin diseases affecting limbs. During treatment with coal tar or dithranol, light cotton bandages (e.g. Tubinet®) are used for occlusion. Light cotton bandages are also used over moisturisers or topical corticosteroids to contain the treatment on the skin, increase absorption, and prevent direct trauma to the skin from scratching. Zinc impregnated bandages are effective for the treatment of atopic eczema and nodular prurigo (Figure 13.4a–c).

Other Treatments Undertaken in Dermatology Day Units

Phototherapy See Chapter 44.

Biological therapy (Chapter 14) One of the biological therapies for severe psoriasis, infliximab, requires intravenous infusions at set time intervals (maintenance 8 weekly) and monitoring of the patient during infusions for adverse drug reactions (Figure 13.5).

Iontophoresis Excessive sweating (hyperhidrosis) of the palms and/or soles can be treated with a course of iontophoresis. This involves passing a small electric current whilst the affected hands and/or feet are immersed in a shallow bowl of tap water (Figure 13.6a and b), sometimes with glycopyrronium bromide.

Cantharidin treatment This is a toxic chemical produced by beetles. Its dilute form is used to treat viral warts that have not responded to conventional treatments (e.g. topical salicylic acid, cryotherapy). As blistering follows application, the treatment should be applied by an experienced nurse (Figure 13.7).

Management of leg ulcers This is discussed in Chapter 52. In some hospitals, leg ulcers are managed by dedicated wound care services, whilst in others ulcers are managed in dermatology day care units.

Radiotherapy

Radiotherapy is occasionally used for skin malignancies as either definitive, adjuvant postsurgical or palliative treatment (Table 13.2). It utilises ionising electromagnetic radiation to damage rapidly dividing tumour DNA. Surrounding normal tissue can also be affected, resulting in potential complications (Table 13.3). Damage to normal tissue is reduced by treating with small divided doses (fractions) of radiation. It is the primary treatment option for skin malignancies in patients unsuitable for surgery (very elderly with multiple co-morbidities) and/or patient preference. It is also used as adjuvant therapy for perineural invasion or lymph node metastases associated with surgically excised squamous cell carcinomas.

Key Points
- Dermatology day care services have an important role in education, treatment, support, and monitoring of patients with a wide range of dermatological diseases.
- Radiotherapy is a non-surgical treatment option for management of skin malignancies.

▶ **Warning**
- A long-term complication of radiotherapy is development of skin malignancies such as squamous cell carcinomas.

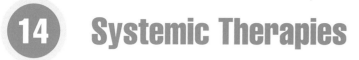

14 Systemic Therapies

Figure 14.1   Mechanisms of action for common systemic therapies. (a) Methotrexate. (b) Glucocorticoids. (c) Azathioprine.
(d) Ciclosporin. (e) Retinoids.

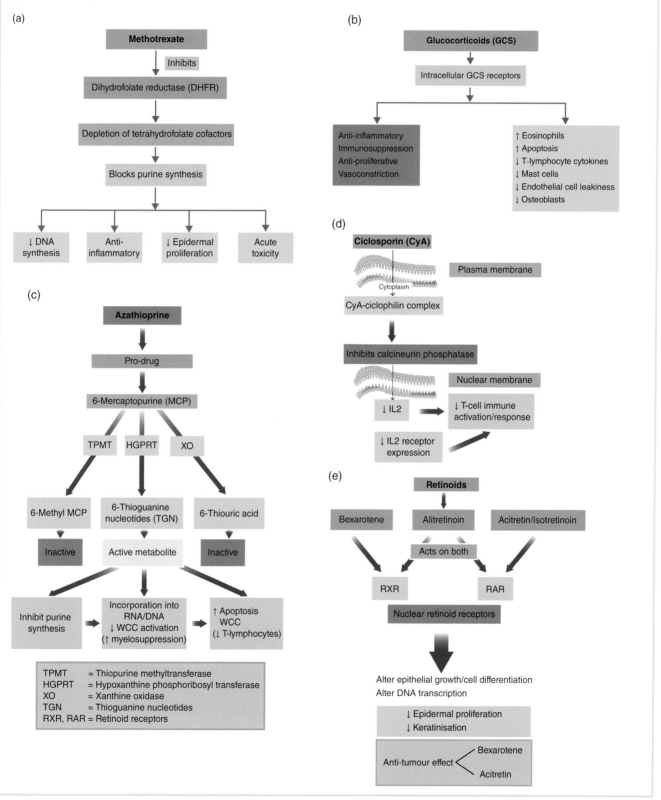

Dermatology at a Glance, Second Edition. Mahbub M.U. Chowdhury, Ruwani P. Katugampola, and Andrew Y. Finlay.
© 2020 John Wiley & Sons Ltd. Published 2020 by John Wiley & Sons Ltd.
Companion website: www.wiley.com/go/chowdhury/dermatology

Figure 14.2 Systemic steroid side effects. Source: Modified from Figure 7.1 with permission from Finlay and Chowdhury (2007).

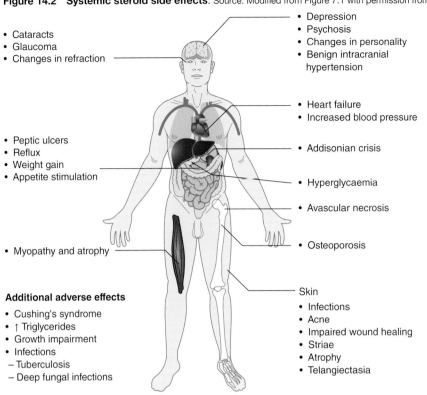

- Cataracts
- Glaucoma
- Changes in refraction

- Peptic ulcers
- Reflux
- Weight gain
- Appetite stimulation

- Myopathy and atrophy

Additional adverse effects
- Cushing's syndrome
- ↑ Triglycerides
- Growth impairment
- Infections
  – Tuberculosis
  – Deep fungal infections

- Depression
- Psychosis
- Changes in personality
- Benign intracranial hypertension

- Heart failure
- Increased blood pressure

- Addisonian crisis

- Hyperglycaemia

- Avascular necrosis

- Osteoporosis

Skin
- Infections
- Acne
- Impaired wound healing
- Striae
- Atrophy
- Telangiectasia

Table 14.1 Common systemic therapies used in dermatology: indications and side effects.

Drug	Indications	Side effects
Corticosteroids	Bullous diseases, connective tissue diseases, vasculitis, atopic eczema and contact dermatitis, lichen planus, inflammatory skin diseases, drug reactions, pyoderma gangrenosum, sarcoidosis	Weight gain, hypertension, pituitary–adrenal axis suppression, cataracts, infections, osteoporosis, growth impairment in children, diabetes, euphoria, gastro-intestinal bleeding (Figure 14.2)
Methotrexate	Chronic plaque, erythrodermic and pustular psoriasis, psoriatic arthritis, cutaneous lupus erythematosus, eczema, sarcoidosis, systemic sclerosis, morphoea	Nausea, mucositis, acute toxicity, bone marrow suppression, macrocytosis, hepatotoxicity, liver and lung fibrosis, nephrotoxicity, teratogenic, reduces spermatogenesis
Azathioprine	Atopic eczema, systemic lupus erythematosus, dermatomyositis, bullous diseases, lichen planus, sarcoidosis	Nausea and vomiting, bone marrow suppression, macrocytosis, hepatitis, acute hypersensitivity, risk of malignancy, e.g. lymphoma, SCC
Ciclosporin	Organ transplant recipients, severe psoriasis and atopic eczema, bullous diseases, pyoderma gangrenosum, chronic urticaria, lichen planus	Nephrotoxicity, hypertension, hyperlipidaemia, hypertrichosis, nausea, gingival hyperplasia, tremor, risk of skin malignancy with previous phototherapy, e.g. SCC, BCC
Apremilast	Moderate to severe psoriasis (and psoriatic arthritis) prior to or when unsuitable for phototherapy or other systemic agents	Diarrhoea, nausea, upper respiratory tract infections, tension headaches and migraine, depression, weight loss
Retinoids: *refer to specific drug*	Acitretin: severe psoriasis, pustular psoriasis, ichthyoses, SCC prophylaxis Isotretinoin: acne, rosacea Alitretinoin: hand eczema Bexarotene: T cell lymphoma	Teratogenic, hyperlipidaemia, hepatitis, mucocutaneous effects, e.g. dry lips and eyes, epistaxis, thyroid defects, photosensitivity, hair loss, palmoplantar peeling, muscle aches, nausea, sweating, mood changes, e.g. depression, benign intracranial hypertension, skeletal defects

Table 14.2 Biologic treatment: indications and uses in dermatology.

Severe psoriasis/psoriatic arthritis
Severe atopic dermatitis
Chronic urticaria
B cell skin lymphoma
Metastatic malignant melanoma
Pemphigus
Hidradenitis suppurativa
Pyoderma gangrenosum
Sarcoidosis
Behçet's disease
Dermatomyositis
Vasculitis e.g. Wegener's granulomatosis

Table 14.3 Biologic treatment: mechanisms of action and indications.

Psoriasis/psoriatic arthritis	Mechanism of action and dosages
Adalimumab	Fully humanised anti-TNF monoclonal Antibody (Ab): 40 mg 2 weekly subcutaneous (S/C)
Infliximab	Chimeric (25% mouse) human–mouse monoclonal Ab; 5 mg/kg infusion every 8 weeks
Etanercept	Fusion protein binds soluble and receptor bound TNF; S/C 25–50 mg twice weekly for 12 weeks.
Secukinumab	Human IgG1 monoclonal Ab selectively binds to and neutralises IL-17a; S/C 300 mg weekly for 4 weeks and then monthly
Ustekinumab	Human monoclonal Ab binds to p40 protein subunit preventing IL-12/IL-23 binding to T cell receptors; S/C 45–90 mg 1–3 monthly
Ixekizumab	Human monoclonal Ab binds IL-17a and blocks pro-inflammatory cytokines and chemokines; S/C 160 mg then 80 mg every 2–4 weeks
Guselkumab	Recombinant human monoclonal Ab binds selectively to IL-23 and blocks pro-inflammatory cytokines; S/C 100 mg 4–8 weekly
Moderate to severe eczema	
Dupilumab	Ab binds IL-4 receptor alpha subunit; inhibits inflammatory response; S/C 300 mg alternate weeks
Urticaria	
Omalizumab	Recombinant humanised monoclonal Ab selectively binds to IgE receptor and inhibits IgE binding to mast cell receptor; S/C 150–300 mg every 4 weeks; also used in asthma
B cell skin lymphomas, pemphigus	
Rituximab	Potent B cell depleting chimeric IgG1 anti-CD20 Ab; infusion dose 375 mg/m^2
Metastatic malignant melanoma	
Ipilimumab	Anti-CTLA-4 protein receptor human monoclonal Ab, blocks cytotoxic T cells which are immune checkpoint inhibitors of T cell activation
Nivolumab, Pembrolizumab	Anti-PD1 (programmed cell death protein-1) receptor protein, downregulates T cells and immune system, used if positive BRAF V600 mutation; used with ipilimumab if no BRAF mutation.
Vemurafenib, Dabrafenib	BRAF protein inhibitor, used if positive BRAF V600 mutation
Trametinib, Cobimetinib	MEK protein inhibitor, used if positive BRAF V600 mutation

Introduction

This chapter discusses systemic therapies that are commonly used in dermatology practice and their indications, mechanisms of action, side effects, and common interactions and contraindications (Table 14.1 and Figure 14.1).

The correct use of systemic therapies requires understanding of basic pharmacological principles, good prescribing skills, and careful monitoring. Multiple factors can influence the choice of systemic therapy including patient preference, prescriber preference and experience, the skin disease to be treated including the severity of the condition, and external factors such as NICE or SIGN guidelines and funding. Patient information leaflets can be helpful to explain the use of the drug, available at www.bad.org.uk/for-the-public/patient-information-leaflets.

Corticosteroids

Systemic corticosteroids are very useful to treat multiple skin conditions such as blistering diseases, connective tissue diseases, vasculitis, dermatitis, lichen planus, and other inflammatory skin diseases. They include oral prednisolone, hydrocortisone, methylprednisolone, and dexamethasone. They can be given orally, intravenously, or intramuscularly. They act on intracellular glucocorticoid receptors to produce anti-inflammatory, immunosuppressive, antiproliferative, and vasoconstriction effects.

Oral prednisolone is usually given once daily in the morning to reduce the suppressive effect on the pituitary–adrenal axis. Typically 0.5–1 mg/kg/day is given and the dosages vary with the disease and patient treated. The dosages are then tapered gradually whilst keeping the disease suppressed. Hydrocortisone can be given intravenously for anaphylaxis and for short-term benefit. Methylprednisolone can be given intravenously or intramuscularly as required.

Steroids can have a range of adverse effects such as weight gain, hypertension, cataracts, infections, osteoporosis, and growth impairment in children (Figure 14.2).

Interactions with aspirin and other non-steroidal anti-inflammatory drugs (e.g. ibuprofen, indomethacin) can include risk of gastro-intestinal (GI) bleeding and so can be prescribed with GI protective drugs such as omeprazole. Corticosteroids can also interact with anticoagulants and methotrexate (MTX), and live vaccines should be avoided. Stopping steroid treatment should be done gradually over one to three weeks, especially with dosages above 10 mg/day, to allow the pituitary–adrenal axis to recover.

Methotrexate

Methotrexate (MTX) is used in the management of chronic plaque, erythrodermic, and pustular psoriasis, psoriatic arthritis, lupus erythematosus, eczema, and sarcoidosis. MTX is derived from folic acid and acts by inhibiting dihydrofolate reductase (DHFR) to reduce DNA synthesis and to reduce epidermal proliferation. It also has anti-inflammatory effects on lymphocytes and neutrophils.

MTX is usually taken orally as a single dose after food once weekly on a specific day. Standard dosages are between 5 and 25 mg once weekly: intramuscular and subcutaneous routes are also possible. In a normal healthy adult an initial test dose of 5 mg is followed with a full blood count at one week to detect any very sensitive patients. Care should be taken in the elderly and in patients with chronic renal disease. Clinical response is expected within six to eight weeks.

The main side effects include nausea, mucositis, bone marrow suppression, and hepatotoxicity. To reduce nausea, folic acid can be added. The 'gold standard' to detect and monitor MTX-induced liver fibrosis is serial liver biopsy. However, monitoring of liver function with procollagen 3 peptide avoids unnecessary liver biopsies. MTX is excreted by the kidneys (need for baseline renal function) and can rarely cause lung fibrosis (baseline chest x-ray). MTX is teratogenic and women of childbearing age should ensure adequate contraception and have regular pregnancy testing.

MTX can interact with aspirin or non-steroidal drugs, ciclosporin, and folate antagonists such as trimethoprim and phenytoin. High alcohol intake should be avoided because this may increase the risk of liver damage. Only 2.5 mg tablets should be prescribed so that there is no risk of confusion with similar looking 10 mg tablets. Patients should be warned to avoid overdosage, which can be fatal. For myelosuppression with mucosal ulceration and skin necrosis, rescue treatment with folinic acid is indicated.

Azathioprine

Azathioprine is an anti-proliferative, corticosteroid sparing immunosuppressant, which inhibits DNA and RNA synthesis. This inhibits proliferation of lymphocytes and pro-inflammatory cells and is a prodrug of 6-mercaptopurine. It is prescribed in oral dosages of between 1 and 3 mg/kg/day and used for lupus erythematosus, dermatitis, dermatomyositis, bullous diseases, lichen planus, psoriasis, and sarcoid.

Current guidelines recommend measuring thiopurine methyltransferase (TPMT), an enzyme involved in azathioprine metabolism. Patients with low or carrier levels of TPMT have reduced ability to metabolise azathioprine and so receive reduced doses of azathioprine with careful monitoring of full blood count and liver function. The usual starting dose is 100 mg/day, with onset of therapeutic benefit within 6–10 weeks.

Main side effects include bone marrow suppression, macrocytosis (enlarged red blood cells with high MCV), nausea and vomiting, hepatitis, and rarely acute hypersensitivity. There is an increased risk of malignancy including non-Hodgkin's lymphoma and squamous cell carcinoma of the skin. Main drug interactions include allopurinol, sulphasalazine, warfarin, live vaccines, and myelosuppressive drugs such as penicillamine and co-trimoxazole.

Ciclosporin

Ciclosporin is a potent immunosuppressant drug that inhibits production of IL-2 by acting on helper T cells. It is used widely to prevent organ transplant rejection, for severe psoriasis and eczema (licensed for short-term use up to eight weeks), and also sometimes used in blistering diseases, pyoderma gangrenosum, and urticaria.

Ciclosporin is used to urgently control disease: it is taken orally twice daily, starting at 2.5–5 mg/kg/day with rapid clinical benefit within one to two weeks. Maintenance dosages are ideally used for up to three months. Main side effects are nephrotoxicity and hypertension: close monitoring including checking liver function and lipids is needed. Other side effects include nausea, hypertrichosis, gingival hyperplasia, tremor, and increased risk of malignancy including skin cancers particularly if exposed to previous phototherapy. Main drug interactions include non-steroidal anti-inflammatory drugs, macrolide antibiotics, ACE inhibitors, MTX, and grapefruit juice. Live vaccinations are contraindicated and care should be taken to avoid excess sun exposure.

Apremilast

Apremilast is an oral non-biologic drug that inhibits phosphodiesterase 4 (PDE4). It is used for moderate to severe psoriasis (and psoriatic arthritis) if patient unsuitable for or when prior to using phototherapy or other systemic oral agents and biological therapies. Apremilast is started at 10 mg daily increasing to 30 mg twice daily and then continued as a maintenance dose taken for six months. Main side effects include diarrhoea, nausea, upper respiratory tract infection, tension headaches and migraines, decreased appetite and weight loss (5–10%), and uncommonly depression and suicidal ideation. Main drug interactions are with rifampicin and carbamazepine.

Retinoids

The main systemic retinoids available are isotretinoin, acitretin, alitretinoin, and bexarotene. They are all biologically active metabolites of retinol (vitamin A), and affect epithelial growth and differentiation. They bind specific nuclear retinoid receptors affecting DNA transcription. These drugs are used orally and are all highly teratogenic and hence tightly regulated. Females should not be pregnant when starting treatment and for up to one month after cessation of isotretinoin and alitretinoin and for up to two years after acitretin. Regular pregnancy tests may be needed. The main side effects are hyperlipidaemia, hepatitis, mucocutaneous effects such as dryness of lips and eyes, thyroid defects, photosensitivity, hair loss, muscle aches, nausea, and sweating. Rarely mood changes including severe depression and suicides, benign intracranial hypertension, and skeletal defects can occur. Main interactions are alcohol, tetracyclines, and vitamin A. Monitoring can include liver function, fasting lipids, and thyroid function.

Acitretin is used for severe psoriasis, pustular psoriasis, and disorders of keratinization including congenital ichthyoses. It can be combined with phototherapy and used long-term if needed at dosages of 0.5–1 mg/kg/day.

Isotretinoin reduces sebum production and is used mainly in the treatment of severe nodulocystic acne or acne resistant to standard treatments such as antibiotics. It is also sometimes used in rosacea, and hidradenitis suppurativa. The optimum dose for efficacy is 1 mg/kg/day for 16 weeks. However this dose is often not tolerated due to mucocutaneous side effects and with lower dosages the treatment period is extended. At the end of their course 80% of patients are clear of acne.

Alitretinoin is used for chronic severe hand eczema not responding to potent topical steroids. It can be very effective, with clearance within three months. Main side effects are headache with less mucocutaneous side effects than other oral retinoids.

Bexarotene is a useful second-line drug for the treatment of cutaneous T cell lymphoma. However it can produce severe hyperthyroidism and hyperlipidaemia and needs close monitoring.

Biologic Treatments

Biological therapies are immunologically active proteins used in severe psoriasis and eczema, urticaria, hidradenitis suppurativa, metastatic melanoma, and other inflammatory skin diseases such as pyoderma gangrenosum (Tables 14.2 and 14.3). They have highly specific structures and functions and are specific monoclonal antibodies, recombinant cytokines, or receptor binding proteins which reduce the relevant molecule or inflammatory response, e.g. tumour necrosis factor or T cell receptors. Due to these highly specific targets and actions there are usually fewer side effects compared to other systemic agents and are therefore preferred by many patients. In order for psoriasis patients to be eligible for treatment they must have severe disease as defined by objective criteria such as DLQI >10, PASI >10 and total body surface area >10%. Pretreatment screening is essential including history of infections, e.g. TB (CXR, blood assay), hepatitis, HIV, and exclusion of demyelinating and heart disease. Main side effects are serious infections, e.g. TB reactivation, injection site reactions, potential cancers, and demyelination and heart disease. They are very expensive and need to be NICE/SIGN approved and hence patients must have first failed on other systemic therapies (including phototherapy) or have had significant side effects.

Key Points
- Always look up dosages, side effects, pregnancy risk, and drug interactions if unsure.
- Give patients written information on systemic drugs and their main side effects.
- New immunologically active biologics need careful screening and monitoring and have revolutionised treatments for severe psoriasis and eczema.

▶ Warning
- Prescribe only 2.5 mg MTX tablets to avoid dose confusion.
- Check TPMT enzyme prior to azathioprine use.
- Document and monitor pregnancy risks with retinoids and other systemic drugs.

Inflammatory Diseases

Part 5

Chapters

15 Psoriasis
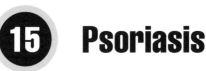

Table 15.1 Systemic treatments and side effects.

Treatment	Side effects
PUVA and UVB	Burning, skin cancer
Methotrexate	Marrow suppression, indigestion, liver damage
Ciclosporin	Hypertension, renal damage, skin cancer
Acitretin	Teratogenic, dry lips, hyperlipidaemia
Mycophenolate mofetil	Gastro-intestinal upset, leukopenia
Apremilast	Diarrhoea, nausea
Biologics	Immune suppression, tuberculosis reactivation

Table 15.2 How to measure psoriasis, to inform decisions and monitor progress.

- **Handprint** – 1% of body surface area (Chapter 12)
- **PASI** – measures redness, scaling, thickness, and area over four body regions. Score range 0–72, but most patients' scores are < 10
- **DLQI** – used to assess how badly the patient's life is being affected (Chapter 5)
- **The Rule of Tens** – If the body surface area > 10%, or the PASI > 10 or the DLQI > 10, this means that the psoriasis is 'severe'. Active therapy, possibly systemic, is required

Figure 15.1 Guttate psoriasis: multiple small lesions.

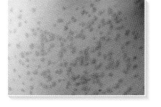

Figure 15.2 Typical plaques of psoriasis.

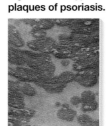

Figure 15.3 Psoriasis plaque on elbow.

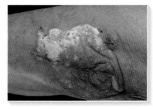

Figure 15.4 Very widespread plaques over the back of a child.

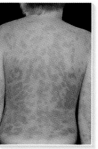

Figure 15.5 Typical sites of psoriasis.

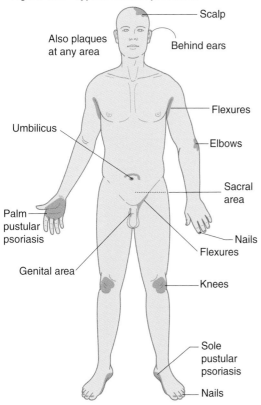

- Scalp
- Also plaques at any area
- Behind ears
- Flexures
- Umbilicus
- Elbows
- Palm pustular psoriasis
- Sacral area
- Nails
- Flexures
- Genital area
- Knees
- Sole pustular psoriasis
- Nails

Figure 15.7 Yellow separation (onycholysis) and pitting of nail.

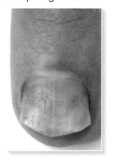

Figure 15.6 Flexural psoriasis: symmetrical shiny red areas with minimal scale in perianal area.

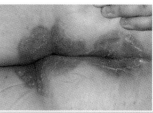

Figure 15.8 Scalp psoriasis: clear red edge and much silvery scale.

Figure 15.9 Scalp psoriasis showing scale adherent to hairs – pityriasis amiantacea (don't confuse with nits).

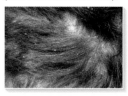

Dermatology at a Glance, Second Edition. Mahbub M.U. Chowdhury, Ruwani P. Katugampola, and Andrew Y. Finlay.
© 2020 John Wiley & Sons Ltd. Published 2020 by John Wiley & Sons Ltd.
Companion website: www.wiley.com/go/chowdhury/dermatology

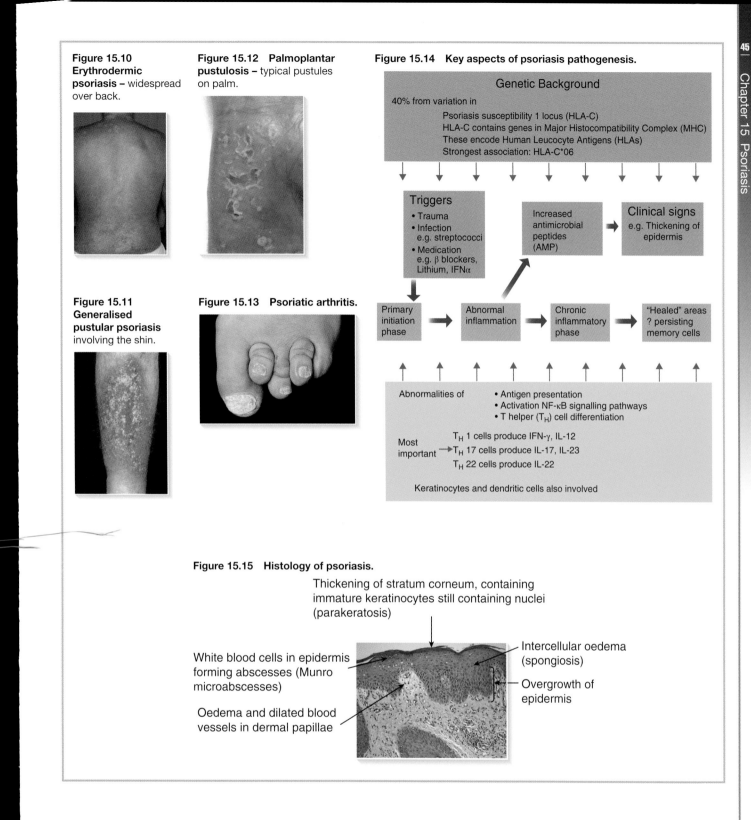

Figure 15.10 Erythrodermic psoriasis – widespread over back.

Figure 15.12 Palmoplantar pustulosis – typical pustules on palm.

Figure 15.11 Generalised pustular psoriasis involving the shin.

Figure 15.13 Psoriatic arthritis.

Figure 15.14 Key aspects of psoriasis pathogenesis.

Genetic Background

40% from variation in

Psoriasis susceptibility 1 locus (HLA-C)
HLA-C contains genes in Major Histocompatibility Complex (MHC)
These encode Human Leucocyte Antigens (HLAs)
Strongest association: HLA-C*06

Triggers
• Trauma
• Infection
  e.g. streptococci
• Medication
  e.g. β blockers,
  Lithium, IFNα

Increased antimicrobial peptides (AMP)

Clinical signs
e.g. Thickening of epidermis

Primary initiation phase → Abnormal inflammation → Chronic inflammatory phase → "Healed" areas ? persisting memory cells

Abnormalities of
• Antigen presentation
• Activation NF-κB signalling pathways
• T helper (T$_H$) cell differentiation

Most important →
T$_H$ 1 cells produce IFN-γ, IL-12
T$_H$ 17 cells produce IL-17, IL-23
T$_H$ 22 cells produce IL-22

Keratinocytes and dendritic cells also involved

Figure 15.15 Histology of psoriasis.

Thickening of stratum corneum, containing immature keratinocytes still containing nuclei (parakeratosis)

Intercellular oedema (spongiosis)

White blood cells in epidermis forming abscesses (Munro microabscesses)

Overgrowth of epidermis

Oedema and dilated blood vessels in dermal papillae

Epidemiology

The incidence of adults receiving a first-ever diagnosis of psoriasis is 2–3 cases per 1000 person-years (Italy): reported prevalence ranges from 1% (China) to 11% (Norway). About 3% of people develop psoriasis at some time in their lives.

Clinical Presentations

Psoriasis can start at any age, although the most common times are in the late teens and in the fifties. There is often a family history. Children may present with 'guttate' (drop-like) psoriasis (Figure 15.1), multiple small, red, scaly areas, a few days after streptococcal throat infection.

There are multiple areas of red, slightly raised and scaly skin 'plaques' (Figures 15.2–15.4). Plaques have a clear edge and are often symmetrical. If scratched, they bleed more easily than normal skin. Knees, elbows, and scalp are often affected, but all areas can be involved (Figure 15.5). Lesions last many months or years, may slowly enlarge and coalesce and can be itchy. Patients are most concerned by the appearance, the scales and the huge impact that the disease can have on their lives.

When the groin, axillae, or other body folds are affected, the scale comes off easily in these moist areas so there is a shiny red appearance (Figure 15.6). Often, the fingernails are affected, with multiple small pits, discoloration, and thickening (Figure 15.7). Toenails are also affected and can look like fungal infection.

Scalp psoriasis (Figures 15.8 and 15.9) can be felt better than seen, although if you part the hair, you see grey matted scale instead of normal scalp skin. Scalp psoriasis has a clear edge, typically with some areas unaffected, in contrast to dandruff that affects the whole scalp.

Rarely, the psoriasis becomes very extensive, with most of the skin becoming red and scaly (erythrodermic, Figure 15.10). This leads to:
- Increased fluid loss through the skin
- Increased protein loss
- Mild heart failure, as 25% of the cardiac output may be diverted to the skin
- Although the skin feels hot, there is great heat loss from radiation, resulting in hypothermia

Very rarely, all areas can become covered by sterile pustules (Figure 15.11). This dermatology emergency, acute generalised pustular psoriasis, should not be confused with chronic localised palmoplantar pustulosis (Figure 15.12) that only affects palms and soles in smokers.

Assessing Co-Morbidities

Psoriatic arthritis affects 30% of patients. There are five types: single large joint arthritis, distal interphalangeal arthritis, arthritis similar to rheumatoid but less severe, arthritis mutilans of fingers and toes (Figure 15.13), and spondylitis and/or sacroiliitis. Screening questionnaires such as the Psoriasis Epidemiology Screening Tool (PEST) may be used to identify psoriatic arthritis.

People with severe psoriasis usually have other problems with their health. Co-morbidities include obesity, hypertension, cardiac problems, diabetes, hyperlipidaemia, and alcohol dependence. Patients should be offered intervention for smoking, alcohol, and high blood pressure, and exercise encouragement. Full cardiovascular risk assessment should be carried out every five years.

Pathogenesis

First, you need to have a genetic susceptibility: the *PSOR1* location on chromosome 9 and other genes controlling inflammatory mediators are likely culprits (Figure 15.14). Once the condition starts, an immune process occurs. T lymphocytes move out of the blood vessels in the skin into the dermis. These spark off the release of chemical messengers, cytokines such as tumour necrosis factor-alpha, which result in the skin becoming inflamed and the epidermis becoming thickened and producing many more keratinocytes than usual, hence the scaliness. Why this process happens in localised often symmetrical areas remains a mystery.

Diagnosis

The diagnosis is usually made clinically from the history and typical appearance. The histology shows massively thickened epidermis, increased thickness of the stratum corneum, increased blood vessels nearer the surface (hence the redness) and inflammation in the upper dermis (Figure 15.15).

Treatment

Topical Treatment

Most people with psoriasis have only a few lesions. Keeping the scale under control is important and frequently applying emollients may be all that is needed. For more active therapy, topical calcipotriol (a vitamin D analogue) is simple to apply and not too messy. Topical corticosteroids can be used alone or in combination with calcipotriol. If they are used over wide areas or continuously over months, there may be localised dermal thinning or even problems from systemic absorption. Scalp psoriasis is best treated with combined topical calcipotriol and corticosteroids.

Topical dithranol (anthralin) is seldom used because it stains the skin (and the clothes) and can cause irritation. However, it is very effective if used carefully. If day care dermatology nursing treatment is available, patients can be helped with their treatment and compliance may improve (Chapter 13).

Ultraviolet Treatment

Widespread psoriasis can be treated with narrow-band UVB (ultraviolet B radiation, wavelength 311 nm) or with PUVA (oral or topical psoralens and ultraviolet A) (Chapter 44). Patients have to attend twice weekly for 8–10 weeks; they get a nice tan but the lifetime number of treatments has to be limited to reduce the risk of skin cancer.

Systemic Treatment

If topical treatments or UV fails, or if the Rule of Tens (Chapter 5; Tables 15.1 and 15.2) is reached, then systemic treatment is probably indicated, even though all systemic therapies have risks of side effects (Chapter 14). Oral methotrexate, ciclosporin, acitretin, mycophenolate mofetil, fumaric acid and apremilast are the first line oral therapies. If these fail, then biologics are used, such as etanercept or adalimumab. However, the most effective biologics are infliximab, ixekizumab, guselkumab, secukinumab, and ustekinumab; they work by specifically targeting key inflammatory messengers. They are given by injection or intravenous infusion and are highly effective, but very expensive. As they are relatively new drugs, their long-term benefits and side effects are not yet fully known.

Obesity, hypertension, cardiac problems, diabetes, depression, and alcohol dependency should be searched for and treated in parallel. For paediatric psoriasis, etanercept is effective and safe.

Key Points
- Match the aggressiveness of intervention to the impact of the disease on the patient's life.
- Compliance with therapy is very difficult in a chronic disease. Make treatment as simple as possible.

▶ Warning
- Erythrodermic psoriasis needs urgent in-patient treatment.

16 Atopic Dermatitis

Table 16.1 Diagnostic criteria for atopic dermatitis (AD).

Must have:

- Itchy skin in the last 12 months

Plus three or more of the following:

- History of flexural involvement
- History of asthma and/or hay-fever (or in children < 4 years, history of atopy in first degree relatives)
- History of a generally dry skin
- Visible flexural eczema
- Onset in the first 2 years of life

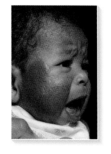

Figure 16.1 Acute infantile AD on the face.

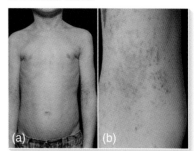

Figure 16.2 (a) Child with widespread acute AD and (b) close-up of the typical erythematous papules at the antecubital fossa.

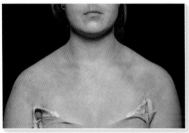

Figure 16.3 AD of the face and upper trunk in an adult.

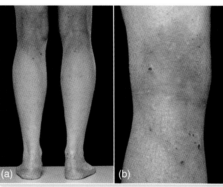

Figure 16.4 (a) Chronic eczema of the legs and (b) close-up of the lichenified plaques at the flexures.

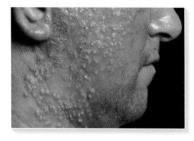

Figure 16.6 Eczema herpeticum on the face.

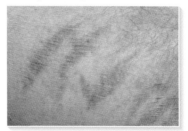

Figure 16.7 Striae due to prolonged use of potent topical corticosteroids.

Table 16.2 Aims of management of AD.

- Patient and parent education about the disease and its management
- Participation of patient and parent(s) in treatment of their AD
- Support patients/parents with psychology input when necessary, care plans for schools
- Restore epidermal barrier function with emollients
- Control skin inflammation and maintenance in remission with topical corticosteroids and calcineurin inhibitors
- Consider second-line therapy for severe disease, e.g. phototherapy, systemic immunosuppressants, biological agents
- Prevent exacerbations secondary to infection, irritants, and allergens
- Maintain long-term disease control

Dermatology at a Glance, Second Edition. Mahbub M.U. Chowdhury, Ruwani P. Katugampola, and Andrew Y. Finlay.
© 2020 John Wiley & Sons Ltd. Published 2020 by John Wiley & Sons Ltd.
Companion website: www.wiley.com/go/chowdhury/dermatology

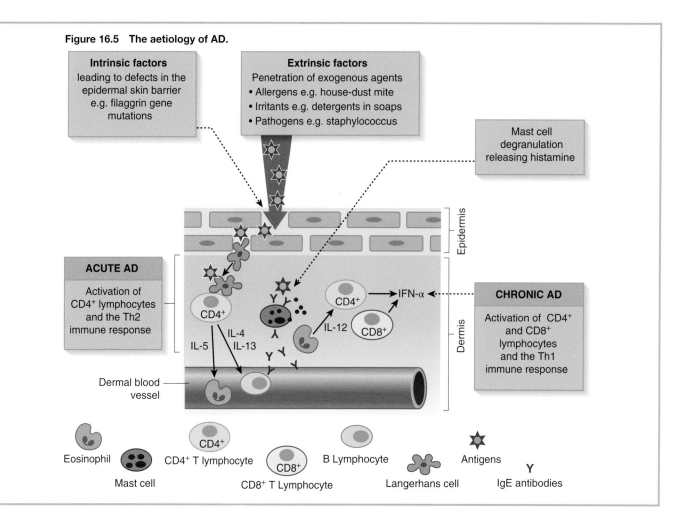

Figure 16.5   The aetiology of AD.

Atopy is the tendency to develop hypersensitivity to allergens as a result of genetic predisposition and environmental factors. Atopic diseases include atopic dermatitis (AD), hayfever, and asthma. Atopic dermatitis is a common, chronic, relapsing, and remitting inflammatory skin disease; its prevalence is about 5–15% in children and 2–10% in adults. The diagnostic criteria for AD are summarised in Table 16.1.

Clinical Patterns According to Age

Infantile AD Onset is within the first six months and persists until the age of two to three years. Usually affects the head and neck (Figure 16.1).

Childhood AD Onset is within the first few years of life and persists until or into puberty. Typically affects flexures (e.g. antecubital and popliteal fossae, neck) (Figure 16.2).

Adult AD Onset is usually in those in their twenties or thirties. It can affect head and neck, flexures of limbs and trunk (Figure 16.3). There is often a previous history of infantile or childhood AD.

Clinical Features

• **Acute** (or acute on chronic) **AD** presents with itchy erythematous papules, patches, and vesicles with or without erosions on the affected areas (Figures 16.1–16.3).

• **Chronic AD** appears as thickened dry skin with prominence of skin markings (lichenification), often with excoriations and postinflammatory pigmentary changes (hyper- or hypopigmentation) (Figure 16.4).

Aetiology and Pathogenesis

In normal skin, keratinocytes and intercellular lipids form the epidermal barrier which retains water and prevents the penetration of

exogenous agents (e.g. allergens and irritants) into the skin. The aetiology of AD is multifactorial, with genetic and environmental influences, epidermal barrier defects, penetration of exogenous agents into the skin and activation of the immune response (Figure 16.5).

Mutations in filaggrin genes have been linked to AD in about 10% of individuals with AD in Europe. Filaggrin is an epidermal skin barrier protein that has a role in the aggregation of the keratin cytoskeleton during epidermal differentiation.

In acute AD, the dermal Th2 immune response is activated by uptake and presentation of antigens by the epidermal dendritic antigen presenting cells (i.e. Langerhans cells) to CD4+ lymphocytes in the dermis and blood vessels. These cells produce Th2 pro-inflammatory cytokines (e.g. interleukin [IL] 4, 5, 13) which recruit eosinophils, B lymphocytes, and induce immunoglobulin E (IgE) production. Immunoglobulin E activates histamine release by mast cells leading to itching. In the chronic phase of AD, eosinophils release IL-12 activating the Th1 immune response leading to release of α-interferon (IFN-α) by CD4+ and CD8+ T lymphocytes.

Complications of Atopic Dermatitis

Bacterial infection The skin of AD patients is colonised with *Staphylococcus aureus*; their exotoxins act as superantigens which activate the inflammatory process in acute AD. *Staphylococcus* also causes superadded infection, leading to flare-ups of AD and impetigo (exudate, yellow crusting, blistering [bullous impetigo]).

Eczema herpeticum (Chapter 24) is localised or widespread herpes simplex infection of skin affected by AD (Figure 16.6). It is a dermatological emergency and presents with grouped vesicles and/or pustules, which progress to superficial erosions and crusting which heal without scarring. Ophthalmology review is essential when the face is involved.

Erythroderma See Chapter 20.

Allergic contact dermatitis including to the patient's own topical treatments (e.g. steroids and/or the preservatives) should be considered in those with treatment-resistant AD (Chapter 35).

Management

- Aims of management of AD are summarised in Table 16.2.
- Patient education on the management of their AD.
- Tailor treatment to the individual patient's disease severity. This can be assessed by clinical examination and objective patient-rated measures such as health-related quality of life questionnaires and clinician-rated measures such as the affected body surface area (Chapter 5) or Eczema Area and Severity Index (EASI) (http://www.homeforeczema.org/documents/easi-user-guide-dec-2016-v2.pdf).
- Regular moisturising breaks the itch–scratch cycle and prevents exacerbations. The choice of moisturiser(s) (Chapter 12) is best decided with the patient to improve treatment adherence. Soap substitute emollients should be used instead of conventional soaps which dry the skin and damage the barrier function, leading to exacerbation of AD.
- First generation oral antihistamines, such as piriton (chlorphenamine), are useful to aid itch relief at night because of their sedative effects.
- Topical corticosteroids are the treatment of choice for controlling the inflammation in AD. The lowest effective potency of topical steroids is used, depending on the patient's age and body site. Steroids are 'weaned off' once clinical clearance has been achieved (Chapter 12). Mild potencies are preferred for the face and flexures; moderate to high potencies for limited periods to other body sites.
- Complications of the long-term use of topical steroids include skin atrophy, striae (Figure 16.7), glaucoma, and growth retardation in children resulting from suppression of the pituitary–adrenal axis (Chapter 12).
- Topical calcineurin inhibitors (tacrolimus and pimecrolimus) are topical immunosuppressants used for maintenance of remission in AD, once the acute flares have been controlled with topical corticosteroids. Their advantage is the lack of steroid-associated complications. However, in view of their immunosuppressant effect, these treatments should not be used on infected eczema.
- Bandaging of limbs affected by AD is often used, either with moisturisers, zinc, or topical corticosteroids (Chapter 13), to protect the skin and enhance absorption.
- Phototherapy (Chapter 44) can be used for widespread AD resistant to topical treatment. Systemic steroids (oral prednisolone) for up to two weeks are occasionally used to control severe widespread AD. Systemic immunosuppressants (e.g. azathioprine, ciclosporin, mycophenolate mofetil) are useful in the long-term control of widespread severe AD unresponsive to the above topical treatments.
- Emerging therapies include the biological agent dupilumab for moderate to severe AD in adults. Dupilumab is a fully human monoclonal antibody against IL-4α receptor subunit on lymphocytes which blocks signalling by IL-4 and IL-13, and thus reduces the inflammatory process leading to AD (Figure 16.5). It is given as a subcutaneous injection once every two weeks.
- Management of superadded infections includes swabbing affected areas for bacterial and viral cultures and prescribing antibiotics (e.g. flucloxacillin) and/or antiviral (e.g. aciclovir) therapy.

Key Points

- Management of AD includes regular moisturising, control of acute flares with topical corticosteroids, and maintaining remission with topical calcineurin inhibitors and avoidance of potential triggers.
- Possible causes for flare-ups of AD include poor treatment compliance, superadded infection, or allergic contact dermatitis.

▶ Warning

- Inappropriate long-term use of super-potent and potent topical corticosteroids can cause serious side effects.

17 Acne and Teenage Skin

Table 17.1 Skin diseases that may affect teenagers.

- **Inflammatory** – acne, eczema (Chapter 16), psoriasis (Chapter 15)
- **Infections** – pityriasis versicolor (Chapter 25)
- **Autoimmune** – vitiligo (Chapter 42), alopecia areata (Chapter 30)
- **Benign skin lesions** – congenital or acquired naevi (Chapter 38), viral warts (Chapter 24)
- **Malignant skin lesions** – malignant melanoma (Chapter 40)
- **Vascular lesions** – vascular malformation (Chapter 31)
- **Self-induced** – dermatitis artefacta (Chapter 49)

Table 17.2 Points to consider when consulting a teenager with a skin disease.

- Impact of skin disease on psychological well-being
- Impact of psychological issues on skin disease
- Impact of chronic disease and its treatment on education and social activities
- Impact of skin disease on major life decisions, e.g. choice of career
- Impact of media and peer pressure to have 'perfect skin'
- Cosmetic issues regarding skin lesions/rashes
- Patient education/disease prevention
- Treatment adherence

Figure 17.1 Severe psoriasis of both palms causing functional and psychological impact.

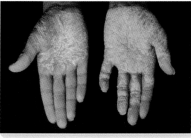

Figure 17.2 Vitiligo of the abdominal wall – note the contrast between the depigmented patches of vitiligo with the darker unaffected skin.

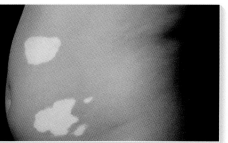

Figure 17.3 Alopecia areata of the scalp.

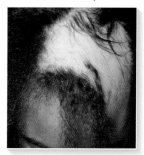

Figure 17.4 Pathogenesis of acne.

- Hair shaft
- Epidermis
- Dermis
- Hyperkeratinisation of infundibulum followed by shedding of keratinocytes into its lumen
- Androgen-stimulated secretion of sebum by sebaceous glands
- Proliferation of *P. acnes*
- Dermal inflammation
- Pilosebaceous unit

Figure 17.5 Open comedones and pustules.

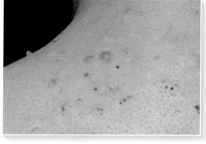

Figure 17.6 Severe nodular, cystic scarring acne.

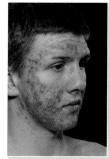

Figure 17.7 Close-up of severe acne – note the comedones, pustules, nodules, and scarring on an inflammatory background.

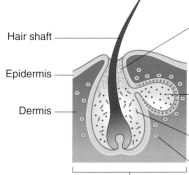

Figure 17.8 Keloid scar formation following severe acne.

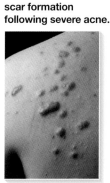

Table 17.3 Mode of action of acne treatments.

Treatment	Mode of action
Topical retinoid	Reduces epidermal hyperkeratinisation, anti-inflammatory
Topical benzoyl peroxide	Anti-inflammatory, anti-bacterial
Topical antibiotics	Anti-inflammatory, anti-bacterial
Oral antibiotics	Anti-inflammatory, anti-bacterial
Anti-androgen	Reduces sebaceous gland hyper-secretion
Oral isotretinoin	Reduces sebaceous gland hyper-secretion and epidermal hyperkeratinisation, anti-inflammatory

Dermatology at a Glance, Second Edition. Mahbub M.U. Chowdhury, Ruwani P. Katugampola, and Andrew Y. Finlay.
© 2020 John Wiley & Sons Ltd. Published 2020 by John Wiley & Sons Ltd.
Companion website: www.wiley.com/go/chowdhury/dermatology

Teenage years can be a stressful period during which many changes occur in the physical and psychological aspects of life. These issues should be borne in mind when consulting a teenager with any form of skin disease.

Points to Consider When Consulting a Teenager with a Skin Disease

Skin diseases are often visible. This can impact on the psychological well-being of affected individuals, exacerbated by media and peer pressure to have 'perfect skin' (e.g. scarring acne, psoriasis, vitiligo or eczema affecting exposed skin) (Figures 17.1–17.3 and 17.6, Table 17.2). Psychological stress from domestic or school issues or the skin disease itself may cause further flares (e.g. psoriasis).

Severe chronic skin diseases (e.g. psoriasis or eczema) may require frequent hospital appointments for day treatment, or in-patient therapy. These may disrupt educational and recreational activities.

Skin lesions on exposed skin may be cosmetically unacceptable for patients. Excision of benign lesions needs to be weighed against the cosmetic effect of the resulting scar. Cosmetic camouflage is beneficial for vitiligo or large vascular malformations.

Education is important in disease prevention and treatment compliance. For example, raising awareness of the skin cancer risk of sunbeds, photo-protection measures, and how to recognise a suspicious skin cancer. Developing a topical treatment regime practical and acceptable to the individual's daily routine can improve treatment compliance in chronic skin diseases.

Acne Vulgaris

This is the most common skin disease affecting teenagers. It is associated with significant impact on psychological well-being. A disease of the pilosebaceous unit in the skin, pathogenesis of acne is multifactorial (Figure 17.4) and includes the following:
• Hyperkeratinisation of the epidermis in the infundibulum of the hair follicles.
• Shedding and accumulation of keratinocytes within the lumen of the infundibulum.
• Stimulation of increased sebum production by androgen hormones.
• Proliferation of *Propionibacterium acnes*, a Gram-positive anaerobic bacterium, within the pilosebaceous units.
• Because of the narrow openings into the skin surface, the shed corneocytes, sebum and *P. acnes* accumulate within the pilosebaceous units which subsequently rupture.
• This leads to dermal inflammation, mainly consisting of neutrophils (early and late stages) and T helper lymphocytes (late stages).
• Upregulation of genes coding inflammatory cytokines including matrix metalloproteinases and interleukin-8.

Diagnosis is made clinically based on the types of lesions described below and the distribution of the rash characteristically affecting the face, back, and shoulders to varying extents. Different stages of clinical severity exist, corresponding to the stages of pathogenesis described above:

• Comedones (Figure 17.5) are non-inflamed early lesions of acne. Closed comedones ('white-heads') are small, approximately 1–2 mm skin-coloured papules. Open comedones ('black-heads') are papules with a central keratin plug consisting of shed keratin. Comedones can lead to subtle 'ice-pick' scars.
• Papules and pustules (Figure 17.5) develop with the onset of inflammation. These erythematous lesions often lead to scarring.
• Nodules and cysts are associated with marked inflammation and tenderness and lead to scarring (Figures 17.6 and 17.7).

Complications of acne include the following:
• Scarring ranging from subtle pitted ('ice-pick') to keloid scars (Figure 17.8).
• Psychological distress due to the disease itself and subsequent scarring.

The aim of treatment is disease control and prevention of scarring (Table 17.3).

Management – Choice of treatment(s) depends on the stage of clinical severity:
• *Mild comedones ± few papules* – topical benzoyl peroxide ± topical antibiotic (e.g. clindamycin), topical retinoid (e.g. adapalene).
• *Moderately severe acne with papules and pustules with mild scarring* – the above topical treatment with a three-month course of oral antibiotics (e.g. lymecycline, doxycycline). In female patients, an anti-androgen combined with oestrogen in the form of the oral contraceptive pill can be used (e.g. Dianette® containing 2 mg cyproterone acetate +35 µg ethinylestradiol).
• *Severe acne with papules, pustules, nodules, cysts, and scarring* – oral isotretinoin 0.3–0.5 mg/kg/day for six months. Isotretinoin is a retinoid and is teratogenic; therefore females of childbearing age commenced on isotretinoin should be counselled and must use reliable contraception (e.g. oral contraceptive pill, intrauterine contraceptive device).

In treatment resistant acne, consider possible underlying causes:
• Polycystic ovarian syndrome in females.
• Ingestion or injection of anabolic steroids.

Key Points
• Skin diseases can have a psychological impact in teenagers.
• Acne pathogenesis includes accumulation of keratinocytes within the pilosebaceous unit, androgen-stimulated increased sebum production and proliferation of *P. acnes* leading to dermal inflammation.
• Treatment of acne depends on disease severity.
• Treatment options include topical anti-bacterials with or without antibiotics, topical retinoids, oral antibiotics, anti-androgens (for females only), and oral isotretinoin.

▶ Warning
• Females of childbearing age with severe acne considered for oral isotretinoin must be counselled regarding teratogenicity. Reliable contraception is needed one month prior to, during and one month post treatment.

18 Hidradenitis Suppurativa

John Ingram

Table 18.1 Diagnostic criteria.

Characteristic lesion types	Inflammatory papules and nodules, open comedones, abscesses, sinus tunnels, rope-like scars
Flexural sites	Axillae, groins, inframammary (women), perineum, posterior auricular, abdominal folds
Chronicity	Recurrent flares, often in same sites

Figure 18.1   Characteristic lesions.

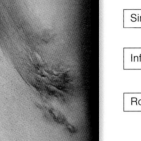

Sinus tunnels

Inflammatory nodules

Rope-like scars

Figure 18.2   Sites affected by hidradenitis suppurativa.

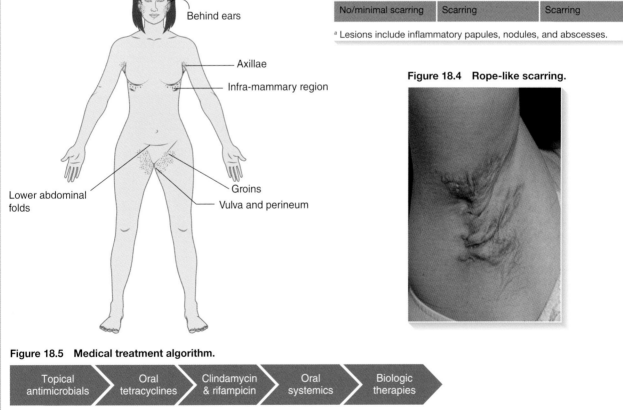

Behind ears

Axillae

Infra-mammary region

Lower abdominal folds

Groins

Vulva and perineum

Figure 18.3   Hurley staging.

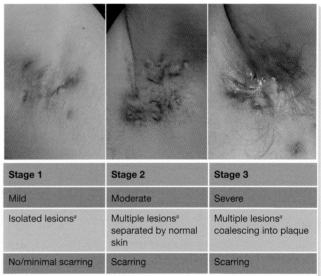

Stage 1	Stage 2	Stage 3
Mild	Moderate	Severe
Isolated lesions[a]	Multiple lesions[a] separated by normal skin	Multiple lesions[a] coalescing into plaque
No/minimal scarring	Scarring	Scarring

[a] Lesions include inflammatory papules, nodules, and abscesses.

Figure 18.4   Rope-like scarring.

Figure 18.5   Medical treatment algorithm.

Topical antimicrobials ▷ Oral tetracyclines ▷ Clindamycin & rifampicin ▷ Oral systemics ▷ Biologic therapies

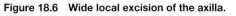

Figure 18.6   Wide local excision of the axilla.

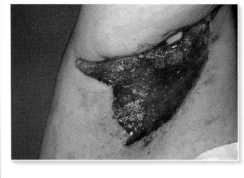

Figure 18.7   Secondary intention wound healing of axillary wound.

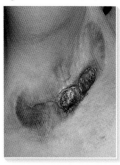

Clinical Features

Hidradenitis suppurativa (HS) is a chronic, painful inflammatory skin disease characterised by multiple skin 'boils' in flexural sites. The diagnosis is made clinically from three features in the history and examination: characteristic skin lesions such as inflammatory nodules, comedones, and skin sinuses, often leading to scarring (Figure 18.1); a predominantly flexural location such as the axillae and groins (Figure 18.2), and frequent flares over time (Table 18.1).

Discharge of pus from lesions, odour, and scarring produce a lot of embarrassment and often result in a large impact on quality of life. About 1% of adults are affected with a 3:1 female: male ratio and disease onset is usually in early adulthood, which means that HS may have a large effect on work absenteeism and formation of intimate relationships. It may be misdiagnosed as 'recurrent boils' or not brought to medical attention due to embarrassment of those affected. Acute flares are typically very painful and, depending on location, may limit basic tasks such as raising the arms, sitting down, or walking.

Disease severity may be classified into mild, moderate, or severe, based on Hurley stages 1, 2, and 3 (Figure 18.3 and Table 18.2). In moderate to severe disease, there is progressive scarring which often has a characteristic 'rope-like' appearance (Figure 18.4).

Co-morbidities

Crohn's disease occurs more frequently in those with HS and there is a higher than average risk of cardiovascular disease, due in part to higher rates of smoking, type 2 diabetes, hyperlipidaemia, and hypertension. In keeping with a chronic, painful, and socially isolating condition, HS is associated with depression. There is also an association with acne and pilonidal sinus.

Aetiology and Pathogenesis

Aetiology is incompletely understood and may involve four factors:
• Genetic – autosomal dominant inheritance is present in about 40% of patients. Although rarely there are pathogenic mutations in the genes encoding gamma secretase, a protein involved in keratinocyte differentiation, there is no genetic test for HS.
• Environmental – there are strong links with smoking and obesity but some people with HS are non-smokers of normal weight.
• Endocrine – this is suggested by onset at or soon after puberty and women may experience flares linked to their menstrual cycle.
• Microbiological – bacteria are often found in deep tissue layers in biopsies from HS lesions but it is unknown whether these are pathological or reflect colonisation of non-sterile sinus tunnels.

In terms of pathogenesis, it has been suggested that HS is due to follicular occlusion because rupture of hair follicles is one of the main histological findings.

Management

Treatment of HS may involve both medical and surgical interventions in parallel. This means that multidisciplinary team (MDT) management is ideal. Pain control for acute flares, as well as support for smoking cessation and weight management, are also important considerations.

Medical Treatment

A stepwise approach is taken, based on disease severity (Figure 18.5). For mild disease, topical antimicrobials, such as clindamycin solution may be of benefit. The next option is usually oral tetracyclines. For moderate to severe HS with a lot of pus formation, a combination of clindamycin and rifampicin antibiotics, taken twice daily for 10–12 weeks may be beneficial. These can cause gastrointestinal disturbance and it is important to consider potential drug interactions, including reduced effectiveness of hormonal contraception. The next step in the algorithm is to consider other oral systemic agents such as acitretin (in men and non-fertile women) and dapsone. For severe HS unresponsive to other therapies, biologic agents such as adalimumab or infliximab may be effective.

Surgical Treatment

As for medical therapy, surgical interventions are tailored to disease severity. Incision and drainage of single active lesions may be performed and electrosurgery is sometimes offered to de-roof sinus tunnels. In terms of the size of surgical procedures, there is a trade-off between recovery time and risk of recurrence. Limited excisions of one or a few lesions offer a shorter recovery time but a relatively high risk of recurrence adjacent to the surgical scar. Wide local excision of an entire skin region, such as all of the hair-bearing axilla (Figure 18.6), provides lower recurrence rates at the expense of extended recovery times. The large skin defects created cannot be closed primarily and may require secondary intention healing (Figure 18.7).

Key Points
• Pain, discharge of pus, scarring, and embarrassment mean that HS has a large impact on quality of life.
• A combination of medical and surgical interventions may be needed, with therapy escalated depending on disease severity.

▶ Warning
• Don't forget adequate pain relief in the management of active HS.

19 Common Inflammatory Diseases

Table 19.1 Inflammatory skin diseases commonly seen in dermatology clinic.

- Psoriasis (Chapter 15)
- Eczema (Chapter 16)
- Lichenoid skin diseases
- Lichen planus
- Drug eruptions
- Pityriasis rosea

Table 19.2 Patterns of lichen planus (LP).

- Mucosal
- Linear
- Annular
- Pigmented
- Follicular
- Bullous
- Atrophic

Table 19.3 Conditions showing Koebner's phenomenon.

- Lichen planus
- Psoriasis
- Vitiligo
- Viral warts
- Molluscum contagiosum
- Sarcoidosis

Table 19.4 Drug causes of lichenoid reactions.

- Mepacrine
- Gold
- Quinine
- Thiazide diuretics
- Isoniazid
- Methyldopa
- Propranolol
- Labetalol
- Enalapril
- Captopril
- Naproxen
- Interferon
- Imatinib
- Leflunomide

Figure 19.1a   LP on ankle.

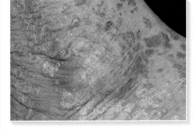

Figure 19.1b   Typical LP shiny papules on wrist.

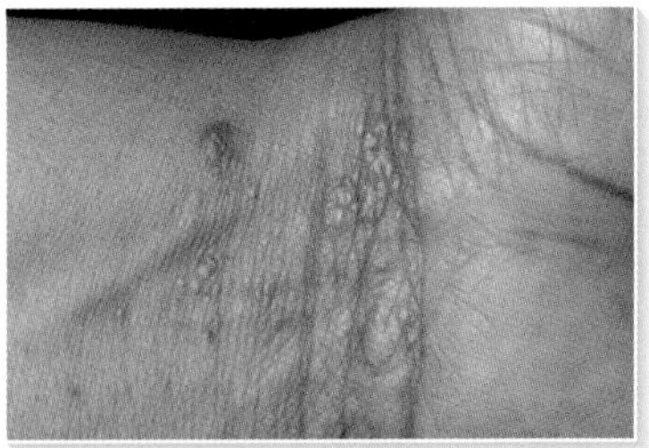

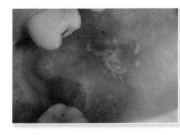

Figure 19.1c   Nail LP.

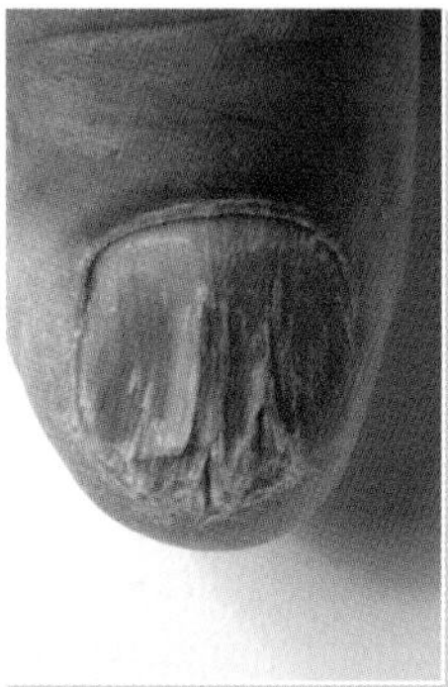

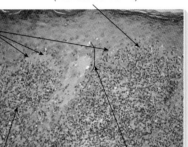

Figure 19.2a and b   Wickham's striae on leg.

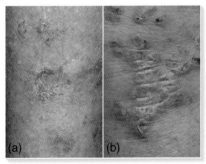

(a)   (b)

Figure 19.3   Mucosal LP with Wickham's striae in mouth.

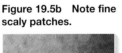

Figure 19.4   Histology of LP (H&E).

lymphocytes in the lower epidermis (interface dermatitis)

necrotic basal epidermal cells (Civatte bodies)

diffuse lymphocytic infiltrate

irregular 'saw-tooth' epidermal thickening (acanthosis)

Figure 19.5a   Typical pityriasis rosea.

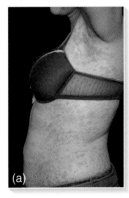

(a)

Figure 19.5b   Note fine scaly patches.

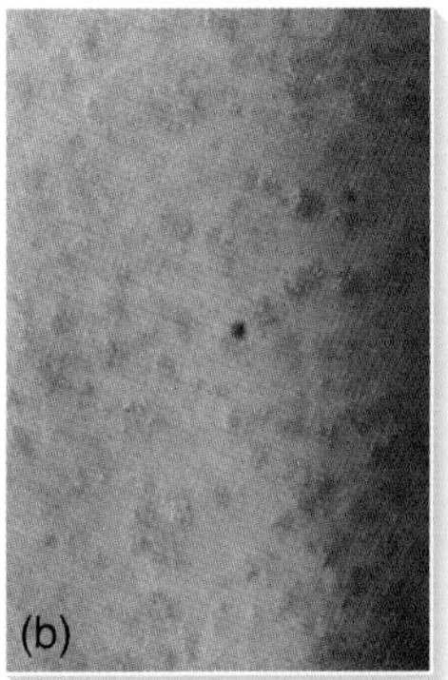

(b)

Figure 19.5c and d   Herald patch.

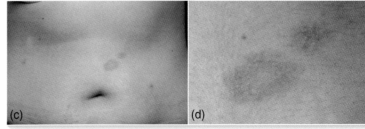

(c)   (d)

Dermatology at a Glance, Second Edition. Mahbub M.U. Chowdhury, Ruwani P. Katugampola, and Andrew Y. Finlay.
© 2020 John Wiley & Sons Ltd. Published 2020 by John Wiley & Sons Ltd.
Companion website: www.wiley.com/go/chowdhury/dermatology

Lichenoid Disorders

'Lichenoid' can describe the appearance clinically of a shiny, flat-topped, papular rash or can suggest histology of band-like inflammatory cell infiltrate in the upper dermis with basal cell necrosis. Lichenoid eruptions can be due to a number of causes including lichen planus (LP), drug eruptions, graft versus host disease (GvHD), and pityriasis lichenoides (Table 19.1).

Lichen Planus

Most people with cutaneous LP (>70%) have oral involvement; 10% present with this. Lichen planus is a T cell mediated autoimmune inflammatory condition. There are possible genetic links and association with hepatitis C. Lichen planus presents as shiny, flat topped, violaceous, polygonal papules on the skin (Figure 19.1). Papules vary in size and many clinical patterns are seen (Table 19.2). In typical presentations, with distribution on the dorsum of the ankles and wrists, a biopsy is not always required; however, LP can occur on any body site including the palms and soles.

The surface white lines with a lace-like pattern are called 'Wickham's striae' (Figure 19.2). Hypertrophy and hyperpigmentation in darker skin types is common and linear lesions can occur along scratch marks or scars (Koebner's phenomenon) (Table 19.3). Itching is common but can be absent.

Mucosal areas in the mouth may cause pain and ulceration (Figure 19.3). Mucous membrane involvement may need patch testing to exclude allergy (e.g. mercury amalgam). The nails are affected (10%) with ridging (Figure 19.1c) and thinning of the nail plate and pterygium (adhesions between the posterior nail fold and nail plate). Scarring alopecia on the scalp with skin atrophy can result in permanent hair loss.

Histopathology

Typical features are an irregular saw tooth thickening of the epidermis (acanthosis) with Civatte bodies (necrotic basal epidermal cells) and a lymphocytic inflammatory infiltrate (Figure 19.4). Specific features are seen in hypertrophic, atrophic, follicular, and mucosal LP. Differential diagnoses include plane warts, eczema, and pityriasis rosea, and lichen simplex chronicus.

Prognosis and Treatment

Lichen planus can clear spontaneously within a few weeks but most acute attacks will last for at least six months if untreated. Mucous membrane lesions may clear more slowly. Resolving lesions generally stop itching. Progression can occur with hypertrophy or hair loss if the scalp is affected.

Potent topical steroids are applied especially if the patient has symptoms of severe itching. Occlusion is used to increase the absorption and effectiveness, particularly with hypertrophic LP. Generalised or LP unresponsive to topical treatments may require systemic therapy such as oral corticosteroids for short periods or retinoids (acitretin), ciclosporin, methotrexate, or oral bath PUVA. Oral lesions may require betamethasone (Betnesol®) mouthwash or triamcinolone in Orabase®.

Other Lichenoid Reactions

Lichen Planus-Like Eruption Due to Drugs

Many drugs are known to cause lichenoid and LP-like changes (Table 19.4). Mepacrine was used as an anti-malarial during the Second World War. Gold has been the most common recent drug causing LP-like eruptions, but this is now used less often for rheumatoid arthritis. Histologically, the pattern of lichenoid changes is similar to idiopathic LP. However, the presence of eosinophils may point more towards a drug reaction. Quinine and thiazide diuretics can cause a lichenoid photodermatitis which can appear more psoriasis-like. Hyperpigmentation and hair loss may be severe.

Previously, 25% of people using photographic colour developers developed acute eczematous and subacute lichenoid changes but automated equipment now minimises this risk.

Graft versus Host Disease

Skin manifestations are prominent in GvHD and can mimic LP. Bone marrow transplantation for severe haematological disorders including acute leukaemias may precipitate GvHD. This is due to lymphoid cells from an immunocompetent donor being introduced into an incompatible recipient who is then incapable of rejecting the lymphoid cells. The threat of GvHD is increased when the genotypes of the donor and recipient are not identical. The reaction varies from mild to severe, with over 70% mortality.

The process may be acute or chronic and most patients with GvHD have skin involvement. This presents one week to three months after transplantation (acute) or after three months (chronic). Patients with GvHD present with fever and erythema of the face, palms, and soles with a generalised papular eruption. Differentials include drug reactions and infections. Chronic GvHD involves the skin, liver, upper respiratory and gastro-intestinal tract. Local or general changes in the skin occur with sclerosis, ulceration, lichenoid changes, and hyper or hypopigmentation with severe poikiloderma. Treatment for skin GvHD includes ciclosporin and phototherapy.

Pityriasis Rosea

Pityriasis rosea is a common, acute, self-limiting disease affecting children and young adults. After being unwell, a typical 'herald patch' follows which is a large, 2–5 cm, inflamed, well-defined, scaly patch. A general eruption with new oval, pink to red, fine, scaly patches occurs one to two weeks later with collarettes of scale surrounding the edges (Figure 19.5). These lesions can occur in a Christmas tree pattern occurring mainly on the trunk, neck, and upper third of the arms and legs. The skin eruption fades within three to six weeks and can usually be diagnosed from the typical history and herald patch. Differentials include seborrhoeic dermatitis, drug eruption, secondary syphilis, urticaria, and guttate psoriasis. Only minimal treatment is needed with topical emollients, mild to moderate strength topical steroids, and, if not responsive, UVB.

Key Points
- Lichen planus has many clinical patterns including mucosal.
- Lichenoid drug reactions can mimic LP.
- Pityriasis rosea is an acute, self-limiting disease in children and young adults; look out for the herald patch.

▶ **Warning**
- Graft versus host disease should be considered in any lichenoid skin eruption in severe haematological conditions.

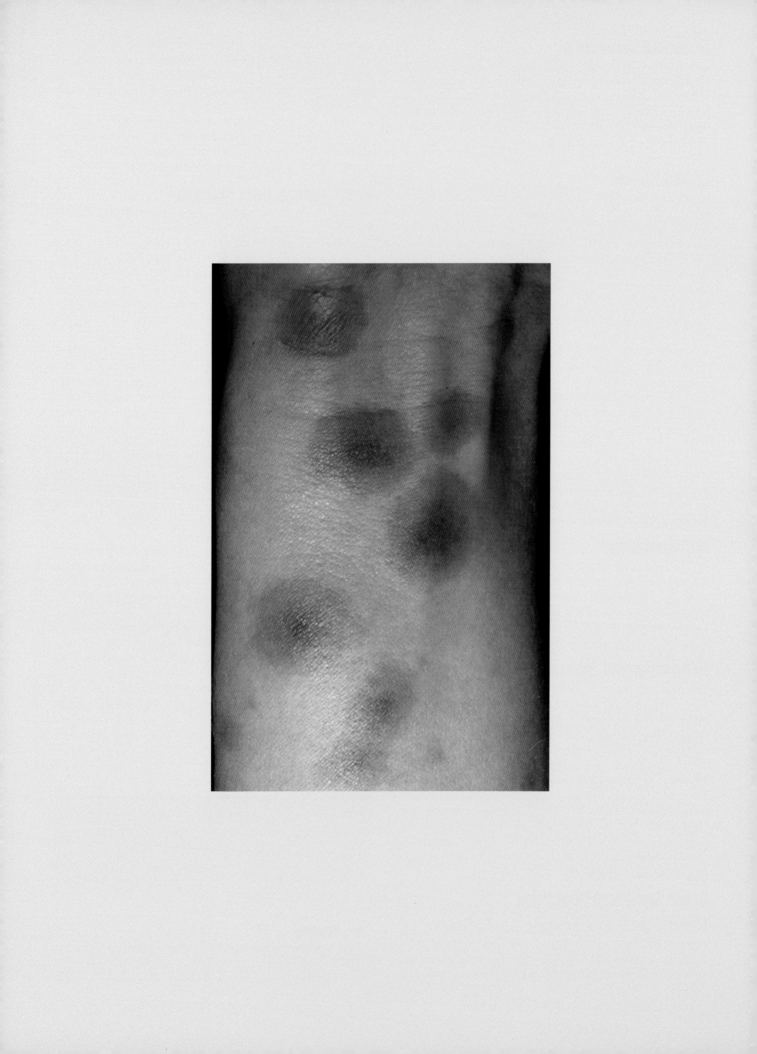

ER Dermatology

Part 6

Chapters

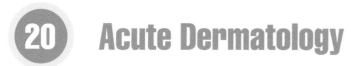

20 Acute Dermatology

Table 20.1 Causes and clinical images of erythroderma.

Causes of erythroderma
• **Inflammatory skin diseases** Atopic dermatitis, allergic contact dermatitis, psoriasis, pityriasis rubra pilaris
• **Drug reaction** Allopurinol, antibiotics (e.g. penicillin, sulphonamides), anti-convulsants (e.g. carbamazepine, phenytoin)
• **Bullous skin diseases** Pemphigus foliaceus, bullous pemphigoid
• **Malignancies** Cutaneous T cell lymphoma, lymphoproliferative malignancies, Sézary syndrome
• **Erythroderma in the neonatal period or infancy** Ichthyosis (e.g. Netherton's syndrome), severe combined immunodeficiency, infections (e.g. staphylococcal scalded skin syndrome, candidiasis)

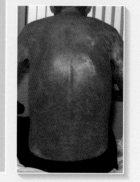

Figure 20.1 Erythrodermic patient.

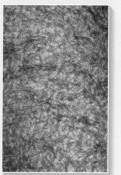

Figure 20.2 Close-up view of erythroderma.

Table 20.2 Pathogenesis and clinical manifestations of Stevens–Johnson syndrome (SJS) and toxic epidermal necrolysis (TEN).

Cutaneous manifestations
• Skin pain • Dusky erythema • Detachment of the epidermis, spontaneously or by sideways pressure (Nikolsky sign) resulting in large areas of denuded skin (resembling a burn)

Extra-cutaneous manifestations
Mucosal exfoliation leads to: • Stomatitis • Oesophagitis • Conjunctival and corneal erosions • Diarrhoea • Painful micturition • Desquamation of respiratory tract

Drug causes of SJS and/or TEN
• Non-steroidal anti-inflammatory medication e.g. ibuprofen • Antibiotics e.g. penicillin • Anti-convulsants e.g. phenytoin • Antiretroviral medication

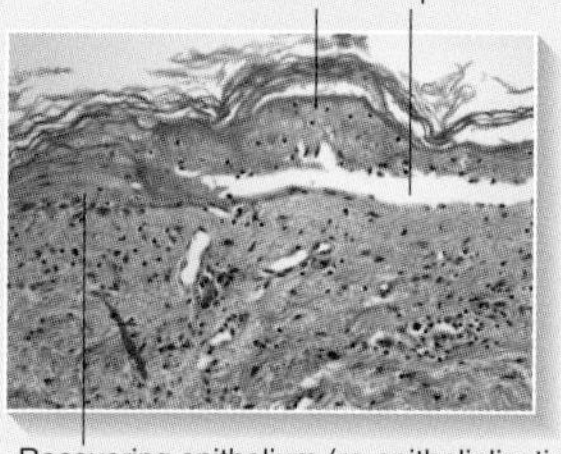

Necrotic roof of blister   Cell free sub-epidermal blister

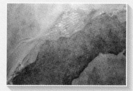

Recovering epithelium (re-epithelialisation)

Figure 20.3 Histology of TEN (H&E ×20), characterised by full thickness epidermal necrosis. Keratinocyte death and apoptosis occurs causing separation at the dermoepidermal junction leading to the clinical manifestations.

Figure 20.4 Detachment of epidermis in TEN.

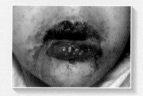

Figure 20.5 Stomatitis due to SJS.

Table 20.3 Causes and pathogenesis of angioedema and anaphylaxis.

Causes of angioedema and anaphylaxis
• Idiopathic • Food, e.g. peanuts, strawberries, shell-fish • Latex • Hereditary C1 esterase inhibitor deficiency (autosomal dominant) • Medication, e.g. non-steroidal anti-inflammatories, aspirin, antibiotics, ACE inhibitors • Contrast medium (radiology procedures) • Bee or wasp sting

Pathogenesis of angioedema and anaphylaxis
• IgE-mediated (type 1 hypersensitivity), e.g. latex and food allergies • Complement-mediated e.g. C1 esterase inhibitor deficiency

Release of vasodilator substances such as histamine ± activation of the complement pathway leading to swelling of dermis and subcutaneous tissue

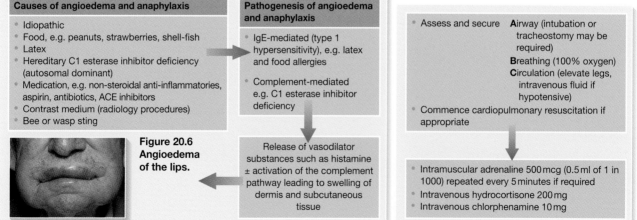

Figure 20.6 Angioedema of the lips.

Table 20.4 Immediate management of anaphylaxis in an adult.

• Assess and secure **A**irway (intubation or tracheostomy may be required)
     Breathing (100% oxygen)
     Circulation (elevate legs, intravenous fluid if hypotensive)
• Commence cardiopulmonary resuscitation if appropriate

• Intramuscular adrenaline 500 mcg (0.5 ml of 1 in 1000) repeated every 5 minutes if required • Intravenous hydrocortisone 200 mg • Intravenous chlorphenamine 10 mg

Dermatology at a Glance, Second Edition. Mahbub M.U. Chowdhury, Ruwani P. Katugampola, and Andrew Y. Finlay.
© 2020 John Wiley & Sons Ltd. Published 2020 by John Wiley & Sons Ltd.
Companion website: www.wiley.com/go/chowdhury/dermatology

Erythroderma

Erythroderma is characterised by generalised erythema, scaling, and exfoliation of the skin affecting at least 90% of the body surface area (Figures 20.1 and 20.2). It has many different causes (Table 20.1). The cause may not be identified in 20–30% of cases (idiopathic).

Complications occur due to skin failure and loss of skin function:
- Skin infections and septicaemia (loss of skin barrier function)
- Hypothermia (loss of thermoregulation)
- Peripheral oedema (loss of albumin)
- Tachycardia and high-output cardiac failure
- Renal failure (loss of fluid and electrolytes).

Management

- Identify and treat or withdraw underlying cause (e.g. drugs)
- Supportive care
- Prevention of complications

The patient should be managed in a warm environment to prevent hypothermia, with regular monitoring of core body temperature, blood pressure, pulse, fluid balance, and for evidence of sepsis.

Treatment includes:
- Fluid and electrolyte replacement, nutritional support
- Sedating antihistamines for itching
- Frequent topical application of emollients
- Systemic antibiotics if evidence of infection
- Systemic steroids (oral prednisolone) may be considered if the underlying cause is likely to be drug induced.

Erythema Multiforme

See Chapter 46.

Stevens–Johnson Syndrome and Toxic Epidermal Necrolysis

This is a disease spectrum, usually drug induced and characterised by potentially life-threatening mucocutaneous exfoliation (Table 20.2; Figures 20.3–20.5). Stevens–Johnson syndrome (SJS) and toxic epidermal necrolysis (TEN) are defined by the affected body surface area (< 10% = SJS, 10–30% = SJS–TEN overlap, > 30% = TEN).

Complications are similar to that of erythroderma. Early diagnosis and management is vital to reduce mortality. SCORTEN is a scoring system used to predict mortality of patients with TEN. This includes indices such as patient's age, co-morbidities, and laboratory markers (e.g. serum creatinine).

Management

Principles of management are similar to that of erythroderma. In addition, patients require non-adherent dressings to denuded skin, regular analgesia, and management of the extra-cutaneous manifestations by ocular, oral, respiratory, and urogenital specialist input. In view of the large surface area of skin loss and life-threatening complications patients with TEN are best managed in a high-dependency or burns unit with strict barrier nursing. Use of systemic steroids is controversial due to increased risk of sepsis. Intravenous immunoglobulins or oral ciclosporin may improve prognosis in TEN.

Angioedema and Anaphylaxis

Different causes can lead to angioedema and anaphylaxis by release of vasodilator substances that result in swelling of dermis and subcutaneous tissue (Table 20.3). Urticaria may or may not be present with angioedema and anaphylaxis (Chapter 37). Angioedema is characterised by painless swelling of the skin, commonly the hands, eyelids, tongue, and lips (Figure 20.6). **Anaphylaxis** is a life-threatening emergency. It is rapid in onset with swelling of the upper airways and throat resulting in difficulty breathing, swallowing and speaking, low blood pressure, and potential loss of consciousness. Anaphylaxis requires urgent intervention (Table 20.4).

Management

- A detailed history to identify the potential cause(s).
- Further investigations may be indicated to identify the causative agent. If IgE-mediated reaction to latex or food is suspected, blood tests for serum IgE and allergen-specific RAST (radioallergosorbent test). If this test is negative, prick-testing should be considered, where full resuscitation facilities are available (Chapter 35). C1 esterase inhibitor, complement C3 and C4 levels should be measured when C1 esterase inhibitor deficiency is suspected.
- Angioedema is treated with a short course of oral steroids and H1 antihistamines. In hereditary angioedema resulting from C1 esterase inhibitor deficiency, C1 inhibitor concentrate infusion has been effective in the management of acute angioedema; danazol, an androgen, has been effective in the long-term prophylaxis of angioedema. Danazol is unsuitable for children and pregnant women because of its androgenic effects (e.g. hirsutism).
- Life-threatening anaphylaxis requires urgent intervention (Table 20.4) followed by a course of oral steroids and an antihistamine. Individuals with a history of anaphylaxis should be advised to wear a MedicAlert® bracelet and carry an EpiPen® (containing 1:1000 adrenaline 300 µg 0.3 ml [adult dose]). The patient and a family member should be taught how to use an EpiPen in the event of anaphylaxis.

Eczema Herpeticum

See Chapters 16 and 24.

Necrotising Fasciitis

Necrotising fasciitis (also called 'flesh-eating disease') is an uncommon, potentially life-threatening, soft tissue infection. The most common causative organism is Group A *Streptococcus*. It is characterised by painful, rapidly progressive skin swelling, colour changes from red to purple–grey, and subsequent necrosis of subcutaneous tissue and fascia. Patients become toxic with fever, tachycardia, and septic shock. Old age, diabetes, non-healing ulcers, penetrating trauma, and surgery predispose to necrotising fasciitis.

Management

- Investigations include full blood count, renal function, C-reactive protein, and wound swabs for bacterial culture.
- Broad-spectrum intravenous antibiotics and urgent surgical debridement of necrotic tissue is the mainstay of treatment.
- Fluid and electrolyte replacement, nutritional support, and analgesia.

Key Points

- Dermatological emergencies can be life-threatening.
- Most common causes are underlying skin diseases or drugs.
- Principles of management include identifying and treating or withdrawing the underlying cause, supportive care in a high-dependency environment, and prevention of complications.
- Individuals with a history of angioedema and anaphylaxis should wear a MedicAlert bracelet and carry an EpiPen.

► Warning

- Patients with TEN are best managed in a high-dependency setting or burns unit.
- Anaphylaxis is a rapid onset, life-threatening emergency that needs urgent intervention to prevent death.

Blistering Skin Diseases

Table 21.1 Possible causes of skin blistering.

- **Inherited**: e.g. epidermolysis bullosa (Chapter 53), bullous ichthyosiform erythroderma (Chapter 53), bullous cutaneous porphyrias (Chapter 45)
- **Acquired**:
  - Drug-induced: e.g. fixed drug eruption (Chapter 22), Stevens-Johnson syndrome, toxic epidermal necrolysis (Chapter 20)
  - Infections: e.g. bullous impetigo, staphylococcal scalded skin syndrome (Chapter 32)
  - Autoimmune: e.g. linear IgA disease (Chapter 32), bullous pemphigoid, pemphigus, dermatitis herpetiformis
  - Other: insect bites, severe sunburn, phytophotodermatitis, contact dermatitis, pompholyx eczema (Chapters 35 and 36)

Figure 21.1   Schematic diagram of the skin basement membrane (BM).

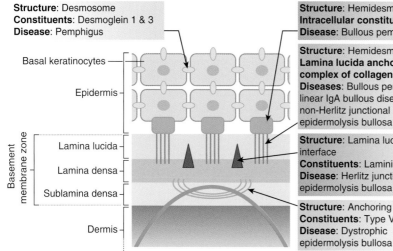

Structure: Desmosome
Constituents: Desmoglein 1 & 3
Disease: Pemphigus

Structure: Hemidesmosome
Intracellular constituent: BP 230
Disease: Bullous pemphigoid

Structure: Hemidesmosome
Lamina lucida anchoring filament complex of collagen XVII: BP180
Diseases: Bullous pemphigoid, linear IgA bullous disease, non-Herlitz junctional epidermolysis bullosa

Structure: Lamina lucida-densa interface
Constituents: Laminin 5
Disease: Herlitz junctional epidermolysis bullosa

Structure: Anchoring fibrils
Constituents: Type VII collagen
Disease: Dystrophic epidermolysis bullosa

Basal keratinocytes

Epidermis

Basement membrane zone

Lamina lucida

Lamina densa

Sublamina densa

Dermis

Figure 21.2   Phytophotodermatitis – note the linear urticated lesions and nearby blisters.

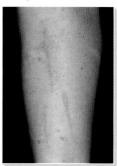

Figure 21.3   Bullous pemphigoid – note the tense blisters, some of which are haemorrhagic, that burst to leave superficial erosions on the skin.

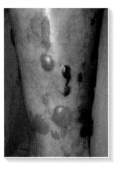

Figure 21.4   Histology of bullous pemphigoid – note the subepidermal blister on this H&E stain ×4.

Epidermis   Unilocular subepidermal blister   Dermal inflammation

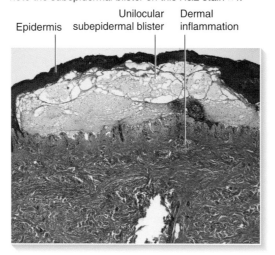

Figure 21.5   Direct immunofluorescence (IMF) of bullous pemphigoid – note the linear deposition of immunoglobulin G (IgG) at the basement membrane.

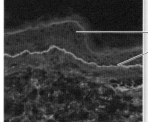

Epidermis

Linear IgG deposition at the basement membrane

Dermatology at a Glance, Second Edition. Mahbub M.U. Chowdhury, Ruwani P. Katugampola, and Andrew Y. Finlay.
© 2020 John Wiley & Sons Ltd. Published 2020 by John Wiley & Sons Ltd.
Companion website: www.wiley.com/go/chowdhury/dermatology

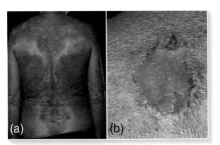

Figure 21.6a and b Pemphigus vulgaris – blisters are fragile and therefore often erosions and crusting are seen rather than blisters.

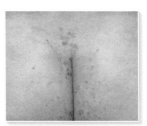

Figure 21.7 Dermatitis herpetiformis – itchy vesicles and small blisters typically develop on the buttocks and extensor aspects of the limbs.

Table 21.2 **Differentiating features between autoimmune bullous skin diseases.**

Disease	Clinical features	Aetiology	Histology	Direct immunofluorescence (IMF)
Bullous pemphigoid	Tense blisters on an urticated base ± mucosal involvement	Immunoglobulin G (IgG) autoantibodies to basement membrane (BM) antigen BP180 or BP230	Subepidermal blisters (Figure 21.4)	Linear IgG at the BM
Pemphigus	Flaccid blisters, skin erosions, and crusting ± mucosal involvement	Autoantibodies to epidermal cell surface proteins desmoglein 1 and 3	Intraepidermal acantholysis ± blisters	Cell surface bound IgG, net-like pattern in epidermis
Dermatitis herpetiformis	Itchy small blisters and vesicles	IgA autoantibodies to gluten tissue transaminase in the gut and epidermis	Subepidermal blisters	Granular IgA in dermal papillary tips
Linear IgA disease (Chapter 32)	Small blisters in an arc pattern ± mucosal involvement	IgA autoantibodies to BM antigen BP180	Subepidermal blisters	Linear IgA deposition along epidermal BM

Table 21.3 **Differentiating features between the types of pemphigus.**

Type of pemphigus	Skin involvement	Mucosal surface involvement	Circulating autoantibodies to	Histology
Pemphigus vulgaris	Fragile blisters and erosions	Always involved	Desmoglein 1 and 3	Suprabasal acantholysis
Pemphigus foliaceus	Superficial scaly erosions	Spared	Desmoglein 1	Subcorneal acantholysis
Paraneoplastic pemphigus	Skin erosions	Severe	Desmoglein 1 and 3, desmoplakin	Suprabasal acantholysis

The skin may blister as a result of different causes (Table 21.1). Disruption of the complex skin basement membrane (BM) at different levels leads to the different blistering skin diseases (Figure 21.1).

Phytophotodermatitis is an uncommon blistering rash caused by a phototoxic reaction following sunlight exposure after contact with plants containing photosensitising chemicals such as psoralen (e.g. giant hogweed, celery, parsnip, and rue). Painful and/or itchy urticated plaques or blisters appear within 24 hours of contact in a streaky pattern at the sites of plant contact (Figure 21.2). Management is with potent topical corticosteroids and antihistamines and avoidance of future contact with offending plants.

Autoimmune Bullous Skin Diseases

Autoantibodies against epidermis or BM components lead to activation of an inflammatory cascade with cleavage of the skin at different levels and blistering (Figure 21.1). Diagnosis is made clinically and confirmed by histology (Table 21.2).

Investigations include serum antibodies to target antigen, biopsy of lesional skin for haematoxylin and eosinophil staining (differentiates level of skin cleavage causing the blister), peri-lesional skin for direct immunofluorescence (IMF), and serum for indirect IMF.

Immunofluorescence

Immunofluorescence helps to differentiate between types of bullous diseases.

Direct IMF A fluorescein-labelled antibody against the suspect disease-causing antibody and/or complement is added to the peri-lesional skin biopsy from the patient. When examined under UV light it demonstrates the deposition pattern of autoantibodies and complement in the skin characteristic of the different bullous skin diseases (Table 21.2).

Indirect IMF The patient's serum containing the disease-causing antibodies is added to an animal tissue (e.g. monkey oesophagus) and incubated. The antibodies are highlighted under UV light using fluorescein-labelled anti-human antibody.

Bullous Pemphigoid

Bullous pemphigoid is an autoimmune bullous disease which is more common in elderly people.

Symptoms and signs Intense pruritus may precede the onset of tense (as the blister wall is the complete epidermis) blisters on an erythematous background which may be localised or widespread

(Figure 21.3). Blisters may also occur on mucosal surfaces (e.g. oral mucosa, Chapter 29). The blisters later burst to leave superficial erosions that heal without scarring.

Aetiology Immunoglobulin G (IgG) autoantibodies to BM antigens BP180 (type XVII collagen) or BP230 result in cleavage of the skin at the dermo-epidermal junction leading to subepidermal blisters (Figures 21.4 and 21.5).

Investigations See above and Table 21.2.

Treatment Localised disease is treated with topical super-potent corticosteroids (e.g. 0.05% clobetasol propionate). Widespread disease requires oral doxycycline or a reducing course of oral prednisolone starting at about 30–40 mg/day combined with an oral immunosuppressant (e.g. azathioprine, mycopheno-late mofetil).There are less side effects with doxycycline.

Pemphigus

Pemphigus comprises a group of rare, potentially life-threatening, autoimmune bullous skin diseases which usually affect middle-aged individuals.

Aetiology IgG autoantibodies to epidermal cell surface proteins desmoglein 1 and 3 lead to loss of cell–cell adhesion (acantholysis) at different levels of the epidermis causing flaccid blisters or scaly erosions of the skin (Figure 21.6) and/or mucous membranes. Blisters are fragile as the blister wall is the thin upper part of the epidermis.

Signs and symptoms The three main types of pemphigus are summarised in Table 21.3. Paraneoplastic pemphigus occurs in association with an underlying lympho-proliferative disease (e.g. non-Hodgkin's lymphoma, Castleman's disease, thymoma).

Investigations See above and Table 21.2. Paraneoplastic pemphigus should prompt investigation for an underlying malignancy (e.g. full blood count, blood film, chest X-ray, further radiological studies such as chest CT scan).

Treatment Systemic therapy with high-dose weaning course of oral steroids (e.g. 60 mg/day prednisolone) in combination with an immunosuppressant (e.g. azathioprine, mycophenolate mofetil). Other treatments include intravenous immunoglobulin, cyclo-phosphamide, and rituximab. Rituximab is a monoclonal antibody against CD20 on B-lymphocytes. The rationale for use of rituximab for pemphigus is to deplete CD20+ B-lymphocytes that are presumed to produce the pathogenic autoantibodies.

Linear IgA Bullous Disease

See Chapter 32.

Dermatitis Herpetiformis

This is an autoimmune bullous skin disease usually affecting young and middle-aged individuals due to IgA autoantibodies (also called IgA anti-endomysial antibodies) to gluten tissue trans-glutaminase in the gut and epidermis. The male:female ratio is 2:1.

Signs and symptoms Itchy vesicles or small blisters, typically on the extensor aspects of limbs and buttocks. Because of the intense itch, excoriations may be the only sign seen (Figure 21.7). Approximately 75% of patients may also give a history of gluten-sensitive enteropathy (coeliac disease).

Investigations See above and Table 21.2. Direct IMF in dermatitis herpetiformis shows granular IgA deposition in dermal papillary tips in contrast to linear IgA disease (Chapter 32) where linear IgA deposition is seen along the epidermal BM.

Treatment Oral dapsone and gluten-free diet. Dapsone rapidly relieves itch. Blood glucose-6-phosphate dehydrogenase level needs to be checked as its deficiency increases the risk of haemolysis due to dapsone. Patients on dapsone require monitoring of full blood count and reticulocyte count (risk of haemolytic anaemia) and liver function (risk of hepatotoxicity).

Key Points

- Intense pruritus may precede the onset of blisters in bullous pemphigoid and dermatitis herpetiformis.
- Immunofluorescence is essential to diagnose autoimmune bullous diseases.
- Mucosal surfaces may be affected in blistering skin diseases.

▶ Warning

- Patients on long-term, high-dose, oral steroids need osteoporosis prophylaxis and monitoring for steroid-induced hypertension and diabetes (glycosuria and raised serum glucose).

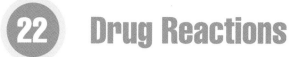

22 **Drug Reactions**

Table 22.1 **Summary of skin reactions to systemic drugs.**

Type of drug reaction	Description	Examples of causative drugs
Lichenoid drug eruption (Chapter 19)	Itchy, violaceous, papular rash similar to lichen planus.	Thiazide diuretics Naproxen
Fixed drug eruption (see text)	Recurrent, well-defined, red–dusky oval plaque(s) or blister(s) at the same site each time the offending drug is introduced	Non-steroidal anti-inflammatory medication Antibiotics (tetracyclines, co-trimoxazole, penicillin) Dapsone
Erythema multiforme (Chapter 46, Figure 22.3)	Red lesions, some target-like	Antibiotics (sulphonamides)
Urticaria (Chapter 37)	Itchy, red-pink, raised swelling (wheals) on the skin of different shapes and sizes. Individual lesions resolve within 24 hours	Non-steroidal anti-inflammatory medication Aspirin Antibiotics Angiotensin converting enzyme (ACE) inhibitors
Angioedema and anaphylaxis (Chapter 20)	Swelling of the skin, especially eyelids, lips, and tongue (angioedema) Mucosal involvement leads to life-threatening swelling of the upper airways and throat (anaphylaxis)	Non-steroidal anti-inflammatory medication Aspirin Antibiotics ACE inhibitors
Erythroderma (Chapter 20)	Generalised erythema and scaling of the skin affecting at least 90% of the body surface area	Allopurinol Antibiotics (penicillin, sulphonamides) Anticonvulsants (carbamazepine, phenytoin)
Acute generalised exanthematous pustulosis (AGEP) (see text)	Widespread sterile pustules on erythematous background associated with fever and neutrophilia	Antibiotics (penicillin, macrolides) Calcium channel blockers ACE inhibitors Anticonvulsants
Drug reaction with eosinophilia and systemic symptoms (DRESS) (see text)	Widespread rash associated with fever, eosinophilia, and multi-organ complications	Anticonvulsants Allopurinol Sulfasalazine Non-steroidal anti-inflammatory medication Dapsone
Stevens–Johnson syndrome (SJS) and toxic epidermal necrolysis (TEN) (Chapter 20)	Potentially life-threatening muco-cutaneous exfoliation with associated skin pain and detachment of the epidermis	Non-steroidal anti-inflammatory medication Antibiotics (penicillin) Anticonvulsants (phenytoin) Anti-retroviral medication

Table 22.2 **Mechanisms underlying skin manifestations of drug reactions.**

Underlying mechanism	Examples
Immediate IgE-mediated	Urticaria Angioedema Anaphylaxis
Immune-complex mediated	Vasculitis Urticaria
Delayed T cell mediated	Photoallergic reaction Fixed drug eruption Contact dermatitis
Idiosyncratic/immune-mediated	Stevens–Johnson syndrome/toxic epidermal necrolysis

Dermatology at a Glance, Second Edition. Mahbub M.U. Chowdhury, Ruwani P. Katugampola, and Andrew Y. Finlay.
© 2020 John Wiley & Sons Ltd. Published 2020 by John Wiley & Sons Ltd.
Companion website: www.wiley.com/go/chowdhury/dermatology

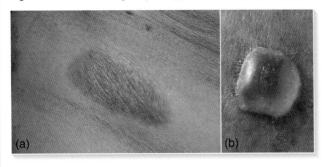

Figure 22.1 **Fixed drug eruption** (a) brown oval plaque (b) blister.

(a)

(b)

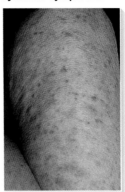

Figure 22.2 **Drug reaction with eosinophilia and systemic symptoms.**

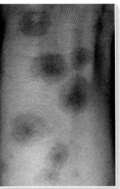

Figure 22.3 **Erythema multiforme** note the erythematous target-like lesions.

A wide range of skin manifestations can result from reactions to medication, either applied topically or taken systemically. Some skin manifestations of drug reactions are benign, localised, and self-limiting once the suspect medication is discontinued. Other reactions can be extensive, associated with systemic complications, and potentially life-threatening.

Reactions to topical therapies are usually irritant or allergic dermatitis and remain localised to application sites. Reactions to systemic therapies are more widespread and may also involve other organs.

Some drug reactions occur immediately or within minutes (e.g. urticaria, angioedema, anaphylaxis) to hours of ingesting the offending medication whilst other reactions may appear after a lag period of up to a week. A detailed clinical history with particular attention to timing between the start of any new medication (prescribed or bought over the counter) and the start of a rash is crucial when a drug reaction is suspected.

Drug Reactions to Topical Treatments

• Topical use of anti-bacterial moisturisers containing benzalkonium chloride can cause an irritant dermatitis, particularly in flexural body sites.
• Topical medication including steroids and antibiotics (e.g. neomycin) can cause an allergic contact dermatitis.
• Side effects of long-term use of potent topical steroids are summarised in Chapter 12 (Topical Therapy). These include skin atrophy, acne, and rosacea. Systemic absorption of excessive use of topical steroids may lead to Cushing's syndrome.

Drug Reactions to Systemic Drugs

Drug reactions to systemic treatments are summarised in Table 22.1. Mechanisms underlying the skin manifestations of drug reactions are summarised in Table 22.2. The underlying mechanism of some skin manifestations remains unclear.

Fixed Drug Eruption

Recurrent, isolated or grouped lesions develop at the same body site each time the offending drug is introduced. The lesions, which may be itchy, are well-defined, red–dusky brown, oval plaque(s) (Figure 22.1a) and may have blisters (Figure 22.1b). Any part of the body can be affected, including mucosal surfaces. Systemic symptoms are absent. The eruption can develop within hours to two weeks after starting the offending medication, and resolve

spontaneously about a week after discontinuing the medication, leaving post-inflammatory pigmentation.

Causative medications include non-steroidal anti-inflammatory drugs, antibiotics (tetracyclines, co-trimoxazole, penicillin), and dapsone. The diagnosis is made based on history and examination. Differential diagnosis includes erythema multiforme and bullous pemphigoid.

Acute Generalised Exanthematous Pustulosis (AGEP)

Widespread, sterile pustules on an erythematous background characterises AGEP. The rash is associated with fever and blood neutrophilia. Symptoms of AGEP develop within hours to days of starting the offending medication and resolve spontaneously with supportive care within one to two weeks of stopping the medication. Causative medication includes antibiotics (penicillin or macrolide based), calcium channel blockers, angiotensin converting enzyme (ACE) inhibitors, and anti-convulsants.

Differential diagnosis of AGEP includes pustular psoriasis and subcorneal pustular dermatosis. The diagnosis of AGEP is made on clinical history and examination, supported by histological findings on skin biopsy of intraepidermal pustules, focal necrosis of keratinocytes, and eosinophils in the pustules and/or dermis.

Drug Reaction with Eosinophilia and Systemic Symptoms (DRESS)

The multi-system drug reaction, DRESS, is characterised by a widespread rash, blood eosinophilia, fever, lymphadenopathy, and multi-organ involvement. High morbidity and mortality of up to 10% is associated with DRESS. The rash can vary from mild, itchy, macular erythema to a widespread papular (Figure 22.2), pustular, blistering rash with skin loss. The severity of skin manifestations does not always correspond with the systemic manifestations; therefore a high index of suspicion is required to make a diagnosis of DRESS and monitor for multi-organ complications including hepatitis, interstitial nephritis, pericarditis, and pneumonitis.

The DRESS reaction develops within two to eight weeks of starting the offending medication and may take several months to resolve following stopping the medication. Management includes supportive care and systemic steroids if there are internal organ complications. Causative drugs include anti-convulsants, allopurinol, antibiotics, and non-steroidal anti-inflammatories.

Management of Drug Reactions

The most important aspects of management of a drug reaction are to discontinue the suspect drug and treat the patient symptomatically. If the rash is itchy, topical cooling emollients containing menthol and an oral sedative antihistamine will provide symptomatic relief. Management of immediate IgE-mediated reactions such as angioedema and anaphylaxis and management of erythroderma, Stevens–Johnson syndrome and toxic epidermal necrolysis are detailed in Chapter 20.

Skin biopsies are undertaken when there is clinical diagnostic uncertainty but histology may not always identify specific diagnoses. Re-challenge with the suspect medication is not recommended in view of the likelihood of a more severe reaction.

Key Points

- A detailed history on use of prescribed or over the counter medication and timing of onset of skin manifestations helps with the diagnosis of drug reactions.
- Patients with a drug reaction should be given written details of suspect medications in order to avoid further use.
- The key to treatment of drug reactions is discontinuing the suspect medication and supportive care.

▶ Warning

- Take urgent action if you suspect DRESS or TEN, which can be potentially life-threatening, with cutaneous and multi-organ failure requiring high-dependency supportive care.

Skin Infections

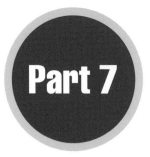

Chapters

23 Bacterial Infections

Table 23.1 Other skin bacterial infections.

- Staphylococcal scalded skin syndrome (Chapter 32)
- Staphylococcal infection in atopic dermatitis (Chapter 16)
- Syphilis (Chapter 29)
- Leishmaniasis (Chapter 27)

Table 23.2 Diseases involving the skin caused by Spirochaetes.

- Syphilis
- Lyme disease
- Yaws

Figure 23.1   Cellulitis: spreading erythema.

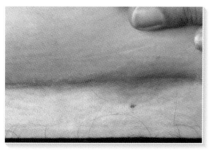

▶ **Warning**
- Differential diagnosis of a hot red leg includes cellulitis, deep venous thrombosis, and lipodermatosclerosis.

Figure 23.2   Erysipelas of face.

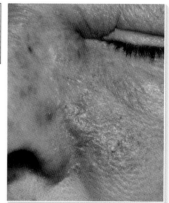

Figure 23.3   Impetigo.

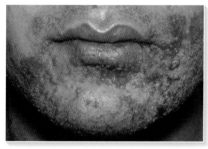

Figure 23.4   Folliculitis.

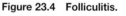
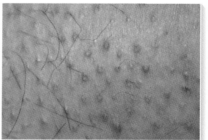

Figure 23.5   Healing furuncle (boil).

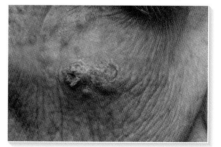

Figure 23.6   Intertrigo: inflammation in skin folds.

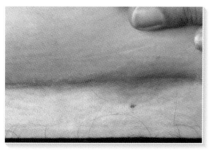

Figure 23.7   Pitted keratolysis: 'moth-eaten' appearance.

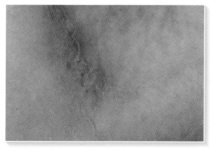

Figure 23.8   Fish tank granuloma between fingers with proximal spread.

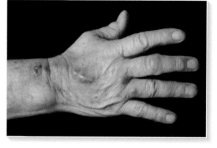

Skin is covered by billions of 'normal' commensal bacteria that prevent pathogenic organisms becoming established. But bacterial skin infections are highly prevalent, and without antibiotics may be fatal. It is important to recognise and treat them early.

Avoidance of infection confers survival advantage: fear of skin disease, 'Is it catching, doctor?' is therefore 'sensible'.

Common bacteria causing infection include *Staphylococcus aureus*, *Streptococcus pyogenes*, *Corynebacterium minutissimum*, *Mycobacterium tuberculosis*, *Mycobacterium marinum* and *Spirochaetes*.

Cellulitis and Erysipelas

- Redness, swelling, heat, tenderness, pyrexia.
- Take swabs for culture from fluid or cracked areas.
- Treatment: 500 mg flucloxacillin four times daily.
- Risks: recurrence, lymphoedema.
- Likelihood of recurrence is reduced by prophylactic low-dose penicillin V.

Cellulitis (Figure 23.1) *Streptococcus* group A or *Staphylococcus aureus* infection of subcutaneous tissue, typically of lower leg. Diffuse edge.

Erysipelas (Figure 23.2) *Streptococcus* group A infection of the dermis. Typically well-defined with red raised edge, on the face, with initial infection around nose or ears.

Impetigo

Superficial infection of epidermis, redness and crusting usually of face in children (Figure 23.3). Easily infects other children. Non-bullous impetigo is usually caused by *Staphylococcus aureus* (*aureus* means 'gold' – the colour of the culture) or by *Streptococcus pyogenes*. *Staphylococcus aureus* causes bullous impetigo with blistering.

Treatment – topical mupirocin or fusidic acid. Second line therapy: systemic flucloxacillin or erythromycin. If undiagnosed impetigo is treated wrongly with topical steroids, it initially improves but then gets worse.

Folliculitis

Very common inflammation around hair follicles resulting in small, itchy, red pustules on scalp or body (Figure 23.4). Pustules may be sterile or may grow coagulase-negative *Staphylococci* or *Staphylococcus aureus*. Predisposing factors include topical irritants and occlusion. Check local and nasal swabs.

Treatment – may settle by itself, but can be persistent and difficult to cure. If severe and *Staphylococci* isolated, topical mupirocin or systemic flucloxacillin. If nasal swabs positive, treat nostrils with mupirocin to reduce nasal carriage.

Boil (Furuncle)

Hair follicle infection from *Staphylococcus aureus* and nasal carriage (Figure 23.5). Like a volcano, if the 'head' is broken pus gushes out.

Treatment – flucloxacillin. If recurrent, check for diabetes, HIV, or Panton–Valentine leucocidin (PVL) toxin strain of *Staphylococcus*.

Erythrasma

Bacterial infection caused by *Corynebacterium minutissimum* (*minutissimum* means 'very small'). Diffuse, persisting, symptomless rash in toe webs, groin, or axillae, that under Wood's light (UVA 365 nm) fluoresces 'coral red'. Differential diagnosis fungal infection.

Treatment – very sensitive to a wide range of topical antibiotics and also sensitive to azoles (e.g. clotrimazole).

Intertrigo (Figure 23.6)

Inflammation of the skin in the body folds (e.g. beneath breasts). Stratum corneum always touching so folds of the skin are moist, creating a warm environment liked by bacteria and fungi. A 'soup' of organisms gives a red, sore, itchy, smelly, oozing rash.

Treatment – keep body folds apart and dry with dressings. Apply topical antibiotic antifungal low potency steroid mixtures.

Pitted Keratolysis (Figure 23.7)

'Moth-eaten' appearance of soles caused by *Corynebacterium* and other bacteria. Smelly, sore, superficial erosions associated with excessive sweating (hyperhidrosis).

Treatment – fucidin ointment and treat the hyperhidrosis.

Trichomycosis Axillaris

Thickening and nodules of hair in axillae, caused by Gram-positive *Corynebacterium*. Not fungal, despite its fungus-sounding name. Common in males, but usually symptom free.

Treatment – anti-perspirant anhydrous aluminium chloride, shave hair.

Lyme Disease

Borrelia burgdorferi infection via tick bites, often from deer, whilst walking in woodland. Named after Lyme, Connecticut, USA. Erythema chronicum migrans, an enlarging red circle, starts a week after the bite and may persist for months. Systemic features: arthritis 50%, neurological 20%, cardiac 10%. Diagnosis by antibody response.

Treatment – 100 mg doxycycline three times daily for two to three weeks. Oral treatment is essential to prevent systemic problems.

Tuberculosis

Direct infection If there is high host immunity: lupus vulgaris ('common wolf'), a single red–brown plaque on head or neck, or warty tuberculosis, a thick warty plaque at area of trauma. If there is poor host immunity: scrofuloderma, an ulcerating nodule over a lymph gland.

Secondary effects Erythema nodosum or erythema induratum (a 'tuberculid'), nodules that may ulcerate over the back of the lower legs in women.

Suspected tuberculosis must be fully investigated locally with skin biopsy for culture and systemically with chest X-ray. In the UK, TB is a notifiable disease. Seek advice from other specialists about investigation and treatment.

Fish tank Granuloma (Figure 23.8)

Tropical fish owners scratch hands on rocks when cleaning their fish tanks. A persistent purple plaque develops after three weeks, because of an 'atypical' *Mycobacterium marinum* infection.

Treatment – biopsy and culture, then doxycycline or clarithromycin.

Key Points

- Correct diagnosis is essential, especially if skin signs of systemic infection.
- Topical steroids make skin infection worse.
- If signs of cellulitis or erysipelas, systemic antibiotics are needed.

24 Viral Infections

Table 24.1 Treatments for post-herpetic neuralgia.

- Analgesics including narcotics
- Amitriptyline and other tricyclic antidepressants
- Gabapentin
- Topical agents e.g. capsaicin or lidocaine patches
- Transcutaneous nerve stimulation

Table 24.2 How to take a viral swab.

- Check transport medium available is for viral culture
- Deroof fresh blister with blade
- Swab the fluid released and blister base
- Insert swab into viral culture medium

Table 24.3 How to do a Tzanck smear.

- Deroof fresh blister and scrape base with blade
- Smear blade material onto glass slide
- Examine microscopically in lab after staining for multinucleated giant cells

Figure 24.1a Warts on fingers.

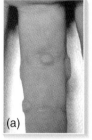

Figure 24.1b and c Plantar warts.

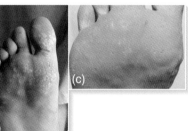

Figure 24.1d Viral wart with bleeding points (capillaries).

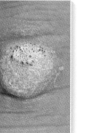

Figure 24.1e Wart on upper lip.

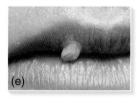

Figure 24.2 Periungual viral wart.

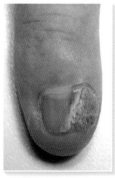

Figure 24.3a and b Herpes simplex virus (HSV) keratitis/ulcers seen with slit lamp.

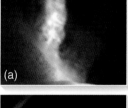
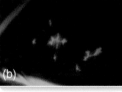

Figure 24.4a Neonatal eczema herpeticum on face.

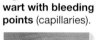

Figure 24.4b HSV infection on adult face.

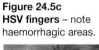

Figure 24.5a HSV around lips.

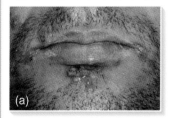

Figure 24.5b HSV on hand.

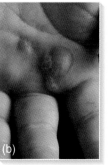

Figure 24.5c HSV fingers – note haemorrhagic areas.

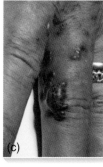

Figure 24.6a Herpes zoster infection on arm.

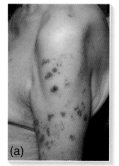

Figure 24.6b Herpes zoster on leg.

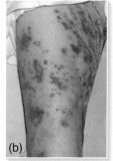
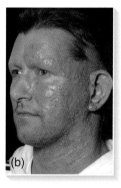

Dermatology at a Glance, Second Edition. Mahbub M.U. Chowdhury, Ruwani P. Katugampola, and Andrew Y. Finlay.
© 2020 John Wiley & Sons Ltd. Published 2020 by John Wiley & Sons Ltd.
Companion website: www.wiley.com/go/chowdhury/dermatology

Viral infections are extremely common and can affect a wide range of ages including young children. They vary in seriousness and how aggressive treatment needs to be depends on the clinical presentation and symptoms. The common viral infections presenting to GPs and dermatologists are discussed here.

Viral Warts

Common viral warts are caused by the human papilloma virus types 1, 2, and 4 and can present on the fingers, hands, and feet (Figure 24.1). Plane (flat) warts may also occur on the dorsum of the hands and face. Typically, warts have dark pinpoint areas which are thrombosed capillaries more obvious when the wart is pared down (Figure 24.1d). This sign is essential to differentiate a wart from an area of callus that could be mistakenly treated as a wart.

Warts are usually asymptomatic and treatment is not essential, particularly in children. Liquid nitrogen therapy is used, working by provoking an inflammatory reaction: the virus is not destroyed by nitrogen. In children, the pain of liquid nitrogen cryotherapy is usually not tolerated (Chapter 9). Warts around the nail folds (Figure 24.2) or plantar warts can be treated with salicylic acid-based preparations which cannot be used on the face.

In adults presenting with multiple warts, immunosuppression should be considered including HIV infection. Patients on long-term immunosuppressives such as azathioprine and ciclosporin can also be affected. Adults are likely to tolerate more aggressive treatment such as cryotherapy or curettage.

Genital warts are treated usually in the genito-urinary department with topical imiquimod or podophyllotoxin.

Hyperkeratotic warts are ideally pared down to remove the thickening prior to any treatments. Topical cantharidin is a toxic chemical derived from beetles which can be used to induce blisters (Chapter 13, Figure 13.7).

Herpes Infections

Herpes simplex

Herpes simplex (cold sore) presents as painful grouped vesicles and erosions caused by human herpes virus 1 or 2. In children, herpes simplex may be asymptomatic or cause fever and regional lymphadenopathy. In neonates, there may be gingivitis, keratoconjunctivitis, or herpes labialis. This will need management with other specialists, particularly for the eyes (Figure 24.3) and genital areas. Differential diagnoses include herpes zoster, impetigo, and other dermatoses.

Eczema herpeticum is a dermatological emergency. It is a widespread infection with herpes simplex in a patient with previous atopic eczema and should always be excluded in an acute severe exacerbation of stable eczema. Patients present with multiple crusted and vesicular lesions, often on the face (Figure 24.4). This can frequently be confused with a bacterial infection or a flare-up of the eczema itself.

In adults, herpes simplex can affect the perioral area and also the fingers (Figure 24.5). It can also provoke erythema multiforme. If herpes simplex is recurrent, prophylaxis with continuous antiviral treatments such as oral aciclovir for three to six months may be required, especially with presentations such as erythema multiforme.

Herpes zoster

Herpes zoster (shingles) is an acute vesicular eruption, usually within a single dermatome, resulting from reactivation of varicella zoster virus from a previous infection with chickenpox (Figure 24.6). The rash heals spontaneously within two to three weeks; however, it may leave scarring. Herpes zoster infection should be considered if there is a painful blistering eruption occurring in one or several dermatomes. You can 'catch' chickenpox from herpes zoster if you have not previously had chickenpox.

Herpes zoster affecting the eye needs to be treated urgently to prevent problems such as keratitis and, if left untreated, blindness.

Investigations

Diagnosis of herpes simplex and herpes zoster is usually obvious clinically but in atypical cases investigations such as herpes serology are necessary.

To diagnose atypical presentations of viral infections, electron microscopy of blister fluid, viral culture from swab of a lesion (Table 24.2), and skin biopsy are essential. For herpes zoster, specific investigations include viral culture, serology, electron microscopy, Tzanck smear (Table 24.3), and checking HIV status if appropriate. Polymerase chain reaction (PCR) testing can detect viral DNA with higher sensitivity and can be useful for quicker urgent results.

Treatment

For herpes simplex, 200 mg oral aciclovir five times per day for five days is used. Herpes zoster is treated with intravenous or oral aciclovir or valaciclovir to prevent progression and reduce risk of post-herpetic neuralgia which can be chronic and extremely painful and debilitating. Oral aciclovir is poorly absorbed (only 20%) and hence high doses are needed for herpes zoster, 200 mg five times daily for at least seven days. Even higher doses are used for eczema herpeticum. Failure to respond to aciclovir may be due to poor absorption or rapid clearance following ingestion or possibly aciclovir resistance. Valaciclovir and famciclovir are alternatives with improved bioavailability. Side effects include headache, nausea, diarrhoea, and renal, hepatic, and neurological dysfunction.

All antiviral agents need to be used within 24–48 hours of eruptions commencing, in either herpes simplex or herpes zoster. Post-herpetic neuralgia treatments such as analgesics and narcotics may not be effective (Table 24.1).

Molluscum Contagiosum

See Chapter 32.

Key Points
- Herpes simplex and herpes zoster need to be treated within one to two days of vesicular lesions.
- Check HIV status in all patients with atypical herpes or viral infections.
- If aciclovir is ineffective remember resistance may occur.

▶ **Warning**
- Beware eczema herpeticum in any acute severe flare-up of eczema presenting with vesicles, especially on the face.

25 Fungal Infections

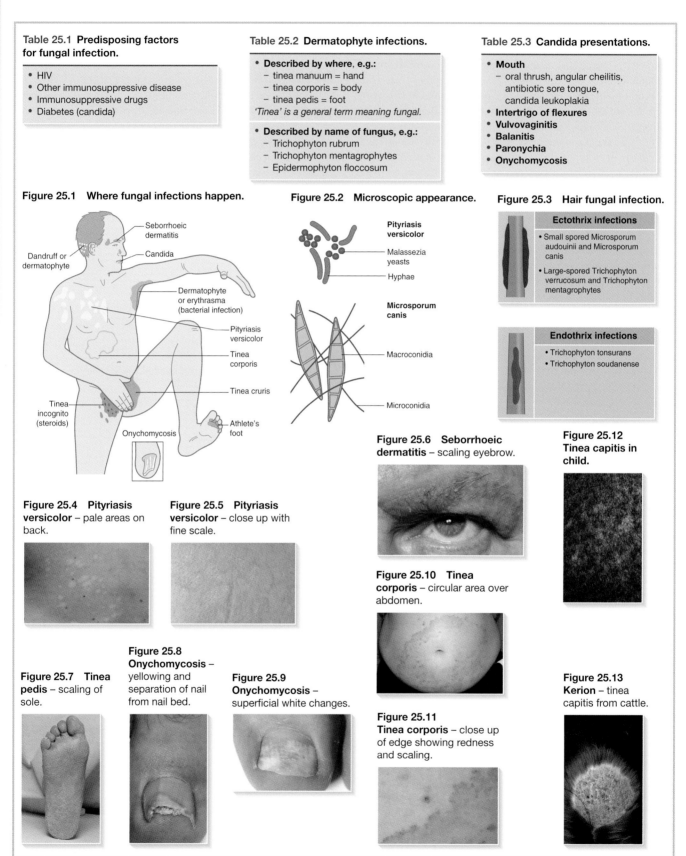

Table 25.1 Predisposing factors for fungal infection.

- HIV
- Other immunosuppressive disease
- Immunosuppressive drugs
- Diabetes (candida)

Table 25.2 Dermatophyte infections.

- **Described by where**, e.g.:
  - tinea manuum = hand
  - tinea corporis = body
  - tinea pedis = foot

  'Tinea' is a general term meaning fungal.
- **Described by name of fungus**, e.g.:
  - Trichophyton rubrum
  - Trichophyton mentagrophytes
  - Epidermophyton floccosum

Table 25.3 Candida presentations.

- **Mouth**
  - oral thrush, angular cheilitis, antibiotic sore tongue, candida leukoplakia
- **Intertrigo of flexures**
- **Vulvovaginitis**
- **Balanitis**
- **Paronychia**
- **Onychomycosis**

Figure 25.1 Where fungal infections happen.

Seborrhoeic dermatitis
Dandruff or dermatophyte
Candida
Dermatophyte or erythrasma (bacterial infection)
Pityriasis versicolor
Tinea corporis
Tinea cruris
Tinea incognito (steroids)
Onychomycosis
Athlete's foot

Figure 25.2 Microscopic appearance.

Pityriasis versicolor
Malassezia yeasts
Hyphae

Microsporum canis
Macroconidia
Microconidia

Figure 25.3 Hair fungal infection.

Ectothrix infections
- Small spored Microsporum audouinii and Microsporum canis
- Large-spored Trichophyton verrucosum and Trichophyton mentagrophytes

Endothrix infections
- Trichophyton tonsurans
- Trichophyton soudanense

Figure 25.4 Pityriasis versicolor – pale areas on back.

Figure 25.5 Pityriasis versicolor – close up with fine scale.

Figure 25.6 Seborrhoeic dermatitis – scaling eyebrow.

Figure 25.10 Tinea corporis – circular area over abdomen.

Figure 25.11 Tinea corporis – close up of edge showing redness and scaling.

Figure 25.12 Tinea capitis in child.

Figure 25.7 Tinea pedis – scaling of sole.

Figure 25.8 Onychomycosis – yellowing and separation of nail from nail bed.

Figure 25.9 Onychomycosis – superficial white changes.

Figure 25.13 Kerion – tinea capitis from cattle.

Dermatology at a Glance, Second Edition. Mahbub M.U. Chowdhury, Ruwani P. Katugampola, and Andrew Y. Finlay.
© 2020 John Wiley & Sons Ltd. Published 2020 by John Wiley & Sons Ltd.
Companion website: www.wiley.com/go/chowdhury/dermatology

There are two main types of fungi. Moulds (e.g. dermatophytes) have long hyphae and grow from the tip. Yeasts (e.g. *Malassezia* and *Candida*) are single-celled organisms, shaped like rugby balls or footballs, that bud to produce new cells (Figure 25.2).

Pityriasis Versicolor

Multiple patches coalesce over upper back, shoulders, and chest in young adults, with light scaling, seen if gently scraped with spatula (Figures 25.4 and 25.5). 'Pityriasis' indicates fine scale, 'versicolor' means variable colour change: some areas become lighter, others darker. Caused by overgrowth of normal skin commensal lipophilic yeasts *Malassezia globosa*, *Malassezia sympodialis*, and *Malassezia furfur*.

Treatment – Topical ketoconazole 2% applied three times or ciclopirox 1%. Topical selenium sulphide 2.5% (Selsun® shampoo) also effective. Oral 200 mg/day itraconazole for five days if widespread.

Malassezia Folliculitis

Itchy papules and pustules on the back and upper body are seen in young adults. The differential diagnosis acne is not itchy.

Treatment – as for pityriasis versicolor.

Seborrhoeic Dermatitis, Dandruff

Superficial scaling in the sternal area, eyebrows (Figure 25.6), ears, nasolabial folds, and diffusely throughout the scalp. Adult seborrhoeic dermatitis is caused by *Malassezia* species.

Treatment – as for pityriasis versicolor.

Dermatophyte Infections

Tinea Pedis ('athlete's foot')

The most common fungal infection, spread by walking in communal changing rooms (Figure 25.7). Skin is macerated between the fourth and fifth toes; it may involve other toe webs, the sole or dorsum of the foot. Vesicles may coalesce, forming bullae because of thick stratum corneum. Usually caused by *Trichophyton rubrum*.

Onychomycosis or Tinea Unguium (Nails)

Yellow–brown, crumbly, thickened nails are seen, infected from tinea pedis (Figures 25.8 and 25.9). The most common organisms are *Trichophyton rubrum*, *Trichophyton mentagrophytes*, or *Epidermophyton floccosum*. If nail clippings show hyphae on microscopy or grow dermatophytes, treat with 250 mg/day terbinafine for 12 weeks.

Tinea Cruris (Groin)

This has superficial, itchy scaling with a well-defined edge. There may be other co-existing infections, such as *Candida* or erythrasma. Topical azoles are also effective against *Candida* so consider using if *Candida* is also suspected.

Tinea Corporis (Body)

Circular lesions are seen, hence 'ringworm' (no worm but remember the ring shape), which may coalesce and show central clearing (Figures 25.10 and 25.11). Scrape slightly scaly edge for microscopy and culture.

Tinea Capitis (Scalp, also including Hair)

The fungus may be on the outside of the hair (ectothrix) (Figure 25.3). It may invade the full shaft thickness (endothrix) making the shaft much weaker and so hairs break easily, giving patchy baldness with black dots, the broken ends (Figure 25.12).

The epidemiology constantly changes. *Trichophyton tonsurans* is now common in the UK and USA urban areas, and *Microsporum canis* is common in some European countries. Treatment is either oral griseofulvin (for *Microsporum*) or terbinafine (for *Trichophyton*, including children with *Trichophyton tonsurans*).

Kerion

An area of severe inflammation, usually on the scalp (Figure 25.13), caused by a zoophilic dermatophyte (i.e. whose host is normally an animal).

As the organism has not evolved on human skin, there is a severe reaction (e.g. *Trichophyton verrucosum* from cattle).

Treatment – 10 mg/kg griseofulvin daily for six weeks.

Favus

Favus is a distinctive type of tinea capitis with yellow, cup-shaped crusts (scutula), caused by *Trichophyton schoenleinii*. Endemic in South Africa and Ethiopia, it may cause scarring alopecia.

Investigations for Fungal Infections

• **Skin** – Scrape edge of active lesions into folded paper or cardboard. Dermatophytes and yeasts may remain alive for weeks.
• **Hair** – Pull out hairs with forceps and culture. Or brush a disposable toothbrush through the affected area 10 times, then press the brush into culture medium in a Petri dish.
• **Nail** – Clip nail, including soft matter beneath protruding edge.
• **Wood's light** – UVA (365 nm) shows extent of pityriasis versicolor. Causes fluorescence of hair in some dermatophyte infections (e.g. *Microsporum canis*), so useful for screening in a school outbreak. But skin dermatophyte infection does not fluoresce.

Dermatophyte Infection Treatment

Terbinafine 1% cream is fungicidal so even one application can cure. If applied daily for five days, less areas will be missed. Terbinafine inhibits squalene epoxidase in fungal cells, so squalene levels build up and they become deficient in ergosterol, essential for fungal (but not human) cell membranes. Other topical treatments for dermatophyte infections include the imidazoles (e.g. ketoconazole, miconazole, clotrimazole) and cheaper treatment such as benzoic acid (Whitfield's) ointment. Nail, hair, and widespread body infection needs systemic therapy with terbinafine, itraconazole, ketoconazole, or griseofulvin.

Candida Infection

Candida albicans is the most common *Candida* species and is a normal commensal in the mouth and gut. *Candida albicans* is Latin for 'white becoming white': a daft name but at least both the cultured yeast and the appearance of thrush look white. Superficial *Candida* infections affect the skin (sometimes with pustules) and nail folds (Candidal paronychia). Infection of the mouth ('oral thrush') may be the presenting sign of HIV. Diabetes may predispose to skin *Candida* infections. Treatment is with topical imidazoles or oral fluconazole or itraconazole.

Key Points
• The key sign of fungal infections is superficial scaling.
• Toe webs are the main site for dermatophyte infections. Check them if fungal infection elsewhere suspected.

► Warning
• Both tinea and Trichophyton are abbreviated to 'T'.
• Do not use steroids in fungal infections. Topical steroids settle itch so seem to be helpful, but fungus grows better, resulting in tinea incognito ('in disguise').

26 Skin Infestations

Figure 26.1   Life cycle of *Sarcoptes scabiei.*

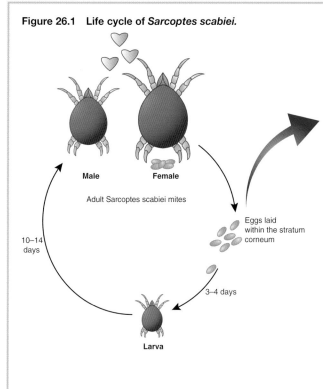

Male

Female

Adult Sarcoptes scabiei mites

10–14 days

Eggs laid within the stratum corneum

3–4 days

Larva

Figure 26.2   Schematic diagram of adult female scabies mite burrowing into the stratum corneum to lay her eggs.

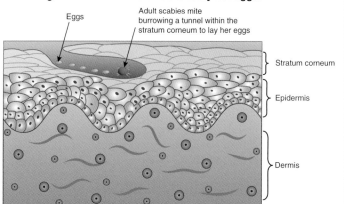

Eggs

Adult scabies mite burrowing a tunnel within the stratum corneum to lay her eggs

Stratum corneum

Epidermis

Dermis

Figure 26.3   Scabetic burrows on the foot of a child.

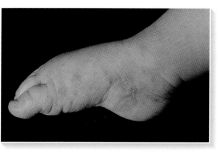

Figure 26.4   Crusted scabies of the foot.

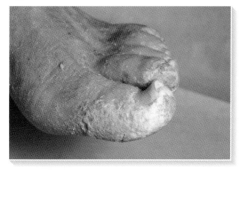

Figure 26.5   Life cycle of *Pediculus humanus capitis* (head lice).

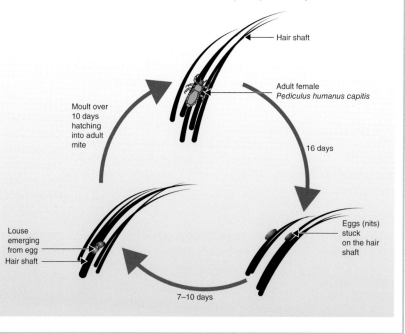

Hair shaft

Adult female *Pediculus humanus capitis*

16 days

Eggs (nits) stuck on the hair shaft

7–10 days

Louse emerging from egg

Hair shaft

Moult over 10 days hatching into adult mite

Dermatology at a Glance, Second Edition. Mahbub M.U. Chowdhury, Ruwani P. Katugampola, and Andrew Y. Finlay.
© 2020 John Wiley & Sons Ltd. Published 2020 by John Wiley & Sons Ltd.
Companion website: www.wiley.com/go/chowdhury/dermatology

Scabies

Scabies is caused by the mite *Sarcoptes scabiei*. Spread is by direct person-to-person contact. The adult female mite burrows into the stratum corneum where she lays her eggs (Figures 26.1 and 26.2). The eggs hatch after a few days in the stratum corneum where the larvae mature into adult mites within two weeks and the female mites lay their eggs to continue the cycle.

The symptoms and signs occur about four weeks after infestation, because of a hypersensitivity reaction to the mites: intensely itchy skin with irregular slightly scaly burrows (seen between the finger webs, wrists, ankles, medial and lateral borders of feet, Figure 26.3) and papules (seen on the penis). In infants, the face is often affected with red itchy papules and hands and feet with vesicles. A secondary eczematous rash is often seen a few weeks after treatment.

Crusted scabies (previously called Norwegian scabies) is severe infestation with scabies resulting in hyperkeratosis of the skin including the subungual skin (Figure 26.4). This is seen in cases of untreated scabies (e.g. elderly individuals with dementia) or those with immune deficiency (e.g. immunosuppression following organ transplantation or in HIV infection).

Diagnosis is based on the clinical features described above. With a magnifying glass or dermatoscope, the mite may be visible as a white dot at the end of the burrow. Close contacts should also be examined for scabies.

Management includes simultaneous treatment of the index case as well as their close contacts (e.g. partner, family members) with topical insecticides, either 5% permethrin cream (Chapter 12) or 0.5% malathion liquid (safer option in pregnant women and children), two applications one week apart. The treatment is applied to the whole body (neck to toes in adults, treat face and scalp as well in infants) and left on for 24 hours. Schools or other institutions (e.g. care homes) attended by the infested individual should be informed as a matter of priority to identify and prevent further spread of the infestation. Children can return to school after their first treatment.

Crusted scabies is treated with oral ivermectin (Chapter 12). Clothing and bed-linen of the index case and their close contacts should be washed at high temperature (50°C).

Head Lice (Pediculosis Capitis)

Head lice are caused by the arthropod *Pediculus humanus capitis*. It is the most common parasitic infestation in school children. The school or nursery attended by the infested child should be informed as a matter of priority, to identify and prevent further spread of the infestation. Infestation is confined to the scalp and is spread by direct head-to-head contact. It can also spread via clothes, hairbrushes, and bed clothing.

The louse has three pairs of clawed legs adapted to grasp the hair shaft (Figure 26.5). The female lice lay their eggs (nits), which are firmly attached to the host's hair. The eggs hatch after about 7–10 days and the cycle continues. The louse feeds on its host's blood whilst injecting its saliva into the host.

Head lice infestation may be asymptomatic. However, some experience intense itching associated with excoriations, eczematous rash, and impetiginisation of the scalp and cervical lymphadenopathy about one month after the initial infestation. This is due to hypersensitivity to the saliva injected by the louse.

Severe untreated head lice infestation may present with marked hyperkeratosis of the scalp with thick scales adherent to the hair shafts (pityriasis amiantacea). The differential diagnoses include severe scalp psoriasis and fungal scalp infection (tinea capitis). Head lice are extremely common in children but less common in adults.

Diagnosis is made clinically, by examination of the scalp aided by a magnifying glass to identify nits attached to the hair shafts, often proximally, and crawling lice. The scalp of close contacts should also be examined for head lice.

Management includes simultaneous treatment of the index case and their close contacts (e.g. family members). Treatment includes wet combing with topical insecticides to kill the lice and nits. Wet combing involves the mechanical removal of lice and nits. The wet hair is combed for about 15–30 minutes with a fine toothed comb daily for two weeks until no further lice are seen.

Topical therapy includes 0.5% malathion lotion (safer in pregnant women and children) which is applied to the hair, washed off after 12 hours and repeated 1 week later. An alternative is 1% permethrin cream (Chapter 12), applied to damp, towel-dried hair and rinsed off after 10 minutes and repeated 1 week later. Clothing and bed-linen of the index case and their close contacts should be washed at high temperature (50°C). Hair combs and brushes of these individuals and toys should be disinfected by soaking them in hot water for 5–10 minutes.

There is no point in keeping children away from school as they should no longer be infectious after first topical treatment.

Body Lice

Body lice are caused by the arthropod *Pediculus humanus corporis* and may be seen in self-neglected individuals. Spread is by direct person-to-person contact. Management is as for scabies.

Key Point
- Topical malathion is the preferred treatment for scabies or head lice in children and pregnant women.

▶ Warning
- Scabies and head lice spread from person-to-person. Treat close contacts at the same time as the patient.

27 Tropical Skin Diseases

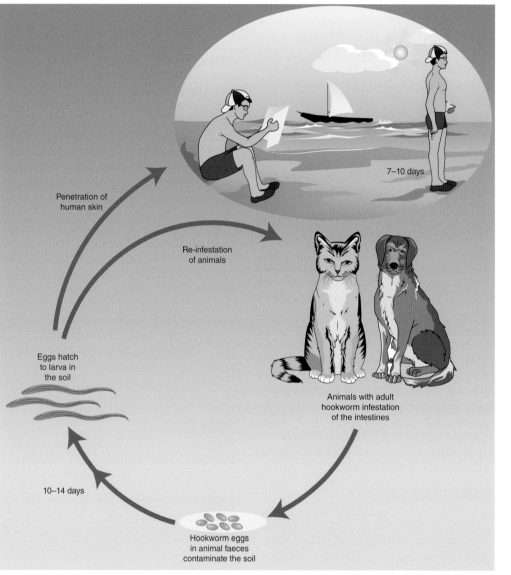

Figure 27.1 Life cycle of hookworms causing cutaneous larva migrans.

Penetration of
human skin

7–10 days

Re-infestation
of animals

Eggs hatch
to larva in
the soil

Animals with adult
hookworm infestation
of the intestines

10–14 days

Hookworm eggs
in animal faeces
contaminate the soil

**Figure 27.3
Cutaneous leishmaniasis.**

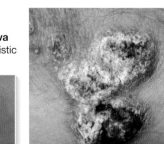

Figure 27.4   Leprosy. (a) Note erythematous plaque on bridge of nose and thickened right supratrochlear nerve. (b) Note anaesthetic hypopigmented macular patch over right deltoid region.

Figure 27.2   Cutaneous larva migrans – note the characteristic extending serpiginous track.

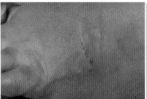

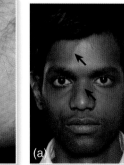

(a)

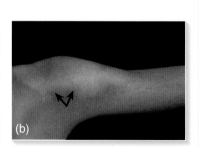

(b)

Dermatology at a Glance, Second Edition. Mahbub M.U. Chowdhury, Ruwani P. Katugampola, and Andrew Y. Finlay.
© 2020 John Wiley & Sons Ltd. Published 2020 by John Wiley & Sons Ltd.
Companion website: www.wiley.com/go/chowdhury/dermatology

Cutaneous Larva Migrans

Caused by the hookworm family Ancylostomatidae, *Ancylostoma braziliense* being the commonest species in the Americas. Domestic pets such as cats and dogs with intestinal hookworm infestation pass the hookworm eggs in their faeces. The eggs hatch into larvae and penetrate and migrate into the human skin, especially via sites in contact with soil contaminated by animal faeces (e.g. feet, buttocks) (Figure 27.1). This is a hazard of sitting on the beach or walking barefoot in an endemic area.

Patients present with an extremely itchy, erythematous, serpiginous track that extends over days due to larval movement (Figure 27.2). The track consists of a combination of papules, vesicles, or blisters. Diagnosis is made clinically. The condition is self-limiting as larvae die within six to eight weeks of penetrating the skin: humans are 'accidental' hosts. Treatment of limited disease is with topical 10% thiabendazole cream for one to two weeks; if widespread disease, oral albendazole or ivermectin.

Leishmaniasis

Caused by different species of the protozoan parasite, Leishmania. It is transmitted by infected female sand-flies who bite human hosts and pass the protozoans into their bloodstream. Incubation period ranges from weeks to a year. There are three main types:
1 **Cutaneous** is the most common form. Patients present with one or more painless ulcers (termed tropical ulcers; Figure 27.3) on exposed skin, often the face or limb, which heal over months with scarring. Regional lymphadenopathy may be present.
2 **Mucocutaneous** form occurs months or years after healing of a cutaneous leishmaniasis lesion. May lead to partial or complete destruction of mucous membranes (e.g. nasopharynx).
3 **Visceral form (kala azar)** is the most severe, due to visceral organ involvement. Patients present with fever, weight loss, hepatosplenomegaly, and anaemia. Mortality in untreated cases is >90%. Also occurs as opportunistic infection associated with HIV infection.

About 90% of visceral leishmaniasis occurs in the Indian subcontinent, Sudan, Ethiopia, and Brazil; 66% of cutaneous leishmaniasis is in Afghanistan, Algeria, Iran, Syria, and South America. Mucocutaneous leishmaniasis is mainly seen in Bolivia and Brazil.

Diagnosis is confirmed by histology and culture of scrapings and/or biopsy of affected skin (cutaneous form); by light microscopic examination or culture of parasites from splenic or bone marrow aspirates (visceral form). Polymerase chain reaction (PCR) of tissue samples is used to identify the species of leishmaniasis, which influences treatment choice.

Treatment is usually with pentavalent antimonial drugs, meglumine antimoniate (first line) or sodium stibogluconate, but depends on species and geographical location. Travellers to endemic areas should use insect repellents and appropriate clothing.

Leprosy

Leprosy is caused by *Mycobacterium leprae*, an intracellular bacterium with a predilection for skin, peripheral nerves, respiratory mucosa, and eyes. The prevalence is falling, but it is still endemic in India, Africa, and South America. It is a notifiable disease in the UK where about 12 new cases are seen each year, all originating overseas.

Mycobacterium leprae causes a chronic granulomatous reaction leading to:
• **Skin** – anaesthetic hypopigmented macules ± erythematous plaques (Figure 27.4a and b).
• **Peripheral nerves** – enlarged peripheral nerves (Figure 27.4a) and peripheral neuropathy.
• **Eyes** – blindness due to direct bacillary infiltration and neuropathy resulting in diminished blinking ± corneal sensation.

It is spread by nasal or oral mucosal droplets from close contact with infected individuals. Incubation period can be up to several years. There are two main subtypes:
1 **Tuberculoid** – strong immune response to *M. leprae*, few skin lesions, low bacterial load (paucibacillary).
2 **Lepromatous** – poor immune response to *M. leprae*, severe disease, with multiple skin lesions and high bacterial load (multibacillary).

Diagnosis is by finding acid-fast bacilli on Ziehl–Neelsen staining in smears and/or biopsies from affected skin or other tissue. Serological tests can detect *M. leprae* antigens or antibodies. Treatment is with rifampicin, dapsone, and clofazimine, depending on disease subtype. Therapy may provoke erythema nodosum leprosum, an immune reaction with red painful skin swelling and fever, for which the treatment is thalidomide.

Tropical Ulcer

This is a rapidly enlarging, painful, foul-smelling ulcer with a raised, thickened, purple edge seen on the lower legs, commonly affecting children living in humid tropical climates. Initial skin trauma leads to papules or blisters which rapidly breakdown to form an ulcer with secondary bacterial infection, often with multiple bacterial species including *Bacillus fusiformis*, *Treponema vincenti*, *Escherichia coli*, and *Enterococci*. As the ulcer enlarges, it can invade deep into muscle and the periosteum.

Diagnosis is made clinically in conjunction with identifying the infective bacterial organisms by swabbing the ulcer. A biopsy for histology may need to be considered to exclude other causes of ulcers. The differential diagnosis includes other infective causes such as cutaneous leishmaniasis, atypical mycobacteria, venous ulcers (Chapter 52) or pyoderma gangrenosum (Chapter 46). Treatment is with antibiotics depending on bacteriology results (penicillin and/or metronidazole) and pain control with analgesics.

Dengue

This is a viral disease prevalent throughout the tropics, transmitted by female mosquitoes mainly of the *Aedes* species. The symptoms develop between 4 and 10 days after the bite from an infected mosquito. These include severe flu-like illness with a high fever, severe headache, myalgia, joint pains, nausea and vomiting, and a rash. The skin manifestations include initial flushing erythema of the face followed by an asymptomatic maculopapular rash that coalesces to a generalised erythema with islands of normal skin.

Severe dengue, also known as dengue haemorrhagic fever, can be potentially life threatening due to severe bleeding complications, plasma leakage, and multi-organ failure. Features also include bleeding evidenced by petechiae, ecchymosis or purpura, bleeding from mucosa, gastro-intestinal tract or other sites, thrombocytopenia (<100 000 cells/mm^3), evidence of plasma leakage such as pleural effusion, ascites, and hypoproteinaemia.

Diagnosis is confirmed by isolation of the dengue virus on serology. There is no specific treatment for dengue. Supportive care is critical to maintain body fluid volume and prevent circulatory failure and progression to hypovolaemic shock. Development of vaccinations to immunise against dengue is underway. At present, prevention of transmission of dengue is aimed at control of the mosquito vector.

Key Point
• A skin biopsy helps confirm the diagnosis of leishmaniasis and leprosy.

▶ **Warning**
• Cutaneous leishmaniasis may progress to mucocutaneous form, leading to mucous membrane destruction.
• Untreated visceral leishmaniasis is potentially fatal.

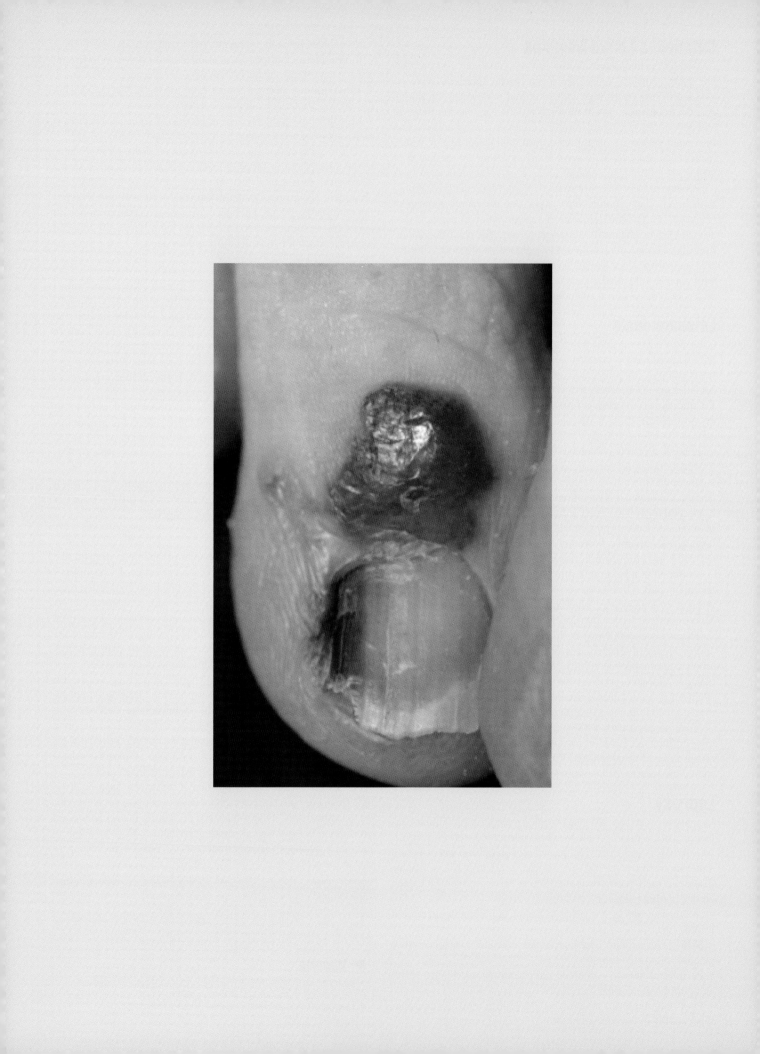

Specific Sites

Part 8

28 The Red Face

Table 28.1 Specific questions and history.

- Where did the eruption start?
- Any history of previous skin disease or family history of skin disease?
- Is this facial eruption itchy?
- Is this facial eruption scaly?
- Any flushing or increased redness (any specific precipitants noted)?
- Any note of allergies or reactions to cosmetics, hair dyes, perfumes?
- Any systemic symptoms such as arthritis or tiredness (anaemia)?

Table 28.3 Specific investigations may be required to confirm diagnosis.

- Skin biopsy: histology and direct immunofluorescence (IMF)
- Autoimmune screen: ANA, anti-Ro/La antibodies
- Full blood count, erythrocyte sedimentation rate (ESR)
- Urea and electrolytes, urine analysis
- Serum IgE
- Patch test
- Skin scrapings for mycology

Table 28.2 Causes of a red face and specific examination clues (Figure 28.8).

Rosacea	Papules, pustules, and no comedones
Perioral dermatitis	Papules particularly around the mouth
Atopic eczema	Flexural erythema and scaling
Seborrhoeic dermatitis	Scaling, erythema particularly on the eyebrows, nasolabial folds, upper chest, and chin
Psoriasis	Well-defined scaly patches and plaques on extensor surfaces of limbs and scalp with nail pitting
Contact dermatitis	Vesicles on face occurring after use of particular products
Discoid lupus erythematosus (DLE)	Diffuse scaling, follicular plugging, atrophy in photosensitive distribution

Figure 28.1a Typical rosacea.

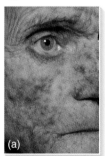
(a)

Figure 28.1b Note marked telangiectasia.

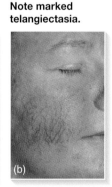
(b)

Figure 28.1c Note central facial distribution.

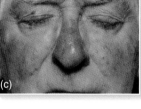
(c)

Figure 28.1d Severe rosacea with marked inflammation.

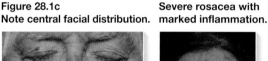
(d)

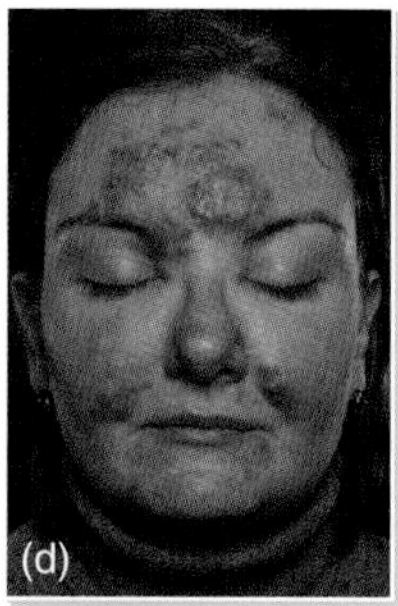

Figure 28.2 Rhinophyma of nose with distortion of shape – can progress gradually.

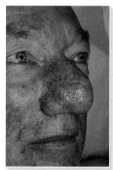

Figure 28.3 Eczema on face.

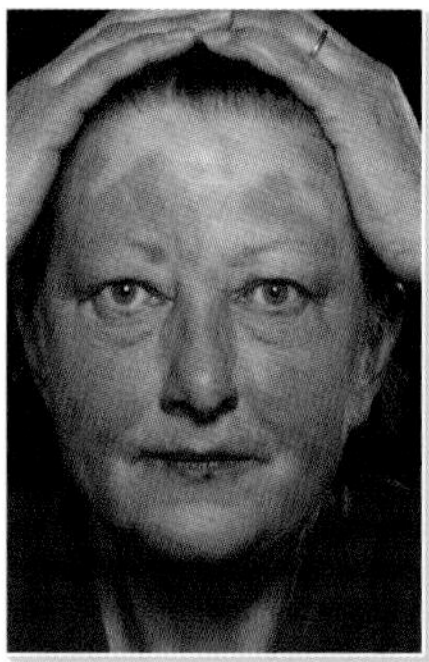

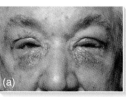

Figure 28.4 Seborrhoeic dermatitis affecting eyebrows.

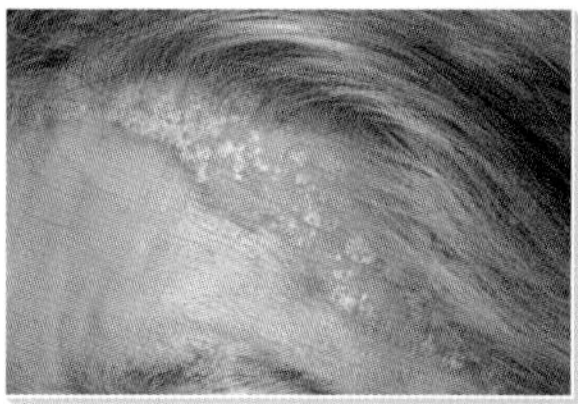

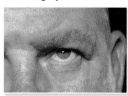

Figure 28.5 Scaly psoriasis plaques, sharp borders near scalp margin.

Figure 28.7a Thick plaques of discoid lupus erythematosus (DLE) confirmed on biopsy – this lady later developed systemic lupus erythematosus (SLE).

Figure 28.7b Telangiectasia and follicular plugging on right cheek.

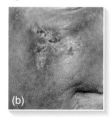
(b)

Figure 28.6a Contact dermatitis to preservatives can affect eyelids.

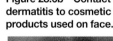
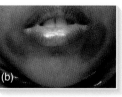
(a)

Figure 28.6b Contact dermatitis to cosmetic products used on face.

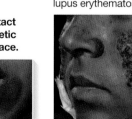
(b)

(a)

Dermatology at a Glance, Second Edition. Mahbub M.U. Chowdhury, Ruwani P. Katugampola, and Andrew Y. Finlay.
© 2020 John Wiley & Sons Ltd. Published 2020 by John Wiley & Sons Ltd.
Companion website: www.wiley.com/go/chowdhury/dermatology

It can be difficult to diagnose the cause of a red face. A good knowledge of differential diagnoses is required. Specific history and full skin examination are needed to differentiate conditions such as rosacea, perioral dermatitis, atopic eczema, seborrhoeic dermatitis, psoriasis, contact dermatitis, and discoid lupus erythematosus (Tables 28.1–28.3, Figure 28.8).

Rosacea

Rosacea is a common inflammatory skin disease seen in adults over 30 years old. It is usually confined to the face, mainly affecting the cheeks, forehead, nose, and chin. Flushing may occur. Papules, pustules, telangiectasia, and erythema are common but no comedones or scaling occur (Figure 28.1). Hypertrophy and lymphoedema of subcutaneous tissue may present with rhinophyma of the nose (Figure 28.2). The cause of rosacea is unknown but it is triggered by spicy foods and alcohol, leading to flushing and then telangiectasia.

Complications of rosacea include conjunctivitis, keratitis, and iritis. Papules and pustules can be treated with antibiotics (topical metronidazole, oral tetracyclines, and oral erythromycin) and topical retinoids. Flushing and telangiectasia may not fully respond even to pulse dye laser. New treatments include ivermectin cream which is anti-inflammatory and kills *Demodex* mites linked with rosacea. Brimonidine gel is an alpha-adrenergic agonist reducing redness by constricting superficial blood vessels.

Perioral Dermatitis

This is a variant of rosacea that occurs in young females around the mouth or sometimes around the eyes. It usually presents with papules and occasional pustules sparing the skin adjacent to the vermillion border. Other features of rosacea such as flushing and telangiectasia are usually absent. Most cases have a recent history of topical steroid usage. This can improve the eruption but it relapses once the treatment is stopped. Topical steroids need to be stopped and other standard treatments for rosacea such as topical metronidazole and oral antibiotics can be helpful.

Atopic Eczema

This can present with facial redness (Chapter 16). Eczema can occur on any area of the face with scaling, itching, and possible vesicles (Figure 28.3). It is important to take a full history including past and family history of atopy and to examine the whole skin looking for other signs of atopic eczema such as flexural eruption on the limbs. Raised total IgE may help to confirm atopy which can coexist in the background with contact dermatitis.

Seborrhoeic Dermatitis

This chronic skin condition affects adults with well-defined, red, scaly patches on the face affecting the eyebrows, nasolabial folds, ears, upper trunk, and scalp (Figure 28.4). This condition relapses intermittently and is associated with *Malassezia* yeast. The key feature of seborrhoeic dermatitis is the distribution and usually the rest of the skin is normal with no history of atopy. If severe, immunosuppression such as HIV infection needs to be considered.

Treatment with topical ketoconazole, oral itraconazole, topical steroids (hydrocortisone), and medicated shampoos containing ketoconazole and selenium sulphide.

Psoriasis (Chapter 15)

Psoriasis commonly affects the face. There may be small patches or plaques particularly along the hairline margin extending from the scalp (Figure 28.5). Patches can be less well defined on the face but signs should be looked for on other areas of the body such as the elbows and knees. The nails can show onycholysis, subungual hyperkeratosis, and nail pitting. A family history of psoriasis may also be useful to point towards the correct diagnosis. The eruption is less likely to be severely itchy in psoriasis than in atopic eczema or contact dermatitis.

Contact Dermatitis (Chapter 35)

Irritant contact dermatitis or allergic contact dermatitis may present with facial redness and scaling with or without vesicles (more common with allergy) (Figure 28.6). History taking needs to be targeted towards any specific reactions such as to cosmetics, shampoos, hair dyes, or perfumes. There may be a background of consistent reactions to these products and patch testing may be required to differentiate between allergy and irritation.

Discoid Lupus Erythematosus

Discoid lupus erythematosus (DLE) can present in sun exposed areas particularly on the scalp, face, upper chest, and upper trunk (Chapter 47). The skin shows well-defined erythematous papules and plaques with thickened scaling (Figure 28.7). Typical features of the lesions are central atrophy with scarring, telangiectasia, and follicular plugging. The lesions can be either hyperpigmented or depigmented, depending on the skin type. Investigations required are skin biopsy (histology and direct immunofluorescence [IMF]), autoimmune screen (antinuclear antibodies [ANA], antiRo/anti-La antibodies), full blood count, erythrocyte sedimentation rate (ESR), urea and electrolytes, and urine analysis.

Five per cent of cases progress to systemic lupus erythematosus (SLE). SLE needs to be considered if there are widespread skin lesions and features such as anaemia, reduced white cell count, and/or positive ANA with high titre of anti-Ro/anti-La antibodies and arthritis.

Management of DLE is sun avoidance and sunscreen use with topical, intralesional, or oral corticosteroid therapies. Hydroxychloroquine (anti-malarial), dapsone, and systemic retinoids may also be useful.

Tinea Faciei

Tinea infection is uncommon on the face but may present with annular scaly patches with central clearing. If topical steroids have been used then the features can be very unusual (tinea incognito). Skin scrapings for mycology are essential to exclude this if suspected.

Figure 28.8 Specific sites commonly affected.

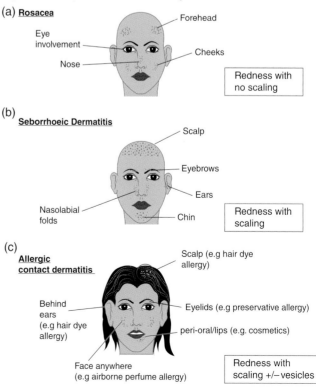

(a) Rosacea — Forehead, Eye involvement, Nose, Cheeks — Redness with no scaling

(b) Seborrhoeic Dermatitis — Scalp, Eyebrows, Ears, Nasolabial folds, Chin — Redness with scaling

(c) Allergic contact dermatitis — Scalp (e.g hair dye allergy), Behind ears (e.g hair dye allergy), Eyelids (e.g preservative allergy), peri-oral/lips (e.g. cosmetics), Face anywhere (e.g airborne perfume allergy) — Redness with scaling +/− vesicles

Key Points

- Look for specific pointers in the history and examination to confirm the diagnosis.
- Consider specific tests for SLE and contact allergy.
- Keep an open mind and review the diagnosis if the skin is not improving.

▶ Warning

- Topical steroids can worsen rosacea, perioral dermatitis, and tinea faciei.

29 Oral and Genital Disease

Table 29.1 Approach to a patient with oral and/or genital disease.

Clinical history
- Onset, duration, symptoms, and functional difficulties due to the genital and/or skin disease, e.g. difficulties swallowing, having sexual intercourse, passing urine
- Skin, nail, hair disease
- Other medical conditions, e.g. Crohn's disease
- Current or previous topical treatment/applications to the affected area, e.g. scented wipes, over-the-counter creams
- Sexual history where appropriate, e.g. high-risk behaviour, previous sexually transmitted infections (STIs)

Clinical examination
- Note the colour, texture of the skin, presence of vesicles, pustules, fissures, ulcers, purpura, discharge, scarring, adhesions of the labia, narrowing of the introitus (females), narrowing of the meatus and difficulty retracting foreskin (males)
- Examine the perineum and perianal skin for extension of the genital rash/lesions to these areas
- Examine the whole skin, nails, and hair for evidence of associated skin disease

Investigations
- Biopsy affected area if diagnosis uncertain or if non-healing ulcers: histology in all cases, direct immunofluorescence (Chapter 21) if bullous diseases suspected
- Swab discharge, ulcers, vesicles, pustules for microbiology, virology, and STI screen (if appropriate)
- Patch test if allergic contact dermatitis suspected

Table 29.2 Causes and examples of genital skin diseases.

- **Inflammatory diseases**
  - Lichen sclerosus (LS)
  - Lichen planus (LP)
  - Zoon's balanitis/vulvitis
  - Psoriasis
  - Eczema (allergic contact dermatitis, lichen simplex)
  - Behçet's disease
  - Aphthous ulcers
- **Pigmentary**
  - Vitiligo
  - Benign vulval melanosis
- **Bullous**
  - Bullous pemphigoid
  - Pemphigus
- **Pre-malignant**
  - Bowen's disease
- **Malignant**
  - Squamous cell carcinoma (SCC)
  - Malignant melanoma (MM)
- **Infections**
  - Viral, e.g. herpes simplex virus (HSV), genital warts
  - Bacterial, e.g. gonorrhoea, syphilis (primary chancre presenting as painless ulcer)
  - Yeast, e.g. candida
  - Infestations, e.g. scabies (itchy papules)
- **Drug-induced**
  - Localised ulceration, e.g. nicorandil, methotrexate
  - Widespread disease, e.g. Stevens–Johnson syndrome, toxic epidermal necrolysis

Table 29.3 Causes and examples of oral diseases.

- **Inflammatory diseases**
  - Lichen planus (LP)
  - Behçet's disease
  - Aphthous ulcers
- **Pigmentation**
  - Benign melanotic macules
  - Addison's disease
- **Bullous**
  - Cicatricial pemphigoid
  - Pemphigus
- **Infections**
  - Viral, e.g. herpes simplex virus (HSV)
  - Yeast, e.g. candida
  - Bacterial, e.g. syphilis – characteristic painless 'snail-track' ulcers
- **Drug-induced**
  - Localised ulceration, e.g. methotrexate
  - Widespread disease, e.g. Stevens–Johnson syndrome, toxic epidermal necrolysis

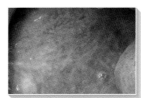

Figure 29.2 Lichen planus of the buccal mucosa – note the typical white reticular network (Wickham's striae).

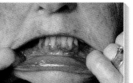

Figure 29.3 Lichen planus of the gingival mucosa – the gums may develop painful erosions in erosive LP.

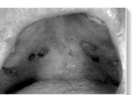

Figure 29.4 Cicatricial pemphigoid of the palate – note the haemorrhagic blisters and the subsequent formation of erosions.

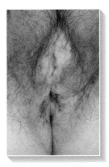

Figure 29.1 Lichen sclerosus of the vulva and perianal skin – note the pallor and haemorrhagic purpura in the figure-of-eight distribution affecting the vulva and perianal skin.

Dermatology at a Glance, Second Edition. Mahbub M.U. Chowdhury, Ruwani P. Katugampola, and Andrew Y. Finlay.
© 2020 John Wiley & Sons Ltd. Published 2020 by John Wiley & Sons Ltd.
Companion website: www.wiley.com/go/chowdhury/dermatology

Genital and oral mucosal diseases may be localised or be part of a generalised skin disease (e.g. Lichen Planus).

Genital Skin Disease

Inflammatory Genital Skin Diseases

Psoriasis presents with symmetrical well-demarcated, erythematous, shiny plaques which may lack the typical scales.

Eczema has ill-defined, itchy, erythematous patches, with hyperpigmentation and lichenification due to chronic scratching.

Contact dermatitis (Chapter 35) on the genital skin can present with itchy, erythematous rash mainly on the external aspect of the genital and/or perianal skin at the points of contact of the allergen or irritant with the skin. Potential allergens in personal hygiene care products such as scented wet wipes include perfumes and preservatives, e.g. methylisothiazolinone. Leave on moisturisers containing antimicrobial chemicals such as benzalkonium chloride can cause irritant dermatitis.

Lichen sclerosus (LS) commonly presents in prepubertal and postmenopausal females with itchy and/or painful erythema, fissures, and erosions of the vulval, perineal, and perianal skin leading to scarring. Atrophic skin with purpura is seen in its quiescent phase (Figure 29.1). In men, similar features are seen on the glans penis. Complications in females include labial adhesions and narrowing of the vaginal introitus leading to difficulty with micturition and sexual function: males may develop phimosis and urethral strictures. There is a < 5% risk of squamous cell carcinoma developing within LS in women; the risk is less in men.

Lichen planus (LP) presents with itchy, shiny, violaceous papules, plaques, or painful erosions on the vulva, shaft, or glans penis. Complications are similar to that of LS.

Zoon's balanitis or vulvitis, also called plasma cell balanitis or vulvitis based on its histological features, presents with asymptomatic, red, shiny plaques on the glans penis or vulva.

Management

- Patients should be examined with sensitivity and due respect.
- Table 29.1 summarises the clinical approach and investigations.
- Reassure patient that inflammatory genital skin diseases are not sexually transmitted.
- Avoid irritant and fragranced products (e.g. scented wipes).
- Use bland emollients as soap substitutes and moisturisers.
- Genital psoriasis, eczema, and Zoon's balanitis/vulvitis generally respond to a few weeks' treatment with mild to moderately potent topical corticosteroids.
- LS and LP require super-potent topical corticosteroids, initially once daily for a month, then alternate days for a further month followed by two to three times per week as required.
- LS or LP unresponsive to topical therapy may require systemic treatment (e.g. methotrexate, acitretin, hydroxychloroquine).
- Circumcision can be curative for Zoon's balanitis.

Infectious Genital Skin Diseases

Genital warts are caused by the human papilloma virus (HPV). They present with small warty papules or larger lesions on the penis, vulva, and perineum, and may extend to the cervix and/or rectum. HPV types 16 and 18 are associated with pre-malignant and malignant transformation of the genital skin. Treatment includes topical 5% imiquimod cream. Topical podophyllin and cryotherapy are also used.

Scabies is caused by the mite *Sarcoptes scabiei* and is transmitted by direct person-to-person contact including sexual contact with an infected individual (Chapter 26). Scabies presents with an intensely itchy rash, scabetic burrows, and itchy papules on the penis. Management of scabies in described in Chapter 26.

Pubic or crab lice are caused by *Phthirus pubis* and transmitted by person-to-person body contact. The female louse lays eggs around the pubic hair shafts, which hatch a week later. Presentation is with itchy, red papules in the pubic area. Treatment is as for scabies (Chapter 26).

Herpes simplex virus (HSV) infection presents with tingling sensation followed by development of grouped vesicles, ulceration, crusting, and healing. Genital HSV is contagious and spreads by direct contact. Treatment is topical and/or oral aciclovir.

Syphilis is caused by the spirochete, *Treponema pallidum*, and acquired as a sexually transmitted infection (STI). Initial presentation is with a painless genital ulcer (primary chancre) associated with inguinal lymphadenopathy two weeks after acquiring the infection. Syphilis serology may not become positive during the appearance of the primary chancre. The spirochetes may be visible on dark field microscopy of the ulcer fluid. The ulcer resolves spontaneously. Secondary syphilis will follow one to three months after the primary chancre characterised by an asymptomatic papular rash with collarette of scale on the palms, soles of the feet, and trunk. Parenteral penicillin is the treatment of choice (doses and duration vary according to stage of disease).

Oral Mucosal Disease

LP presents as a white, net-like, reticular pattern (Wickham's striae) and erosions on the buccal and gingival mucosa (Figures 29.2 and 29.3).

Aphthous ulcers are the most common type of mouth ulcers. These painful ulcers are well demarcated with a yellowish centre and erythematous edge. They occur as an isolated episode or may recur, precipitated by stress and trauma.

Behçet's disease is a chronic multi-system vasculitis leading to recurrent oral and genital ulcers, arthritis, and skin lesions (e.g. erythema nodosum).

Cicatricial pemphigoid (mucous membrane pemphigoid) presents with blisters of the oral and/or ocular mucosa, leading to erosions and scarring (Figure 29.4). Other mucosal and skin surfaces may be involved (e.g. oesophagus, nasal and genital mucosa, scalp skin).

Management

- Potent to super-potent topical corticosteroids, in ointment form for better mucosal adhesion. Oral LP and aphthous ulcers can also be treated with hydrocortisone oral mucosal pellets held in contact with lesions. Steroid inhalers (e.g. beclometasone) can be sprayed on to gingival LP.
- Anaesthetics (e.g. lidocaine gel) can be used for pain relief.
- Cicatricial pemphigoid affecting the eyes and oesophagus requires early intervention to prevent scarring and associated complications of visual impairment and dysphagia. Use systemic steroids with azathioprine or intravenous cyclophosphamide. The biologic rituximab is effective in severe cases.
- Oral colchicine, dapsone, and thalidomide have been effective in managing the systemic manifestations of Behçet's disease.

Key Points

- Differential diagnosis of recurrent mouth and/or genital ulcers includes Behçet's disease, cicatricial pemphigoid, pemphigus, infections (e.g. syphilis), or drug-induced causes.
- Sexual contacts of those with STIs should be traced and treated.

▶ **Warning**

- Non-healing oral and/or genital ulcers and lesions should be biopsied to exclude pre-malignant or malignant disease.

30 Nail and Hair Disease

Table 30.1 Approach to a patient with nail disease.

Clinical history	Clinical examination	Investigations
• Underlying skin disease • Underlying systemic diseases • Dietary history, e.g. severe iron deficiency causing koilonychia • Current and relevant previous medication and treatment, e.g. prolonged illness, chemotherapy causing Beau's lines (horizontal ridges on nail plates)	• Examine all 20 nails, taking note of their shape, colour, texture, and surface changes • Examine the whole skin including oral mucosa for associated skin disease • Physical examination for evidence of underlying disease, e.g. cardiac disease (clubbing of nails)	• Nail clippings for mycology (fungal nail infections) • Nail biopsy (Chapter 10), (subungual melanoma) • Serum ferritin (koilonychia)

Table 30.2 Approach to a patient with hair disease.

Clinical history	Clinical examination	Investigations
• Underlying skin disease • Underlying systemic diseases • Menstrual history, e.g. amenorrhoea or irregular periods in polycystic ovarian syndrome associated with hirsutism, heavy periods resulting in iron deficiency, and diffuse non-scarring alopecia • Current and relevant previous medication and treatment, e.g. radiotherapy for ringworm infection (pre-1940s) or skin cancer resulting in localised scarring alopecia of the scalp	• Examine the scalp skin for evidence of scarring, erythema and scaling, texture and strength of hair shaft, distribution and volume of hair • Distribution of hair in other parts of the body, e.g. face, limbs, axillae • Examine the whole skin including oral mucosa for associated skin disease • Physical examination for evidence of underlying disease, e.g. virilisation (hirsute woman)	• Scalp skin scraping for mycology (tinea capitis) • Microscopy for hair shaft abnormalities (bamboo-shaped hair in Netherton's syndrome) • Serum ferritin (diffuse non-scarring alopecia) • Serum luteinising and follicular stimulating hormones, testosterone, androstenedione (hirsutism), thyroid function (diffuse alopecia, alopecia areata) • Ultrasound scan of pelvis (polycystic ovaries) • Other: porphyria screen, pituitary hormone profile • CT/MRI scans of the pituitary gland (pituitary tumour), abdomen or pelvis (adrenal or ovarian tumours)

Table 30.3 Causes and examples of nail disease.

Pitting
• Psoriasis, lichen planus, alopecia areata

Subungual hyperkeratosis
• Psoriasis, fungal infections, viral warts, squamous cell carcinoma

Onycholysis
• Psoriasis, fungal infections

Longitudinal ridging of nail plate
• Darier's disease, lichen planus

Shape of nail plate
• Koilonychia, e.g. iron deficiency
• Clubbing, e.g. cystic fibrosis, endocarditis

Colour changes of the nail
• Black – e.g. racial melanonychia, subungual haematoma, melanoma
• Yellow – e.g. yellow nail syndrome, jaundice
• White – e.g. chronic renal failure, hypoalbuminaemia

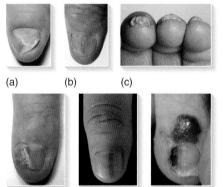

(a) (b) (c)

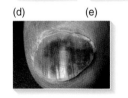

(d) (e) (f)

(g)

Figure 30.1a–g Nail diseases:
(a) Nail psoriasis: Note the pitting of the proximal nail plate and onycholysis of the distal nail plate.
(b) Lichen planus affecting the nail: Note the longitudinal ridging of the nail plate and adhesions between the posterior nailfold and nail plate (pterygium).
(c) Subungual hyperkeratosis.
(d) Subungual viral wart affecting nail growth.
(e) Longitudinal melanonychia: Normal finding in racially pigmented individuals.
(f) Subungual melanoma: Note the pigmentation of the surrounding skin due to the melanoma (Hutchinson's sign).
(g) Subungual haematoma: Note the normal cuticle.

Dermatology at a Glance, Second Edition. Mahbub M.U. Chowdhury, Ruwani P. Katugampola, and Andrew Y. Finlay.
© 2020 John Wiley & Sons Ltd. Published 2020 by John Wiley & Sons Ltd.
Companion website: www.wiley.com/go/chowdhury/dermatology

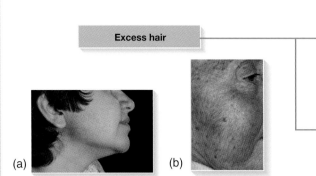

Table 30.4 Causes and examples of diseases leading to excess hair growth.

Hirsutism in women
- Endogenous androgens, e.g. polycystic ovary syndrome, androgen-secreting ovarian, or adrenal tumours
- Pituitary disorders, e.g. Cushing's disease

Hypertrichosis in children, men, or women
- Medication, e.g. minoxidil, ciclosporin, long-term systemic steroids
- Systemic diseases, e.g. porphyria cutanea tarda
- Endogenous androgens, e.g. ovarian or adrenal tumours
- Pituitary disorders, e.g. Cushing's disease

Figure 30.2 a and b   Diseases causing excess hair:
(a) Hirsutism: Dark, coarse, shaven hair in the beard distribution in a female with polycystic ovary syndrome.
(b) Hypertrichosis: Diffuse fine hair on the face of a patient with porphyria cutanea tarda.

Table 30.5 Causes and examples of hair loss (alopecia).

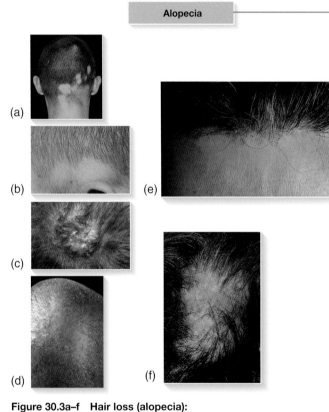

Non-scarring
- Telogen effluvium
- Androgenetic alopecia
- Alopecia areata
- Self-induced (trichotillomania)
- Inflammatory, e.g. psoriasis
- Hair shaft disorders, e.g. bamboo shaped hair (trichorrhexis invaginata) in Netherton's syndrome
- Drug-induced, e.g. warfarin, retinoids
- Infections, e.g. tinea capitis
- Systemic diseases, e.g. hypothyroidism, iron deficiency

Scarring
- Inflammatory skin diseases, e.g. lichen planopilaris (LPP), lupus erythematosus, folliculitis decalvans
- Neoplastic, e.g. basal cell carcinoma
- Treatment-related, e.g. radiotherapy

Figure 30.3a–f   Hair loss (alopecia):
(a) Alopecia areata.
(b) Alopecia areata (close up view): Note the regrowth of short hairs within the patches of alopecia.
(c) Scaly plaque on the scalp with underlying inflammation: The differential diagnosis includes psoriasis, tinea capitis.
(d) Scarring alopecia of the scalp: This patient had previously treated folliculitis decalvans.
(e) Lichen planopilaris (LPP): Note the perifollicular erythema and scaling on the frontal hairline.
(f) LPP: Note the perifollicular erythema and scaling and the atrophic scarring alopecia.

Hair and nail diseases are congenital or acquired. They may be seen in isolation and independent of each other or associated with skin or systemic disease (e.g. lichen planus of the skin, nails, and scarring alopecia). A systematic approach to nail and hair diseases will help identify the cause and aid treatment (Tables 30.1 and 30.2).

Nail Diseases

Different presentations, causes, and examples of nail diseases are summarised in Table 30.3 with examples illustrated in Figure 30.1. Trauma is by far the most common cause of a black or red subungual lesion, but **subungual melanoma** should be considered in subungual hyperpigmentation. A diagnostic clue is the (often variable) pigmentation of the posterior nail fold (Hutchinson's sign). A longitudinal nail biopsy will confirm the diagnosis (Chapter 10). The whole lesion should be surgically excised with adequate surgical margins. The patient should be followed up regularly for monitoring of recurrence or metastatic disease (Chapter 40).

Management

• Fungal nail infections require three to four months of oral antifungal treatment with terbinafine or itraconazole.
• Specific treatment of nail changes due to skin or systemic diseases is difficult. Systemic treatment given for the underlying skin disease may improve the nail changes (e.g. methotrexate or biological treatments for psoriasis).
• Practical management advice includes keeping nails cut short and moisturised to reduce trauma and breakage of nails. In onycholysis, nail lacquer may improve the cosmetic appearance.

Hair

The human skin has three types of hair. Fine, soft, fair, **lanugo hair** covers most of the foetus's skin in utero and is shed prior to a full-term birth. Fine **vellous hair** develops on most of the skin after birth, except for the palms and soles of feet. Coarse, darker, **terminal hairs** occur on the scalp. During puberty, terminal hairs also develop in the axillae, pubic area, and beard area in men.

Each human hair goes through a cycle: active growth phase (**anagen**), which may last a few years, followed by cessation of cell division in the hair bulb (**catagen**), and hair shedding (**telogen**) (Chapter 4).

Excess Hair

Hirsutism is increased growth of terminal hair in women in a male pattern androgen-dependant distribution, e.g. beard, moustache, and chest. These women need to be investigated for an underlying cause of increased androgens before concluding idiopathic hirsutism. **Hypertrichosis** is increased growth of terminal hair in a non-male distribution, which may be localised or generalised. Causes, examples, and investigation of hirsutism and hypertrichosis are summarised in Tables 30.2 and 30.4.

In addition to treatment of the underlying cause, the following are aimed at decreasing excess hair: plucking, shaving, waxing, electrolysis, topical eflornithine (slows the rate of hair growth by inhibiting ornithine decarboxylase), laser (Chapter 51) and intense pulsed light (IPL) therapy, and anti-androgen for hirsutism due to polycystic ovary syndrome (e.g. Dianette®).

Hair Loss (Alopecia)

Hair loss may be localised or diffuse, scarring or non-scarring. Causes, examples, and investigation of alopecia are summarised in Tables 30.2 and 30.5. Wigs should be discussed for individuals distressed by diffuse alopecia, in particular the scarring type.

Telogen Effluvium

This is diffuse, sudden, hair loss a few months after a significant illness or pregnancy. Explanation and reassurance of hair regrowth in a few months is all that is required.

Male Pattern Hair Loss (Androgenetic Alopecia)

This is common in men, but also occurs in women. There is often a family history of male pattern alopecia. The scalp skin is normal. The common hair loss patterns are the frontal–temporal region

and vertex (men and women) and diffuse hair loss sparing the parietal and occipital scalp (usually men). Exclude other causes of diffuse hair loss (Table 30.5).

Treatment – topical 5% minoxidil, oral finasteride (for men), and hair transplant (specialist centres).

Alopecia Areata

The aetiology is unknown but possibly due to autoimmune destruction of hair follicles. There may be a personal or family history of other autoimmune diseases such as Hashimoto's thyroiditis or vitiligo.

Presentation and progression can range from a single or several round patches of hair loss on normal scalp skin (Figure 30.3a and b) to complete hair loss on the scalp (totalis) or whole body (universalis). Hair may regrow spontaneously (initially depigmented) without scarring. Poor prognostic features include childhood onset, alopecia totalis or universalis, and presence of exclamation mark hairs (short hairs that are dark distally, and thin and depigmented towards the scalp) suggesting continuing disease activity.

Treatment – topical or intralesional steroids, topical irritants (dithranol) and sensitizers (dinitrochlorobenzene), phototherapy (PUVA) and, rarely, oral steroids or immunosuppression with oral ciclosporin.

Alopecia Associated with Inflammatory Skin Diseases

Psoriasis and eczema cause localised or diffuse non-scarring alopecia with erythema of the scalp. As there is no scarring, the prognosis for hair regrowth is good once the disease has been treated. Local treatment for psoriasis and eczema of the scalp includes topical steroid application, the topical vitamin D analogue calcipotriol (psoriasis only), and tar-based shampoo.

Discoid lupus erythematosus (DLE) and lichen planus (LP) can affect the scalp resulting in scarring, destruction of the hair follicles, and permanent hair loss. In addition to systemic treatments (Chapters 14 and 47), local treatment includes potent topical corticosteroids to control the inflammation.

Lichen planopilaris (LPP)

This is lichen planus (Chapter 19) of the hair follicle resulting in progressive scarring alopecia affecting the scalp; other hair-bearing sites such as eyebrows may also be affected. LPP presents with perifollicular erythema, scaling, and itchy, violaceous papules leading to atrophic scarring alopecia (Figure 30.3e and f). A scalp biopsy will confirm the clinical diagnosis.

Treatment – super-potent topical or intralesional steroids, antimalarials such as hydroxychloroquine, oral retinoids, and, rarely, short course of oral steroids.

Key Points
• Consider an underlying systemic cause for nail or hair diseases.
• Spontaneous hair regrowth is common in alopecia areata; poor prognostic factors predict progression of alopecia.

▶ **Warning**
• Subungual melanoma should be considered if subungual hyperpigmentation is present.

Specific Ages

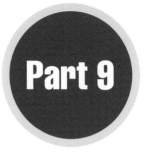

Chapters

31 The Newborn Infant

Table 31.1 Skin manifestations of the newborn.

- **Benign physiological phenomenon and skin pigmentation**, e.g. cutis marmorata, Mongolian blue spots
- **Transient rashes**, e.g. neonatal acne, miliaria, toxic erythema of the newborn, transient neonatal pustular melanosis
- **Persistent and/or progressive rashes or skin diseases**
  - Hereditary – epidermolysis bullosa, disorders of keratinisation (e.g. ichthyosis vulgaris)
  - Acquired – inflammatory (e.g. seborrhoeic dermatitis, atopic eczema), transplacental transfer of maternal auto-antibodies (e.g. neonatal lupus erythematosus)
- **Skin lesions**
  - Vascular malformation, haemangioma
  - Melanocytic naevi

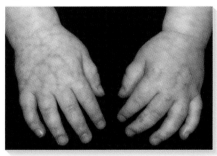

Figure 31.1   Cutis marmorata.

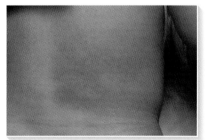

Figure 31.2   Mongolian blue spot on the lower back.

Figure 31.3 Vascular malformation (port wine stain).

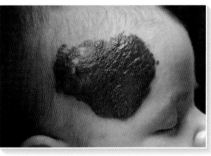

Figure 31.4   An infantile haemangioma.

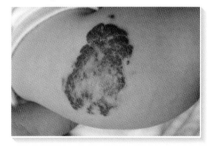

Figure 31.5   A regressing infantile haemangioma.

Figure 31.6   Congenital melanocytic naevus – note the hair and variable pigmentation within the naevus.

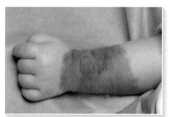

Table 31.2 Differentiating features between vascular malformations and infantile haemangiomas.

	Vascular malformation	Infantile haemangioma
Onset	Present at birth	Within the first few weeks/months of life
Clinical course	Grows with the child (does not regress)	Rapid proliferation in the first few months followed by spontaneous regression over years
Histological features	Combination of one or more of mature capillary, arterial, venous, and lymphatic channels	Endothelial hyperplasia (proliferative phase) followed by fibrosis (regression phase)

The skin of newborn infants may be covered by vernix caseosa, a white lipid-containing material. The skin barrier function is normal at full-term birth, but impaired if premature. Table 31.1 lists skin conditions seen in newborn infants.

Benign Physiological Phenomenon

Cutis marmorata is a transient, net-like, mottled, violaceous discoloration caused by a normal physiological response to a cool environment (Figure 31.1). Persistent cutis marmorata may be associated with limb hypertrophy and macrocephaly.

Dermatology at a Glance, Second Edition. Mahbub M.U. Chowdhury, Ruwani P. Katugampola, and Andrew Y. Finlay.
© 2020 John Wiley & Sons Ltd. Published 2020 by John Wiley & Sons Ltd.
Companion website: www.wiley.com/go/chowdhury/dermatology

Benign Skin Pigmentation

Mongolian blue spots are slate-grey to blue flat patches on the lower back or buttocks in neonates of Asian, Oriental, or Afro-Caribbean origin (Figure 31.2). They are benign and disappear with time.

Transient Rashes

Neonatal Acne

Infants present with papules and pustules on the cheeks which resolve after a few months. The condition results from stimulation of neonatal sebaceous glands by transplacental transfer of maternal adrenal androgens. Acne cysts may develop, requiring systemic antibiotics such as erythromycin to prevent scarring.

Miliaria

Miliaria are multiple clear to yellowish vesicles seen on the face of neonates, especially in warm and humid environments, caused by blocked and/or immature sweat ducts. They resolve spontaneously.

Toxic Erythema of the Newborn

This is an erythematous macular rash with yellow papules containing eosinophils. It occurs on the face, trunk, and limbs in the first few days of life and resolves spontaneously over a few days.

Transient Neonatal Pustular Melanosis

This is an asymptomatic rash of unknown aetiology which appears on the first day of life. It consists of vesicles and pustules on the trunk, palms, and soles which then rupture to form pigmented macules. It resolves spontaneously over a few months.

Persistent and/or Progressive Rashes

Seborrhoeic Dermatitis

One of the most common, often self-limiting skin diseases seen in infants. The exact cause is unknown.

Infants present with an asymptomatic, red, ill-defined, scaly rash affecting the scalp ('cradle cap'), face and napkin area including skin folds (in contrast to napkin dermatitis, which spares skin folds).

Treatment – emollients and mild steroids (e.g. 1% hydrocortisone) to control inflammation and olive oil to loosen scalp scaling.

Neonatal Lupus Erythematosus

Infants present with erythematous scaly macules and plaques on the face and trunk which resolve spontaneously within months. Caused by transplacental transfer of maternal auto-antibodies (anti-Ro antibodies) which can lead to congenital heart block. Management of the skin includes photoprotection and topical mild corticosteroids. Heart block requires cardiology care and possible pacemaker.

Skin Lesions

Table 31.2 summarises the differentiating features between vascular malformations and infantile haemangiomas.

Vascular Malformations

These vary in size, can occur anywhere on the body and be cosmetically distressing for children and parents (Figure 31.3). They are initially flat, but become raised and darker with age.

Treatment – pulsed dye laser, cosmetic camouflage.
Complications – glaucoma, if overlying an eye.
• **Naevus flammeus** – flat pink telangiectatic mark seen in up to 50% of newborn infants on the back of the neck ('stork mark') or forehead ('angel's kiss'). Usually fades with time.
• **Sturge–Weber syndrome** – capillary malformation (port-wine stain) in segment(s) of the trigeminal nerve distribution with underlying intracranial angiomas, associated with epilepsy.

• **Klippel–Trénaunay syndrome** – triad of vascular malformation of a limb associated with venous varicosities and overgrowth of the underlying soft tissues and bone.

Infantile Haemangiomas

The most common benign tumours of infancy. Vary in size, body site, and number and appear as well-demarcated, bright red plaques or nodules during the proliferative stage (Figure 31.4). When regressing, the lesions flatten and become purple and grey (Figure 31.5). Haemangiomas regress spontaneously: about 50% by 5 years of age, and the remainder by 10 years. Most do not require treatment unless they develop complications or interfere with function (e.g. haemangioma on the lip or anogenital region).

Complications – bleeding, ulceration, infection.
Treatment – bleeding can be controlled with direct pressure. Ulcerated haemangiomas require wound care, analgesia, topical and/or oral antibiotics, and pulsed dye laser. Topical timolol applied daily for six months reduces the size and visibility of superficial haemangiomas: systemic propranolol is effective for large, rapidly proliferating lesions. Propranolol is given in liquid form, up to 2 mg/kg in two to three divided doses per day up to 12 months of age. As propranolol is a non-selective beta-blocker, the infants need to be monitored for potential side effects including hypotension, bradycardia, bronchospasm, and hypoglycaemia. Infants with > 5 (or rarely hundreds) haemangiomas may have extra-cutaneous haemangiomas in one or more of the following: liver, heart, brain, gastrointestinal tract, or eyes. Depending on the organs involved, the infant is at risk of potential life-threatening haemorrhage and must be managed by a specialist multi-disciplinary team.

Congenital Melanocytic Naevi

Present at birth and vary in size from a few millimetres to several centimetres across. Often deeply pigmented, usually flat but may be palpable, contain terminal hair, and show colour variation (Figure 31.6). Giant naevi (> 20 cm diameter) may have surrounding multiple smaller satellite naevi.

Complications of giant congenital naevi – cosmetic issues, risk of malignant transformation to melanoma at a young age. Naevi overlying the head, neck, and spine may rarely be associated with melanosis of the meninges and central nervous system and neurophysiological abnormalities.

Management – monitor naevi with serial photographs, excise suspicious areas, large naevi may require multi-step surgery with use of tissue expanders and skin grafts. If naevi overlying the head, neck, and spine in infants, a practical approach is for regular neurological examination with magnetic resonance imaging (MRI) based on clinical findings.

Key Points
• Vascular malformations in trigeminal distribution may have glaucoma and intracranial complications.
• Giant congenital melanocytic naevi are associated with a small but significant risk of malignant melanoma.
• Most infantile haemangiomas regress spontaneously and do not require intervention unless complications.

▶ **Warning**
• Skin barrier function is impaired in premature neonates, so increased risk of systemic absorption of topical steroids.

32 The Child with a Rash

Table 32.1 Approach to a child with a rash.

Clinical history	Clinical examination	Investigations
• Onset: acute or chronic • Systemic symptoms (fever) • Duration of rash • Change in rash over time (intermittent, progressive) • Symptoms of rash (itching, pain) • Family history of skin disease • Recent contact with individuals with a rash (scabies, chickenpox) • Drug history • Other medical history (atopy: asthma, hay-fever) • Other history: insect bites, contact with plants	• Distribution of the rash (generalised, localised, extensor or flexor aspects of limbs) • Morphology of the rash/lesions (Table 32.2) • Involvement of nails, scalp, mucosal surfaces (e.g. tinea corporis and psoriasis may both involve the nails and scalp) • Systemic manifestations (fever in infectious causes)	• Skin scrapings from scaly lesion or rashes for mycology • Swab for microbiology (e.g. impetigo) • Skin biopsy (blistering rashes or when diagnosis uncertain) • Blood investigations depending on diagnosis: blood cultures (bacterial meningitis), viral serology, full blood count (FBC), coagulation screen, renal function for purpuric/petechial rashes • Blood pressure and urine dipstick for evidence of haematuria in purpuric/petechial rashes

Table 32.2 Clues to diagnosis based on the morphology of the rash in a child.

- **Macular (+/– papular) rash** – viral exanthem (e.g. measles, rubella), drug-induced (e.g. penicillin, phenytoin), Kawasaki disease
- **Papular rash** – scabies (Chapter 26), molluscum contagiosum
- **Papulovesicular rash** – chickenpox
- **Scaly rash** – eczema (Chapter 16), psoriasis (Chapter 15), tinea corporis, pityriasis versicolor, pityriasis rosea
- **Blistering rash** – insect bites, bullous impetigo (Chapter 23), linear IgA bullous disease, epidermolysis bullosa (Chapter 53), staphylococcal scalded skin syndrome, Stevens–Johnson syndrome/toxic epidermal necrolysis (Chapter 20)
- **Urticarial rash** – idiopathic urticaria (Chapter 37), urticaria pigmentosa (UP)
- **Petechial/purpuric rash** – meningococcal septicaemia, Henoch–Schönlein purpura, haemorrhagic oedema of infancy, haematological disease (leukaemia, idiopathic thrombocytopaenic purpura), non-accidental injury

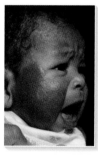

Figure 32.1 Atopic eczema.

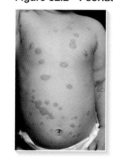

Figure 32.2 Psoriasis.

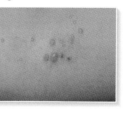

Figure 32.3 Molluscum contagiosum.

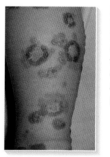

Figure 32.4 Linear IgA bullous disease – note the distribution of blisters in an arc-like pattern.

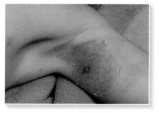

Figure 32.5 Staphylococcal scalded skin syndrome (SSSS).

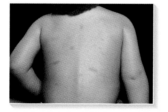

Figure 32.6 Urticaria pigmentosa (UP).

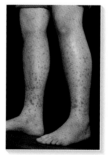

Figure 32.7 Henoch–Schönlein purpura.

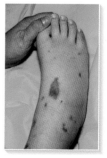

Figure 32.8 Meningococcal septicaemia – note the petechiae and purpura.

Dermatology at a Glance, Second Edition. Mahbub M.U. Chowdhury, Ruwani P. Katugampola, and Andrew Y. Finlay.
© 2020 John Wiley & Sons Ltd. Published 2020 by John Wiley & Sons Ltd.
Companion website: www.wiley.com/go/chowdhury/dermatology

There are many causes of children's rashes (Tables 32.1 and 32.2).

Macular (± Papular) Rash

Measles presents as an erythematous maculopapular rash starting on the face, spreads to the trunk, and fades over a few days. Koplik's spots (transient clusters of white papules with red halo) on the buccal mucosa, fever, cough, and lymphadenopathy occur. Incidence of measles in the UK has risen because of some children missing their measles, mumps, and rubella (MMR) vaccination, following a now discredited *Lancet* article falsely linking MMR with autism. Treatment is symptomatic with monitoring for complications (e.g. pneumonia). Diagnosis is clinical but viral DNA may be identified on blood culture.

Papular Rash

Molluscum contagiosum (Figure 32.3) is a common self-limiting poxvirus infection. Skin-coloured papules with central umbilication develop on the trunk, face, or limbs. Lesions are self-limiting but treatments include cryotherapy, curettage, or topical potassium hydroxide solution or 5% imiquimod cream.

Papular–Vesicular Rash

Chickenpox is a highly contagious airborne disease caused by varicella zoster virus. Patients present with general malaise, fever, and an itchy papular–vesicular rash on the head and trunk; lesions scab and crust and heal over within a week with or without scarring. Different stages of the rash may be seen at one time. Diagnosis is usually clinical. Treatment is symptomatic with monitoring for complications (e.g. pneumonia); antiviral treatment (e.g. aciclovir) started within 48 hours of the rash onset may decrease the disease severity. Reactivation of the varicella zoster virus causes shingles (herpes zoster).

Blistering Rash

Linear IgA Bullous Disease (Chronic Bullous Disease of Childhood)

This is caused by IgA auto-antibodies against the bullous pemphigoid antigen on the basement membrane (Chapter 21, Figure 21.1). Blisters develop in an arc pattern (Figure 32.4) and may occur in the mouth and eyes. Skin biopsy shows a subepidermal blister; direct immunofluorescence of peri-lesional skin shows linear IgA deposition along the epidermal basement membrane. The disease resolves over a few years, but may recur.

Treatment – topical steroids and oral steroids with dapsone.

Staphylococcal Scalded Skin Syndrome

Staphylococcal scalded skin syndrome (SSSS) is caused by disruption of epidermal keratinocyte adhesion by circulating exfoliative toxins produced by specific phage-types of *Staphylococcus aureus*. The child presents with pyrexia and tender erythema followed by superficial blistering, desquamation, and re-epithelialisation over two weeks (Figure 32.5). Flexures are often affected.

Investigations – swab possible sources of primary *S. aureus* infection (nose, throat, skin) for culture and sensitivity, blood cultures, full blood count (FBC), and renal function.

Management – analgesia, systemic flucloxacillin, emollients, non-adherent dressings for eroded skin, and pressure-relieving mattress to minimise friction and skin blistering. Diagnosis is clinical but a skin biopsy may be required to exclude other diagnoses (e.g. Stevens–Johnson syndrome and toxic epidermal necrolysis; Chapter 20). Mucosal surfaces are spared in SSSS and there is no epidermal necrosis on skin biopsy.

Urticarial Rash

Urticaria Pigmentosa

Urticaria pigmentosa (UP) is a cutaneous mastocytosis caused by increased mast cells. Multiple brown macules are seen, with or without papules, often on the trunk (Figure 32.6). Lesions itch and urticate when rubbed (Darier's sign), or if the child is active or warm. Mutations in *c-kit* gene can cause UP.

Management – oral antihistamines and avoiding triggers that may result in massive release of histamine such as physical triggers (heat, vigorous rubbing, exertion), medication (aspirin, non-steroidal anti-inflammatory drugs, codeine, morphine), radio-contrast media, and some general anaesthetics. UP resolves spontaneously by adulthood in about 50% of children. If lymphadenopathy with or without hepatosplenomegaly investigate for systemic mastocytosis (rare in childhood).

Petechial and Purpuric Rash

These result from disorders of blood vessels (e.g. vasculitis) or blood (e.g. idiopathic thrombocytopenic purpura, leukaemia).

Henoch–Schönlein Purpura

This is a self-limiting, IgA-mediated vasculitis associated with preceding infection (e.g. streptococcal upper respiratory tract infection). Characterised by a palpable purpuric rash of buttocks and lower legs, with some necrotic and ulcerated lesions, and resolving over one month (Figure 32.7). The vasculitis may affect the kidney and/or gastro-intestinal tract.

Investigations – throat swabs, serum anti-streptolysin O titres, ESR, CRP, FBC, serum electrolytes, urea and creatinine, urine for haematuria, proteinuria, and blood pressure. Skin biopsy is rarely needed, as the diagnosis is clinical.

Treatment – non-steroidal anti-inflammatory analgesia, rest, and penicillin (if streptococcal infection). Renal involvement determines prognosis and may need systemic steroids.

Important Conditions Not to Miss

Meningococcal Septicaemia

The child develops flu-like symptoms, high fever, headache, neck stiffness, and a widespread macular erythematous rash that changes into petechiae with or without purpura (Figure 32.8). The petechiae do not blanch when a glass tumbler is pressed on the skin. There may be rapid progression to septicaemic shock with brain damage or death. Suspected meningococcal septicaemia should be treated with intravenous or intramuscular benzylpenicillin or cefotaxime immediately.

Kawasaki's Disease

An acute multi-system vasculitic disease that usually affects children aged under five years. It is characterised by fever for at least five days, cervical lymphadenopathy, conjunctival injection, strawberry tongue, red fissured lips, maculopapular rash, oedema, erythema, and desquamation of hands and feet. Prompt management is essential to prevent complications (e.g. myocardial infarction).

Investigations – FBC, ESR, CRP, ECG, echocardiography, angiography, and CT (to detect coronary aneurysms).

Treatment – intravenous immunoglobulins with high-dose aspirin and systemic steroids until resolution of inflammatory markers and cardiac complications.

Key Points

- In urticaria pigmentosa avoid trigger factors that risk massive endogenous histamine release and shock.
- Treat suspected Kawasaki's disease promptly with intravenous immunoglobulins and high-dose aspirin to minimise cardiovascular complications.

▶ **Warning**

- A febrile child with a non-blanching petechial and/or purpuric rash should be treated promptly with systemic antibiotics for presumed meningococcal septicaemia.

33 Skin Problems in Pregnancy

Table 33.1 **Skin problems in pregnancy.**

Physiological skin changes in pregnancy

- Increased pigmentation, e.g. areola of breast, melasma (usually face)
- Spider naevi (commonly chest wall)
- Striae on the abdominal wall
- Diffuse non-scarring alopecia postpartum with subsequent normal regrowth of hair (telogen effluvium)

Pregnancy-related dermatoses

- Intrahepatic cholestasis of pregnancy
- Polymorphic eruption of pregnancy
- Pemphigoid gestationis

Skin lesions in pregnancy

- Benign skin tags
- Thickening or increased pigmentation of pre-existing melanocytic naevi
- Pyogenic granuloma
- Malignant melanoma

Table 33.2 **Differentiation between pregnancy-related dermatoses.**

Characteristic features	Intrahepatic cholestasis of pregnancy	Polymorphic eruption of pregnancy[a]	Pemphigoid gestationis
Clinical features	Severe generalised itching +/− jaundice	Extremely itchy urticated papules and plaques	Extremely itchy blistering eruption
Characteristic distribution	Mainly palms and soles of feet	Abdominal wall with periumbilical sparing	Widespread, including periumbilical area
Timing of presentation	Any trimester, but commonly third trimester	Third trimester or immediate postpartum period	Second or third trimester
Risk to foetus	Foetal distress, prematurity, stillbirth	None	'Small for dates' foetus
Prognosis	Could recur in subsequent pregnancies or in association with oral contraceptive pill	Usually does not recur in subsequent pregnancies; less severe if recurs	Recurs more severely in subsequent pregnancies, menstrual cycle or with oral contraceptive pill

[a] Also termed Pruritic Urticarial Papules and Plaques of Pregnancy (PUPPP).

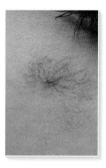

Figure 33.1 Spider naevus – benign telangiectasia with a central arteriole that blanches on pressure. Seen in children, pregnant women, and multiple lesions in association with liver disease.

Figure 33.3 Benign skin tags.

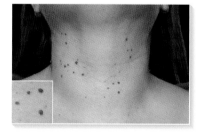

Figure 33.5 Malignant melanoma.

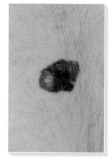

Figure 33.2 Melasma on the face – hyperpigmentation, commonly seen on the face, in association with high oestrogen states (e.g. pregnancy, use of the oral contraceptive pill).

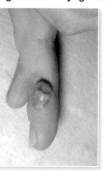

Figure 33.4 Pyogenic granuloma.

Figure 33.6 Polymorphic eruption of pregnancy – note the characteristic periumbilical sparing.

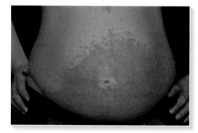

Physiological Skin Changes in Pregnancy

Physiological skin changes occur in women during pregnancy (Table 33.1). Patients require reassurance regarding the benign nature of these changes. For example, in **telogen effluvium** (Chapter 30) the hair will regrow a few months postpartum. Some changes may persist and may later require treatment to improve the cosmetic appearance. For example, **spider naevi** (Figure 33.1) may be treated with pulsed dye laser and **melasma** (Figure 33.2) with depigmentation treatment (topical hydroquinone, tretinoin, and hydrocortisone), sunblock, and advice on sun protection.

Skin Lesions in Pregnancy

The vast majority of skin lesions that change or occur during pregnancy are benign (Figure 33.3) and do not require any active treatment. The differential diagnosis of a rapidly growing lesion during pregnancy is either a pyogenic granuloma or a malignant melanoma, although these are not specifically 'pregnancy-related'.

Pyogenic granulomas (Figure 33.4) commonly occur on fingers, but can develop at any body site. Usually, there is a history of a preceding injury followed by the development of a nodular lesion that bleeds on contact. Pyogenic granulomas are treated by curettage of the lesion followed by cautery of the base of the lesion.

Malignant melanoma (Figure 33.5), although rare, is one of the most common malignancies presenting during pregnancy and may metastasise to the placenta and foetus. A melanoma may arise from a pre-existing naevus or develop de novo at any body site. Clinically suspicious lesions should be completely excised promptly for a histological diagnosis (for details on melanoma see Chapter 40).

Pregnancy-Related Dermatoses

Differentiating between pregnancy-related dermatoses is important because of their effect on the outcome of the pregnancy (Table 33.2).

Polymorphic Eruption of Pregnancy

This develops in the third trimester or in the immediate postpartum period with extremely itchy urticated papules and plaques. The rash may be widespread or confined to the abdominal wall with characteristic periumbilical sparing (Figure 33.6).

Diagnosis is made clinically, it has a benign course and therefore does not require further investigation.

Treatment is aimed at symptomatic relief and consists of topical antipruritic treatment (e.g. 1% menthol in aqueous cream), topical corticosteroids, and sedative oral antihistamines (e.g. chlorphenamine).

Pemphigoid Gestationis

Pemphigoid gestationis usually develops in the second or third trimester with a widespread, extremely itchy, blistering rash. It is thought to occur due to presence of tissue of paternal genetic origin (foetus, hydatidiform mole, choriocarcinoma) and changes in maternal oestrogen and progesterone levels. May recur in subsequent pregnancies with the same partner.

Maternal autoantibodies against the bullous pemphigoid antigen BP180 in the skin basement membrane results in blistering. These autoantibodies may also target the placental basement membrane resulting in placental insufficiency and a 'small for dates' foetus.

Diagnosis is confirmed by skin biopsies for routine histology and direct immunofluorescence (Chapter 21). Serum pemphigoid antigen BP180 antibody levels can be used to assess disease severity and monitor the disease.

Management – topical antipruritic treatment (e.g. 1% menthol in aqueous cream), oral antihistamine (e.g. chlorphenamine), and topical and systemic steroids (oral prednisolone).

Intrahepatic Cholestasis of Pregnancy

This can develop during any trimester, commonly the third trimester. Patients present with severe generalised itching and jaundice. Due to the potential adverse effects on the foetus (foetal distress, prematurity, stillbirth), the mother requires close monitoring with measurement of serum bile salts and bilirubin.

Treatment – topical antipruritic treatment (e.g. 1% menthol in aqueous cream), oral ursodeoxycholic acid or cholestyramine, or narrowband ultraviolet B (UVB) phototherapy (Chapter 44).

Effect of Pregnancy on Pre-existing Skin Diseases

The effect of pregnancy on pre-existing skin diseases is variable. Psoriasis and acne generally improve, whereas atopic eczema worsens. However, psoriasis and acne may worsen postpartum.

Management of Skin Diseases During Pregnancy

Consideration of the potential risk to the foetus is required when managing any form of skin disease in pregnancy. Bland emollients can be used liberally to moisturise any dry skin condition and provide symptomatic relief from itching. Topical corticosteroids are safe when used sparingly, under medical supervision, for treatment of certain skin diseases during pregnancy (e.g. severe eczema, pemphigoid gestationis, polymorphic eruption of pregnancy).

Narrowband UVB phototherapy is considered safe for the treatment of severe psoriasis, eczema, and pruritus from intrahepatic cholestasis during pregnancy.

Use of systemic treatment for skin diseases is limited because of the potential risk to the foetus during pregnancy. Systemic steroids (e.g. oral prednisolone) may be used, under close supervision, for severe skin diseases during pregnancy such as severe eczema and pemphigoid gestationis.

Erythromycin is the safest systemic option for the treatment of severe acne during pregnancy.

Key Points
- Pemphigoid gestationis and intrahepatic cholestasis of pregnancy can be associated with adverse foetal outcome.
- Risk–benefit ratio to the mother and foetus should be considered in consultation with the obstetrician when using systemic therapy for skin diseases during pregnancy.

▶ Warning
- A rapidly growing lesion during pregnancy should be surgically excised for histological examination to exclude malignant melanoma.

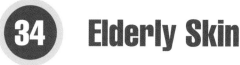

34 Elderly Skin

Table 34.1 Skin diseases in the elderly.

• **Benign skin lesions**
  – Seborrhoeic keratoses (Chapter 38)
  – Campbell de Morgan spots
  – Solar keratoses (Chapter 38)
 	
• **Malignant skin lesions**
  – Non-melanoma skin cancer (basal cell carcinoma, squamous cell carcinoma) (Chapter 39)
  – Melanoma (Chapter 40)
  – Cutaneous T cell lymphoma (Chapter 41)
	• **Skin rashes and other skin manifestations**
	  – Xerosis
	  – Stasis eczema
	  – Seborrhoeic dermatitis (Chapters 25 and 28)
	  – Psoriasis (Chapter 15)
	  – Drug-induced rashes (Chapter 22)
	  – Skin manifestations due to systemic causes (Chapter 46)
	  – Bullous skin diseases (bullous pemphigoid) (Chapter 21)
	  – Skin infections/infestations (tinea pedis, onychomycosis, scabies) (Chapters 25 and 26)
	  – Leg and pressure ulcers (Chapter 52)

Figure 34.1 Multiple skin lesions including basal carcinomas and solar keratoses on the nose and cheeks.

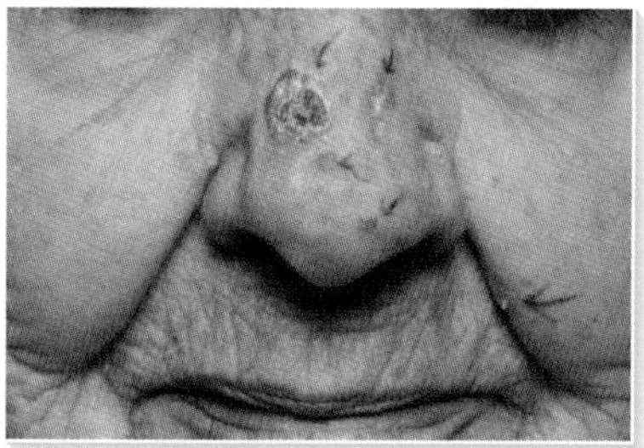

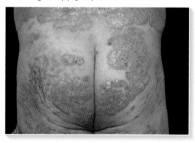

Figure 34.2 Delayed presentation of a large squamous cell carcinoma on the right temple.

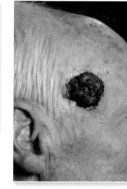

Figure 34.3 Chronic venous ulcer with surrounding stasis eczema of the lower leg.

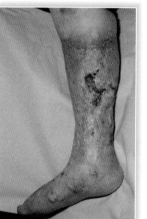

Figure 34.4 Eroding nodular basal cell carcinoma of the nose due to delayed presentation.

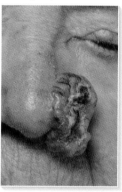

Figure 34.5 Large plaque psoriasis on the buttocks where the patient had difficulty reaching to apply topical treatment.

Figure 34.6 Multiple Campbell de Morgan spots.

Figure 34.7 Delayed presentation of a nodular malignant melanoma on the forearm.

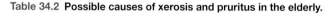
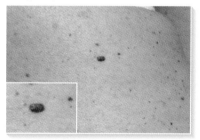
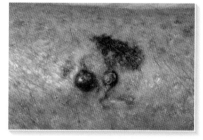

Table 34.2 Possible causes of xerosis and pruritus in the elderly.

• **Age** – age-related xerosis and pruritus (Chapter 50) • **Drug-induced** – diuretics, non-steroidal anti-inflammatory medication, antiseptic washes • **Skin diseases/infestations** – eczema, lichen planus, cutaneous T cell lymphoma, scabies • **Nutritional deficiencies** – iron deficiency (causing anaemia) • **Haematological diseases** – lymphoma, myelodysplasia, multiple myeloma • **Metabolic or endocrine diseases** – renal impairment, liver disease, hypothyroidism, diabetes

Figure 34.8 Xerosis.

Dermatology at a Glance, Second Edition. Mahbub M.U. Chowdhury, Ruwani P. Katugampola, and Andrew Y. Finlay.
© 2020 John Wiley & Sons Ltd. Published 2020 by John Wiley & Sons Ltd.
Companion website: www.wiley.com/go/chowdhury/dermatology

Skin diseases affecting elderly individuals are summarised in Table 34.1. Elderly patients may present with multiple skin lesions, either benign, malignant, or a combination (Figure 34.1).

Attitudes to Skin Diseases in the Elderly

Some elderly patients 'put up' with skin diseases that they consider non-life-threatening. Patients may delay seeking medical attention until the rash or lesion becomes symptomatic (e.g. bleeding basal cell carcinoma or squamous cell carcinoma) (Figure 34.2).

Co-Morbidities Impacting on Skin Disease in the Elderly

Co-morbidities may be the primary cause, contribute to the skin disease or impact on its management (e.g. impaired mobility due to arthritis may result in stasis eczema or chronic venous leg ulceration) (Figure 34.3).

Memory or visual impairment can also delay presentation until the rash or tumour is more extensive or advanced (Figure 34.4).

Elderly individuals are often on multiple systemic medications, some of which may cause skin diseases (e.g. perianal ulceration due to nicorandil). Potential interactions with other medications and exacerbation of other co-morbidities should be borne in mind when starting elderly individuals on systemic treatment for their skin disease (e.g. worsening diabetes with the use of oral steroids).

Factors to Consider When Managing Elderly People with Skin Diseases

Practicalities of applying topical treatment – elderly patients living alone or those with co-morbidities such as arthritis or poor vision may not be able to apply topical treatments to difficult to reach and/or see body sites (e.g. back) (Figure 34.5). Family members or carers may need to be involved and educated about the topical treatment.

Skin diseases such as eczema or psoriasis require several topical treatments: moisturisers to be applied frequently and all over the skin, and an 'active' treatment such as a topical corticosteroid or vitamin D analogue to be applied for a limited period only to affected skin. A clear, written, treatment plan to include the name, application site, frequency, and duration of specific treatments is helpful. Try to keep it simple.

Those living alone or unable to comply with treatment may benefit from dermatology day care or inpatient treatment (Chapter 13).

Benign Skin Lesions

Common benign skin lesions including those seen in the elderly are described in Chapter 38.

Campbell de Morgan Spots

This is one of the most common benign skin lesions occurring in the elderly consisting of dilated capillaries (Figure 34.6). Multiple lesions develop on any body site, often the trunk. They appear as small, red (hence the term cherry angiomas), non-blanching macules or papules. Lesions are usually asymptomatic and therefore treatment is not required. Larger lesions, which may be prone to repeated trauma and bleeding, can be treated with electrocautery.

Malignant Skin Lesions

These are discussed in Chapters 39–41. Malignant lesions in the elderly may be larger and more advanced because of delay in presentation (Figure 34.7).

Xerosis and Pruritus

Xerosis (dry skin) (Figure 34.8) and pruritus (Chapter 50) are common with many possible underlying causes (Table 34.2).

Management of xerosis and pruritus includes a detailed clinical history, with particular attention to the drug history.

In addition to examination for underlying skin diseases or infestation (e.g. scabies), the patient should have a full physical examination, including palpation for lymphadenopathy and hepatosplenomegaly (lymphoma, myelodysplasia). Blood investigations should include a full blood count, renal and liver function, thyroid function, glucose, ferritin, serum immunoglobulins, and electrophoresis.

Further investigations include a blood film, urine Bence Jones proteins, creatinine clearance, ultrasound scan of the liver, spleen, and kidneys, and biopsy of skin, lymph node, or bone marrow.

In addition to treating the underlying cause, symptomatic treatment for xerosis and pruritus includes topical emollients (especially with urea or lactic acid base), topical antipruritic agents (e.g. 1% menthol in aqueous cream), avoidance of soap and use of soap substitutes, bath emollients (caution elderly patients about the risk of slipping in the bath), and oral antihistamines.

Bullous Pemphigoid

Bullous pemphigoid is an autoimmune bullous skin disease that mainly affects elderly individuals and is described in Chapter 21.

Pre-bullous pemphigoid can present as intense pruritus in an elderly patient prior to the development of the tense blisters.

Localised disease can be managed with super-potent topical corticosteroids such as clobetasol propionate. Widespread disease requires either systemic doxycycline or a tapering dose of systemic steroids (e.g. prednisolone starting at 40 mg/day) with an immunosuppressant such as mycophenolate mofetil or azathioprine.

Key Points

- Elderly individuals may present with advanced skin malignancies because of delayed presentation.
- Underlying malignancy needs to be excluded in patients presenting with xerosis and pruritus.
- Elderly patients on prolonged systemic steroid treatment should be monitored for hypertension and diabetes, and given prophylaxis for osteoporosis and gastritis.

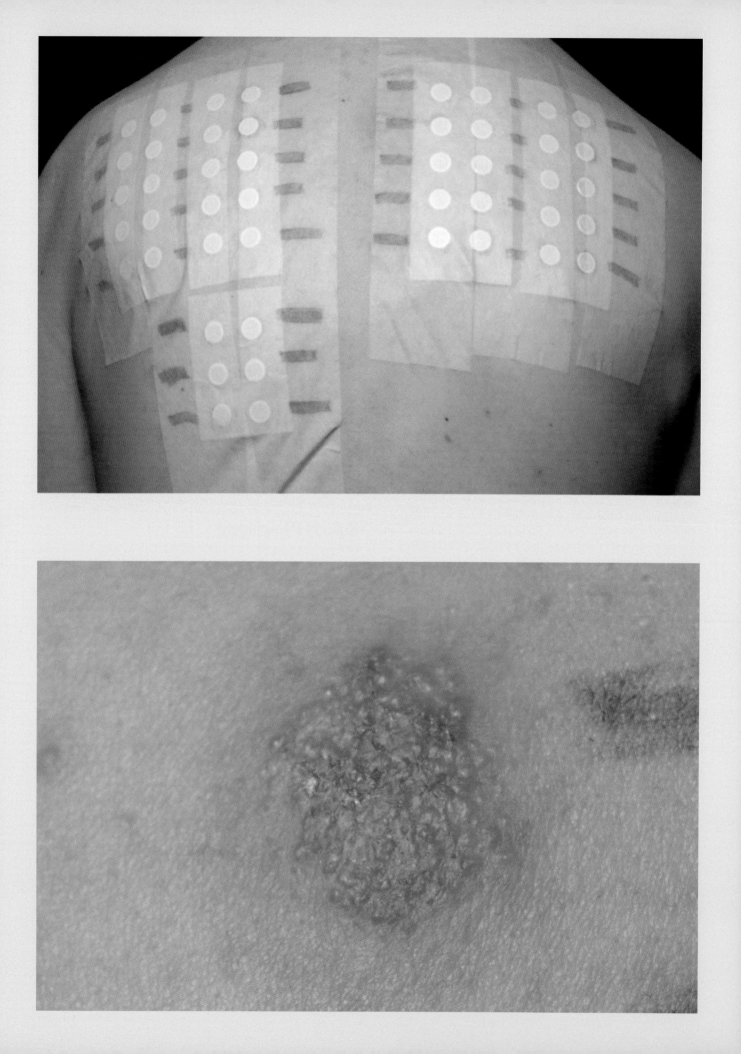

Skin Allergy

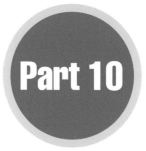

Part 10

35 Cutaneous Allergy

Table 35.1 Indications for patch testing.

- Atopic dermatitis
- Hand dermatitis
- Other dermatoses, e.g. discoid, stasis, seborrhoeic
- Specific site dermatitis, e.g. eyelids, foot, perineal
- Occupational dermatitis
- Cosmetic and hair dye allergy

Figure 35.1   Mechanisms of type I and type IV allergy.

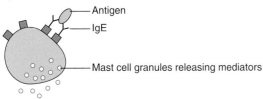

- Antigen
- IgE
- Mast cell granules releasing mediators

(a) Type I allergy is due to mast cell degranulation releasing mediators such as histamine

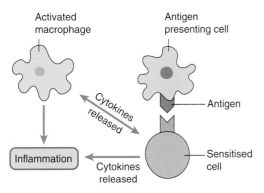

Activated macrophage

Antigen presenting cell

Cytokines released

Antigen

Inflammation

Sensitised cell

Cytokines released

(b) Type IV allergy requires antigen-presenting cells to bind the antigen and to present this to T-cells inducing allergen-specific T-cells. Further contact with the antigen will release cytokines to activate macrophages, leading to inflammation and further proliferation of allergen-specific memory T-cells

Table 35.2   Common examples of allergens tested.

Potassium dichromate	Leather, cement
4-Phenylenediamine base	Hair dye
Thiuram mix	Rubber accelerator
Nickel	Metal, jewellery
Colophony	Pine resin, adhesives, printing ink
Methylisothiazolinone	Preservatives in creams, wipes, shampoos
Wool alcohols	Ointment base in creams
Epoxy resin	Resin in adhesives
Balsam of Peru	Perfumes and flavouring agent
Mercaptobenzothiazole	Rubber chemical
Formaldehyde	Disinfectant, cosmetic preservative
Fragrance mix, limonene, linalool	Perfumes
Sesquiterpene lactone mix	Plants, e.g. chrysanthemum
Tixocortol-21-pivalate	Topical steroids (hydrocortisone)

Figure 35.2   Overlap of dermatitis types.

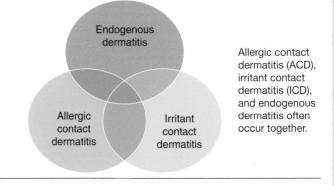

Endogenous dermatitis

Allergic contact dermatitis

Irritant contact dermatitis

Allergic contact dermatitis (ACD), irritant contact dermatitis (ICD), and endogenous dermatitis often occur together.

Figure 35.3 Hand eczema.

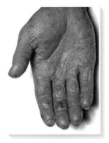

Figure 35.4   Irritant contact dermatitis (ICD) – note scaling in web spaces.

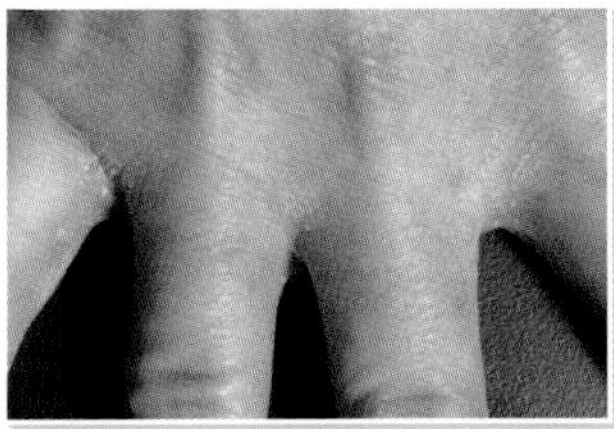

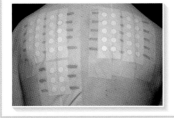

Figure 35.5 Severe pompholyx with vesicles.

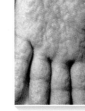

Figure 35.6 Patches ready to apply.

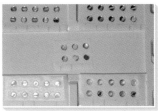

Figure 35.7 Patches applied to back.

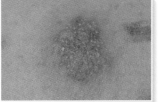

Figure 35.8 Nickel allergy with vesicles.

Figure 35.9   Strong hair dye allergy with blisters.

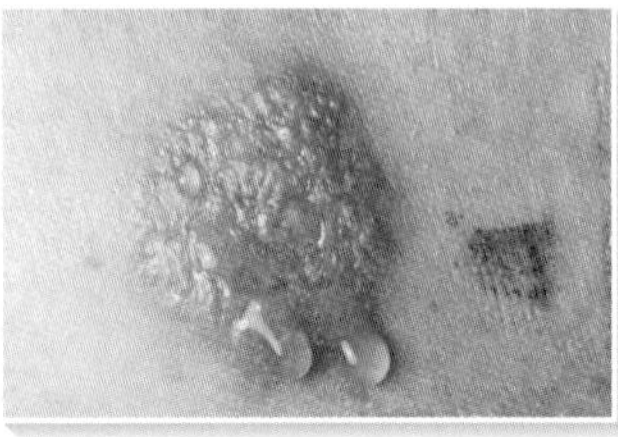

Figure 35.10 Multiple positive skin prick test reactions (circled).

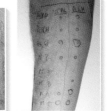

Dermatology at a Glance, Second Edition. Mahbub M.U. Chowdhury, Ruwani P. Katugampola, and Andrew Y. Finlay.
© 2020 John Wiley & Sons Ltd. Published 2020 by John Wiley & Sons Ltd.
Companion website: www.wiley.com/go/chowdhury/dermatology

Contact dermatitis can be irritant or allergic and occurs when a substance or chemical comes into contact with the skin.

- 5% of all dermatology presentations are due to contact dermatitis.
- 50% of occupational disease may be due to dermatitis.

Hairdressers, beauticians, florists, machine operators, printers, and metalworkers are more prone to contact dermatitis.

Hand eczema is very common and up to 25% of women will have this at some time during their life (Figure 35.3).

Irritant Contact Dermatitis

Irritant contact dermatitis (ICD) is the result of localised toxic effects of an irritant on the skin.

ICD accounts for approximately 80% of all contact dermatitis, whilst allergic contact dermatitis (ACD) accounts for only 20%. This is often in contrast to the patient's suspicions as they frequently link skin eruptions with an allergy.

Patients with ICD present with redness, scaling, and fissures on the skin, especially the dorsal and palmar surfaces of the hands, but it may occur mainly in the finger web spaces (Figure 35.4). The definitive diagnosis of ICD needs confirmation by exclusion of ACD with patch testing.

Allergic Contact Dermatitis

ACD is a type IV or delayed (T-lymphocyte mediated) hypersensitivity reaction. Type IV allergy requires antigen presenting cells (APC) in the epidermis (e.g. dendritic Langerhans cells) to bind the antigen to major histocompatibility complex (MHC) class II proteins. APC travel to the draining lymph nodes via lymphatics and activate T cells by presenting this complex. These T cells then release cytokines (e.g. IL-2) to activate macrophages leading to proliferation of allergen-specific memory T cells (sensitisation) (Figure 35.1b). On further encountering the same antigen (allergen) these T cells will migrate to the site of skin contact to release further cytokines and cause inflammation (elicitation).

ACD occurs much less frequently than ICD but is of great importance as it can frequently force a worker to change jobs as protective measures often fail to work. When chronic, ICD and ACD can look quite similar clinically; however, vesicles are more common in ACD. Vesicles can also occur in endogenous pompholyx eczema, especially on the sides of fingers (Figure 35.5). ACD and ICD can be difficult to differentiate and may co-exist (Figure 35.2).

Treatment of ACD consists of identifying the relevant allergen, treating the current problem with topical or systemic treatment (e.g. oral prednisolone), and educating the patient to avoid contact with the allergen.

Patch Testing

Patch testing is a specialised technique where allergens are applied to the patient's back to detect delayed hypersensitivity (Tables 35.1 and 35.2).

The test involves three visits in one week, with patches containing known allergens applied on Day 0 (Monday), patches removed and first reading on Day 2 (Wednesday), and final reading on Day 4 (Friday).

The allergens (chemicals) tested are usually placed in Finn chambers. These 8 mm aluminium pots are placed on an adhesive tape in strips of 10 (Figure 35.6).

A standard patch test series was put together in the 1980s in order to standardise patch testing and is regularly updated. This series aims to test an individual patient to the most common allergens (around 40 allergens) encountered in the environment. Additional series (e.g. hairdresser or cosmetic series) can be added if the investigator feels this is necessary. Up to 60–80 allergens can be tested on the backs of most adults (Figure 35.7).

Reactions are graded by intensity of papules, vesicles, and blisters under the applied patch test allergen. Stronger reactions indicate the specific allergen is more likely to be relevant to the patient's current skin problem. Common examples are nickel and hair dye allergy (Figures 35.8 and 35.9).

Prick Testing

Type I allergy is caused by mast cell degranulation releasing mediators such as histamine (Figure 35.1a). Prick testing is primarily used to detect allergens causing type I (IgE-mediated) or acute hypersensitivity reactions. Antihistamines should be stopped two to four days prior to the test.

In this test a small needle is used to gently prick the skin through a drop of fluid containing a known allergen. This allows a small quantity of allergen into the dermis (Figure 35.10).

A positive control (histamine) and negative control (saline) are used to compare skin reactivity. Reactions (at 15 minutes) larger (2–3 mm greater in diameter) than the saline reaction or at least 50% of the histamine reaction diameter are taken as positive.

Solutions containing antigens are available commercially for many allergens including latex, house dust mite, animal fur, trees, grasses, and various food products, e.g. peanut.

Management and Prognosis of Contact Dermatitis

- Skin protection with suitable gloves, regular emollients, and hand care is essential.
- Avoidance of irritants and allergens causing the dermatitis.
- Allergen avoidance needs to be strict and it can take up to six weeks to see any benefit in the skin.
- If any improvement occurs then continued avoidance is essential and indicates a good prognosis.

Key Points
- ICD is more common than ACD.
- Always think of contact allergy in non-resolving dermatitis.
- Overlap of ICD, ACD, and endogenous eczema is common.

▶ Warning
- Prick test with care (resuscitation facilities) if the patient has a history of anaphylaxis.

36 The Working Hands

Table 36.1 Types of hand eczema and other differentials.

- **Psoriasis** – sharp, well demarcated edges of silvery scaly patches or plaques, symmetrical and slight itch, worse with friction. Other clues include scaly scalp, nail pitting, extensor surface of elbows and knees affected (Figure 36.1)
- **Hyperkeratotic hand eczema** – increased itching compared to psoriasis. Can be difficult to distinguish as can have sharp margins with fissures also (Figure 36.2)
- **Tinea manuum** – may be unilateral on palms. Can affect manual workers, e.g. with wet work. Scaly, inflamed leading edge (with or without tinea pedis) (Figure 36.3)
- **Pompholyx** – vesicles can be extremely itchy on lateral sides of fingers and palms, healing with scaling (Figure 36.4)
- **Irritant contact dermatitis** – scaling in web spaces and dorsum of hands with no vesicles (Figure 36.5)
- **Allergic contact dermatitis** – vesicles can be present (not diagnostic) (Figure 36.6)
- **Atopic hand eczema** – atopy including asthma and hay-fever. Previous history in childhood of atopic eczema affecting flexures. Apron pattern of eczema at the base of the fingers (Figure 36.7)

Table 36.2 Occupations predisposed to hand irritation (and causes).

- **Hairdressers** (due to handwashing, shampoos) (Figure 36.5)
- **Nurses** (handwashing, alcohol gels)
- **Mechanics** (oils, detergents)
- **Chefs** (raw vegetables, fish)
- **Butchers** (handwashing, meats)

Table 36.3 Occupations predisposed to allergy (and causes).

- **Construction workers** (chromium in cement)
- **Hairdressers** (hair dyes, nickel)
- **Florists** (plants, e.g. chrysanthemum) (Figure 36.6)
- **Aromatherapists** (perfumes, essential oils)
- **Rubber workers** (natural latex, preservatives in processing)
- **Metal workers** (nickel, cobalt, chromium)

**Table 36.4
Treatment for hand eczema.**

- **Topical corticosteroids** (with occlusion)
- **Oral corticosteroids**
- **Hand PUVA**
- **Immunosuppressants** (e.g. azathioprine, ciclosporin, methotrexate)
- **Retinoids** (e.g. alitretinoin)

Figure 36.7 Apron pattern in endogenous eczema, i.e. like an 'apron on two legs'.

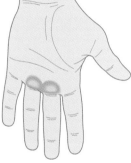

Figure 36.1a Thickened, sharp edged, scaly psoriasis plaques on palms.

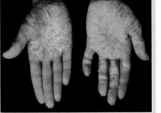

Figure 36.1b Note painful fissures on hand.

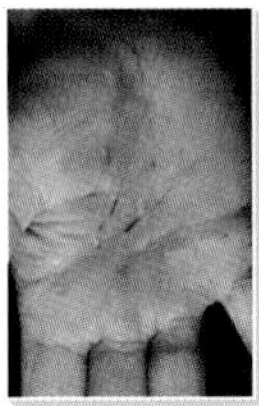

Figure 36.1e and f Severe pustulosis with brown macules.

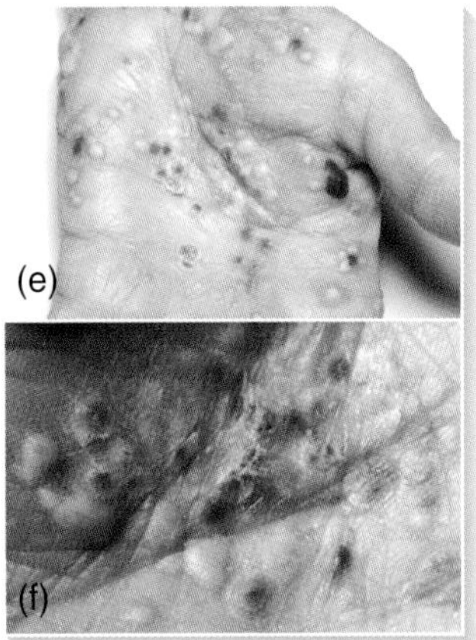

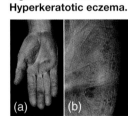

(e)

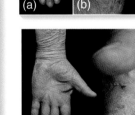

(f)

Figure 36.2a and b Hyperkeratotic eczema.

(a) (b)

Figure 36.3a and b Tinea manuum in manual worker.

(a) (b)

Figure 36.1c Hyperkeratotic psoriasis at friction sites.

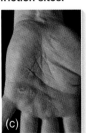

(c)

Figure 36.1d Typical silvery scaling on dorsum hand.

(d)

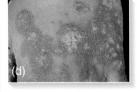

Figure 36.4 Note itchy vesicles on palm.

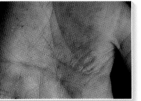

Figure 36.5 Irritant contact dermatitis in a hairdresser.

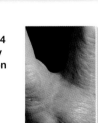

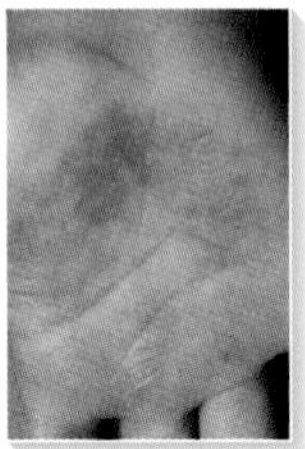

Figure 36.6 Dominant hand of florist with chrysanthemum allergy.

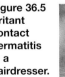

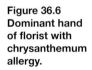

Dermatology at a Glance, Second Edition. Mahbub M.U. Chowdhury, Ruwani P. Katugampola, and Andrew Y. Finlay.
© 2020 John Wiley & Sons Ltd. Published 2020 by John Wiley & Sons Ltd.
Companion website: www.wiley.com/go/chowdhury/dermatology

Problems with the skin on the hands are very common, accounting for 90% of all occupational skin diseases. Hand dermatitis has a prevalence of 5–10% in the population with an incidence of around 5% per year. Psoriasis, tinea infections, and atopic eczema including pompholyx affect the hands (Table 36.1). Endogenous dermatitis, allergic contact dermatitis (ACD), and irritant contact dermatitis (ICD) need to be differentiated by detailed history, examination, and investigations such as patch testing (Chapter 35).

Hand Eczema

Patients with chronic hand eczema tend to have prolonged sick leave, increased health costs, and decreased quality of life. Each year 60% of people with hand eczema visit their GP and up to 20% visit a specialist. Twenty-five percent of chronic hand eczema is caused by ACD.

Poor prognosis for hand eczema is associated with atopy (especially respiratory), contact allergy, older age, increased severity and longer duration (> one year) of eczema. Other factors are patient exposure to wet work, increased frequency of handwashing, and wearing gloves for long periods of time (>four to six hours per day).

Thirty percent of nurses develop hand eczema. Senior nurses with atopy, multiple handwashes during the day, and wearing gloves for prolonged periods of time are particularly at risk. This is mainly due to ICD; however, ACD needs to be excluded with patch testing.

Apprentice hairdressers have a high risk of hand eczema because of excess wet work and exposure to irritant and potentially allergenic chemicals (e.g. nickel, hair dyes). Up to 35% develop hand eczema within two years. Up to 30% of people in occupations at high risk of hand eczema (e.g. food industry, builders, hairdressers) may need to change their occupation, leading to a better prognosis medically.

Intervention with correct diagnosis and early treatment within one year of presentation leads to a better prognosis.

Prevention of Hand Eczema

The focus of any prevention should be at early stages for those at risk.

Primary and secondary prevention involves education of skin care for professions with increased risk. Important factors include elimination of relevant contact factors such as irritants and potential allergens.

Maintenance of the skin barrier function is essential with skin care education and skin protection. Skin protection includes personal protection equipment such as gloves and gauntlets (long gloves with forearm protection). Simple measures, such as reducing the amount of handwashing, are very effective.

Occupational hand eczema due to natural latex allergy in health care workers can be prevented by using low allergenic, powder-free, latex gloves. Alternatives that can be used instead of latex gloves are vinyl or nitrile gloves. Prognosis in health care workers with latex or rubber allergy can be very favourable with these simple measures.

Certain occupations are predisposed to problems with 'working hands' with regards to irritant and allergic contact dermatitis (Tables 36.2 and 36.3). Specific treatment for other hand diseases is determined by the diagnosis (e.g. psoriasis or tinea manuum).

Treatment

The hands need to be protected with regular use of emollients and soap substitutes and strict avoidance of irritants (Table 36.4). Topical or oral corticosteroids can be used for other causes of hand eczema including pompholyx.

Topical steroids may need to be used at very high potency for a short period of time (e.g. clobetasol propionate [Dermovate®] for six weeks). Topical steroids can be used under occlusion to get adequate absorption using cling film or cotton gloves. Oral steroids can be used but there is a risk of rebound flare once they are stopped.

Topical PUVA therapy can be used for the hands for a period of 8–10 weeks (20–30 treatments).

Any infection confirmed with skin swabs should be treated with systemic and topical antibiotics. Systemic therapies such as alitretinoin (oral retinoid) are recommended by the National Institute for Health and Care Excellence (NICE) to be used after potent topical steroids (e.g. clobetasol propionate [Dermovate®]) if Dermatology Life Quality Index (DLQI) is > 15 and the physician's assessment indicates severe hand eczema.

Immunosuppressants used include azathioprine, ciclosporin, and methotrexate. These can be effective in selected patients even though they are not licensed for use in hand eczema.

Key Points
- Hand eczema accounts for 90% of all occupational skin disease patients.
- Hand eczema has a poorer prognosis in atopic individuals especially if severe with a long history.
- Contact allergy to allergens such as chrome may lead to persistent hand eczema even after avoidance of the allergen.
- Hand psoriasis can look similar to hyperkeratotic hand eczema.
- Consider all differentials for work-related hand skin disease and review the diagnosis if there is no improvement.

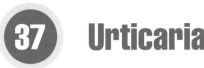

37 Urticaria

Table 37.1 Causes of urticaria.

- **Drugs** – aspirin, non-steroidal anti-inflammatory drugs (NSAIDs), angiotensin converting enzyme (ACE) inhibitors, omeprazole, and simvastatin
- **Antibiotics** – penicillins, cephalosporins, and tetracyclines
- **Foods** – fish, milk, potatoes, carrots, spices, bananas, shellfish, and hazelnuts
- **Food additives** – tartrazine and azo dyes including sunset yellow, benzoates, sulphites
- **Infections** – viral and bacterial such as dental sepsis, sinusitis, gall bladder, and urinary tract

Table 37.2 Enquiries for history taking in urticaria.

- **Comprehensive history required** – onset, disease course, duration of individual wheals, presence of purpura or angioedema
- **Systemic symptoms** – malaise, headache, abdominal pain, wheezing, and syncope
- **Precipitating factors** – heat, cold, pressure, friction, sunlight, latex
- **Drug history** – aspirin, non-steroidal anti-inflammatory drugs, antibiotics, over the counter medication
- **Other history** – association with any recent infection, foods, family history of angioedema

Table 37.3 Investigations in urticaria.

- Exclude associated conditions including full blood count, ESR, thyroid function (abnormal in 5% of chronic urticaria patients), urinalysis
- Skin biopsy if urticarial vasculitis suspected
- Food diary, specific IgE to foods (if strongly suspected)
- Chart of frequency and severity on scale 0–10 (to monitor any change)

If angioedema prominent:
- C1 esterase inhibitor level and complement C2, C4 (may be reduced in hereditary angioedema)
- Complement C3, C4 (may be reduced in urticarial vasculitis)

Table 37.4 Drug treatments.

- **Urticaria:**
  - Classic H1 antihistamines – chlorphenamine, hydroxyzine
  - Second generation H1 antihistamines – cetirizine, loratadine, fexofenadine
  - Anti-leukotrienes – montelukast
  - Immunomodulators – ciclosporin, mycophenolate mofetil
  - Omalizumab (Chapter 14)
  - Corticosteroids
- **Non-hereditary angioedema:**
  - Epinephrine (EpiPen®)
  - Ciclosporin
  - Intravenous immunoglobulins
- **Hereditary angioedema:**
  - Androgens – danazol and stanozolol
  - Epsilon (aminocaproic acid)
  - Tranexamic acid
  - Fresh frozen plasma

Table 37.5 Types of physical urticaria.

- Dermographism
- Delayed pressure
- Vibration
- Exercise, heat, cold
- Cholinergic
- Sun exposure
- Aquagenic urticaria
- Contact urticaria

Eosinophil rich inflitrate

Lymphocyte

Separation of the collagen by oedema

Neutrophil

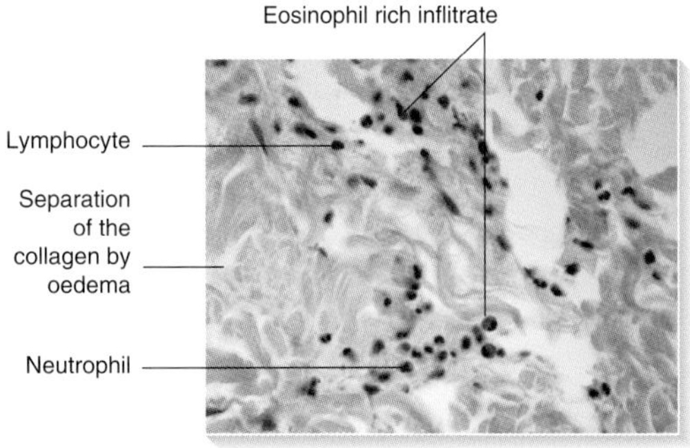

Figure 37.1 Histology (H&E ×60).

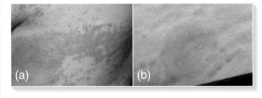

Figure 37.2 a and b Typical urticaria on trunk.

(a) (b)

Figure 37.3 Annular urticaria.

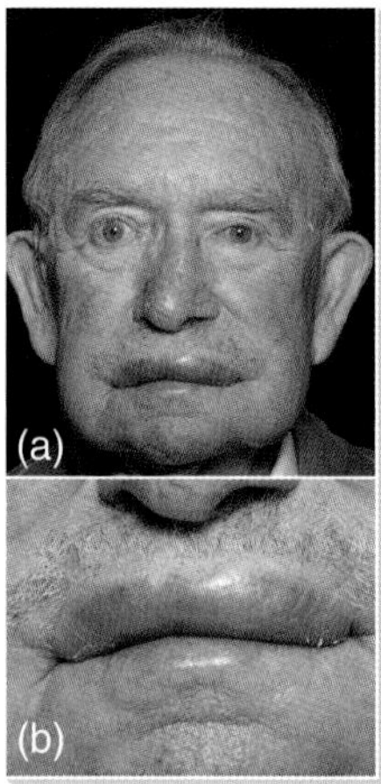

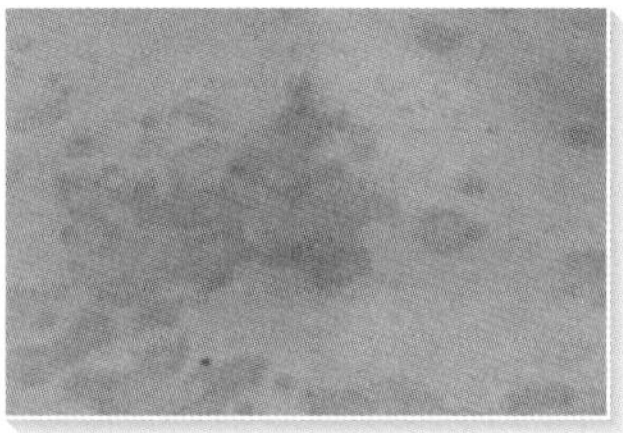

Figure 37.5 Angioedema of eyelids.

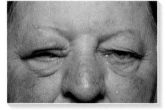

Figure 37.4a and b Angioedema of upper lip with marked swelling.

(a)

(b)

Urticaria is a common condition which can present to dermatologists, immunologists, and GPs.

Urticaria is known as 'nettle rash', itchy hives, or wheals. It is a temporary eruption of erythema and oedema with swelling of the dermis and is usually itchy. Urticaria and angioedema (deeper dermal and subcutaneous swellings) may occur together.

Classification

Urticaria can be classified as ordinary urticaria consisting of acute or chronic urticaria. Urticaria is defined as chronic if lasting more than six weeks. A cause is less likely to be found than for acute urticaria. Other types include physical and cholinergic, contact urticaria, and immune complex urticaria such as urticarial vasculitis.

Dermatology at a Glance, Second Edition. Mahbub M.U. Chowdhury, Ruwani P. Katugampola, and Andrew Y. Finlay.
© 2020 John Wiley & Sons Ltd. Published 2020 by John Wiley & Sons Ltd.
Companion website: www.wiley.com/go/chowdhury/dermatology

Histology and Pathophysiology

Histology of ordinary urticaria wheals shows oedema and perivascular mixed cellular (eosinophils, lymphocytes, neutrophils) dermal infiltrate with vascular and lymphatic dilatation (Figure 37.1). Electron microscopy may show dermal mast cell degranulation.

Pathophysiology of urticaria includes increased capillary and venous permeability. Cutaneous mast cell activation releases mediators including histamine leading to activation of H1 receptors which induces itching, erythema, and whealing.

Other histamine releasing factors involved include tryptase and neuropeptides (substance P). Plasma mediators (bradykinin) and complement may play a part in angioedema with complement activation leading to immune complex urticaria and urticarial vasculitis.

Clinical Features

Urticaria presents as itchy, erythematous macules and wheals with pink, swollen, raised areas with a surrounding flare (Figure 37.2). The sites affected are variable and can include the palms and soles. The number, shape, and size of the lesions vary with bizarre shapes including annular patterns (Figure 37.3). In ordinary urticaria the individual wheals resolve within 24 hours and may last only a few hours. They leave no skin change.

Fifty percent of patients with urticaria may have angioedema of the face, lips (Figure 37.4), eyelids (Figure 37.5), hands and genitalia (Chapter 20). Mucosal swellings can occur inside the mouth (e.g. tongue, pharynx, and larynx). Occasionally, systemic symptoms associated with urticaria include vomiting, general malaise, headache, and abdominal pain with syncope and, in severe forms, anaphylaxis.

In urticarial vasculitis, lesions last > 24 hours and can leave bruises. Skin biopsy is essential to confirm this diagnosis.

Causes

Acute urticaria has no identifiable cause in 30% of patients (Table 37.1). Acute allergic urticaria may be caused by an IgE-mediated mast cell degranulation. The most common causes are drugs, foods, and, rarely, food additives.

Chronic urticaria has wheals that still occur over six weeks or more and 40% may have physical urticaria (e.g. delayed pressure urticaria). Most are idiopathic as only 10–20% have an identifiable cause. Chronic urticaria affects 0.5–1% of individuals (lifetime prevalence) with significant reduction of quality of life.

Potential exacerbating factors of urticaria include drugs such as aspirin or non-steroidal anti-inflammatory drugs (NSAIDs) and viral or bacterial infections, but treatment of these infections does not always clear the chronic urticaria.

Prognosis

Acute urticaria attacks may last for a few hours a day and then fade. Chronic cases, particularly if idiopathic, may last for months or even years. Fifty percent of patients with urticaria can be clear within 6–12 months.

Management

Detailed history and some investigations may be necessary (Tables 37.2 and 37.3).

Reassurance regarding the diagnosis is needed. Reducing stress and alcohol, and avoidance of aspirin, salicylates, NSAIDs, and opiates is helpful.

Diets may need to exclude food additives, colourings, or preservatives if these substances are detected as causative agents.

Drug Management (Table 37.4)

As urticaria is histamine mediated, H1 receptor blockers (antihistamines) can reduce itch, whealing, and erythema. Second generation H1 antihistamines (e.g. loratadine) are the treatment of choice with low levels of sedation and minimal anti-cholinergic side effects and can be used safely up to four times standard dosages. Antihistamines may need to be used regularly for long periods to gain satisfactory control of the urticaria. Next treatment steps include classic antihistamines such as chlorphenamine which has side effects of sedation and anti-cholinergic properties but are useful for night-time sedation and to reduce itching. Anti-leukotriene drugs, e.g. montelukast, can be helpful prior to progressing to immunomodulators, e.g. ciclosporin, mycophenolate mofetil. Omalizumab (Chapter 14) has transformed treatment of refractory severe chronic urticaria.

Corticosteroids are effective in patients with severe urticaria and short courses of oral steroids are often prescribed for acute exacerbations. However, prolonged use must be avoided because of the risk of side effects and also instability of the urticaria once the prednisolone is stopped. This makes further control of the urticaria extremely difficult.

Non-hereditary angioedema with respiratory involvement may require epinephrine (adrenaline) which causes rapid vasoconstriction. Treatment may need to be repeated if there is no improvement within 10–20 minutes and self-administration of epinephrine (EpiPen®) may be required in the future (Chapter 20).

Physical and Cholinergic Urticarias

This is a distinct group of patients with a physical cause for the whealing (Table 37.5). Cholinergic urticaria can be linked with heat and sweating. Approximately 20% of urticaria patients have physical urticaria with dermographism which is the triple response arising from firm stroking of the skin. This involves local erythema with capillary vasodilatation followed by oedema and surrounding flare. This is normal in 5% of people and if exaggerated is called dermographism. Clinically, this may present as whealing and itching at sites of trauma and friction with clothing and gloves (e.g. on hands). These types are less common and management requires avoidance of the cause, oral antihistamines, and further treatment as above for chronic urticaria.

Hereditary Angioedema

This is very rare (5% of angioedema) and occurs without urticaria. A family history is usually present (autosomal dominant trait on chromosome 11). The condition starts in childhood but can be delayed into late adult life. Recurrent swellings of the skin and mucous membranes occur with nausea, vomiting, abdominal colic, and urinary symptoms. Swelling of the pharynx, larynx, and bronchial tree can occur leading to death. Results of therapy with conventional antihistamines are poor. Androgens may be effective but replacement therapy with fresh frozen plasma may be needed for short-term prophylaxis and for urgent treatment (Table 37.4).

Key Points
- Acute urticaria usually lasts less than six weeks.
- Chronic urticaria can be long lasting (years) with no cause found in 80% of patients and can severely affect quality of life.
- Management of urticaria can be difficult requiring combination of antihistamines progressing to immunomodulators such as ciclosporin and omalizumab.

► Warning
- Corticosteroid therapy makes further control of urticaria extremely difficult.

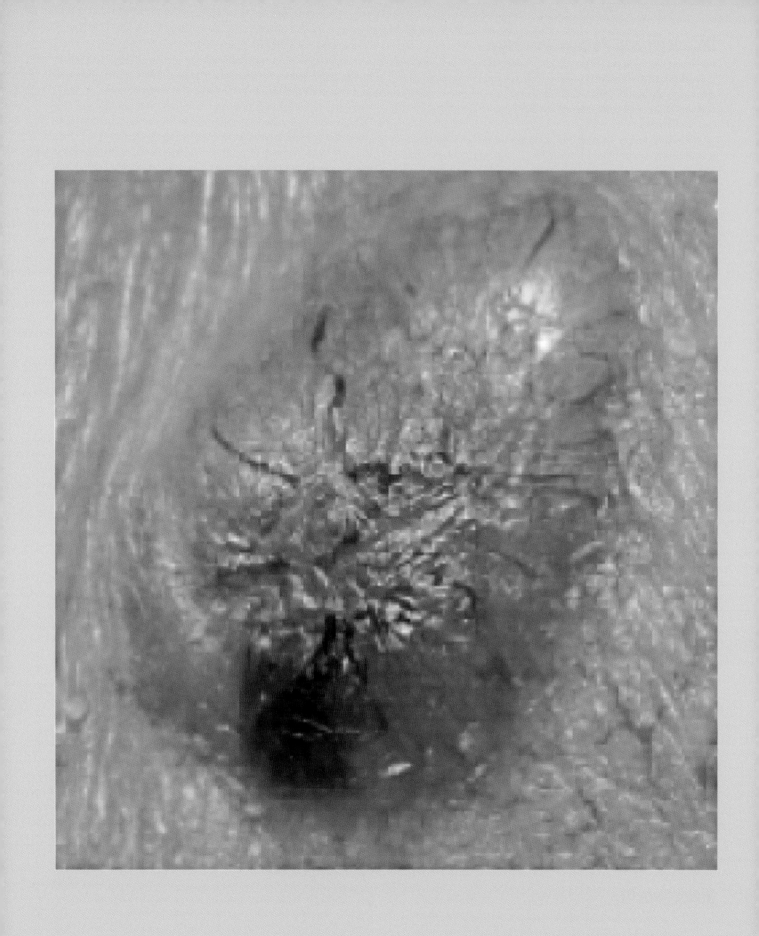

Skin Tumours

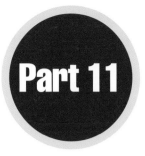

Part 11

Chapters

38 Benign Skin Lesions

Table 38.1 Classification of benign lesions based on derivation.

- **Epidermis** – seborrhoeic wart, solar keratosis, Bowen's disease
- **Melanocytes** – freckle, lentigo, melanocytic naevus
- **Hair follicles** – epidermoid cyst
- **Fibroblasts** – dermatofibroma

Figure 38.1
Junctional naevus
– flat and dark.

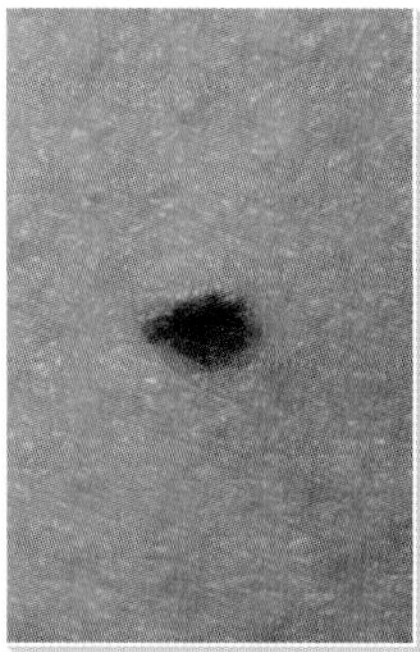

Figure 38.2
Compound naevus
– raised and dark.

Figure 38.3
Intradermal naevus
– raised and skin coloured.

Figure 38.4 **Freckles.**

Figure 38.6
Lentigo maligna
– irregular pigmented
area. Needs skin
biopsy.

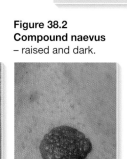

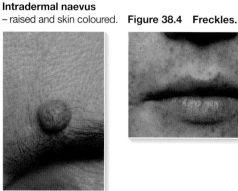

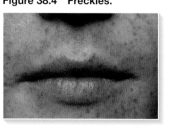

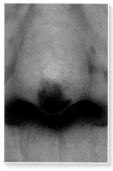

Figure 38.5
Solar lentigo – regular shaped
pigmented macule.

Figure 38.7
Seborrhoeic wart.

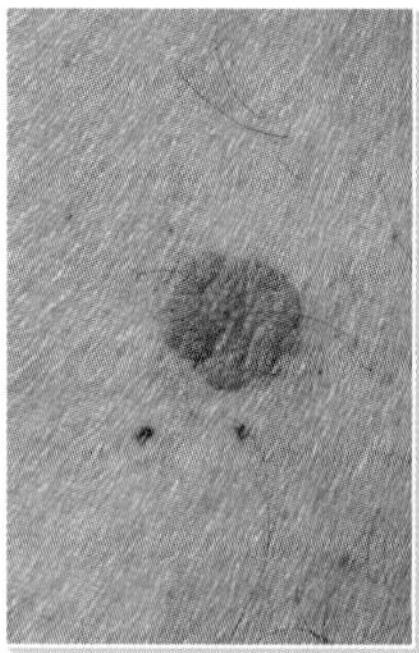

Figure 38.8
**Pigmented seborrhoeic
wart.**

Figure 38.9a
**Epidermoid cyst with
punctum.**

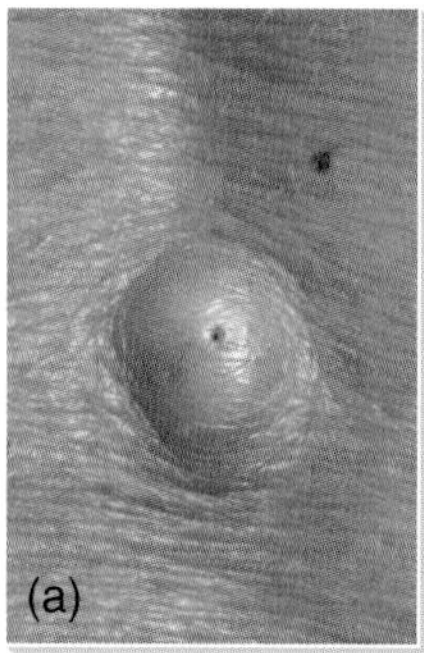

Figure 38.9b
**Large pilar cyst on
scalp.**

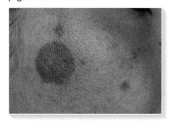

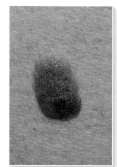

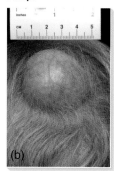

(a)

(b)

Figure 38.10
Dermatofibroma
– can be pigmented.

Figure 38.11a and b
Skin tags.

Figure 38.12a
Cutaneous horn on cheek.

Figure 38.12b
Cutaneous horn on ear.

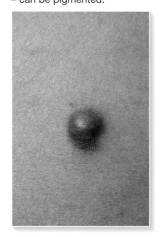

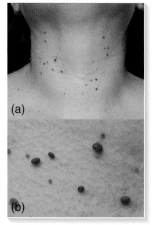

(a)

(b)

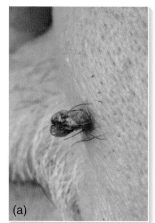

(a)

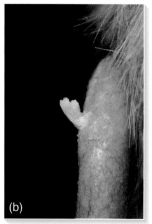

(b)

Dermatology at a Glance, Second Edition. Mahbub M.U. Chowdhury, Ruwani P. Katugampola, and Andrew Y. Finlay.
© 2020 John Wiley & Sons Ltd. Published 2020 by John Wiley & Sons Ltd.
Companion website: www.wiley.com/go/chowdhury/dermatology

Figure 38.13a and b   Solar keratoses on scalp and closeup.

Figure 38.14a and b   Bowen's disease.

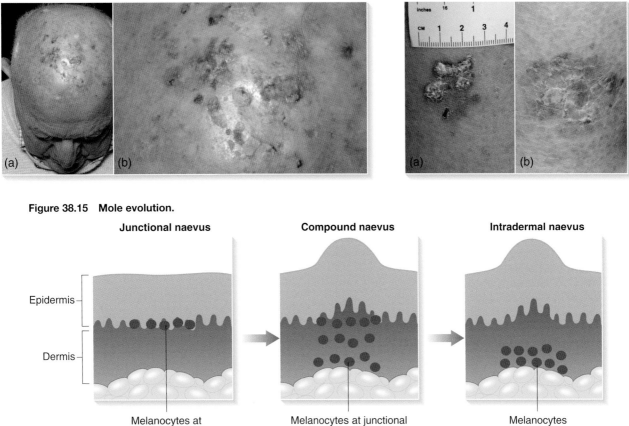

Figure 38.15   Mole evolution.

Benign Melanocytic Naevi

enign skin lesions are very common and constitute a large number of skin consultations in general practice. It is important to be able to make a confident, correct, clinical diagnosis to reassure the patient or to suggest further appropriate management, which may include surgical removal.

It is essential that the patient understands the lesion is likely to be benign prior to embarking on a procedure that may lead to a less than ideal cosmetic appearance, risking patient dissatisfaction.

When considering these lesions it is important to think about their derivation (Table 38.1).

Benign Melanocytic Naevi

These consist of three main types: junctional, compound, and intradermal melanocytic naevi. These are all benign and are called moles. These are common and appear in childhood and puberty and can become smaller in later life. It is not unusual to see up to 30 naevi in sun exposed areas. However, those with fair skin, a family history of moles, and increased sun exposure are likely to have larger numbers (> 40).

A melanocytic naevus can change through the three stages from a junctional naevus (usually flat and dark) to a compound naevus (raised and usually dark) to an intradermal naevus (usually flesh coloured) (Figures 38.1–38.3 and 38.15).

• As a **junctional naevus** is flat and brown, a new mole may be difficult to differentiate from malignant melanoma and hence may need to be excised for histology (Figure 38.1). If confident that it is a mole, it can be left alone or excised with a narrow 2 mm margin.

• A **compound melanocytic naevus** is raised, pigmented, and can be hairy. Again, if the diagnosis is confident, it can be left alone (Figure 38.2). A shave excision is better cosmetically than a full ellipse excision for these moles. The patient should be warned regarding the likely cosmetic result of a flat scar and that pigmentation and hairs can regrow within the area.

• An **intradermal naevus** is usually raised and non-pigmented (Figure 38.3) and needs to be differentiated from a basal cell carcinoma (BCC) (Figure 39.1).

• Red flag signs for any suspicious changes in moles include change of size, shape, colour, and symptoms such as bleeding and itch (Table 40.1).

Freckles and Lentigos

Freckles are common benign lesions that usually occur on sun exposed areas and consist of multiple pigmented macules that darken after sun exposure (Figure 38.4). These start in childhood and do not have an increase in melanocytes but the melanosomes within the melanocytes produce increased melanin in response to sun exposure.

A **lentigo** can also be a small pigmented macule but the pigmentation is the result of an increase in the number of melanocytes in the basal layer and does not darken significantly after sun exposure (Figure 38.5). They are solitary, occur on sun exposed skin, and can be termed solar lentigines. Lesions that are larger may need to be excised for diagnosis to exclude a lentigo maligna (Hutchinson's freckle). This is a pre-malignant melanocytic lesion that usually occurs on the face and can transform to a lentigo maligna melanoma (Figure 38.6).

Seborrhoeic Keratosis (Basal Cell Papilloma)

Seborrhoeic keratoses (warts) are benign and very common, especially on the trunk of elderly patients. They are multiple, superficial, crusted lesions with a greasy appearance, with new lesions developing over time. Size can vary from few millimetres up to 3 cm in diameter. The lesions have a 'stuck-on' appearance and seem to be superficially attached to the dermis (Figure 38.7). The crusted surface can fall off but usually recurs and can be of variable dark colours causing confusion with malignant melanoma (Figure 38.8). They are asymptomatic but can be very itchy and become inflamed or irritated after trauma. Follicular plugged areas can be seen with a dermatoscope which can be extremely helpful for diagnosis (Chapter 11). They are best managed with reassurance and explanation of the diagnosis. Usually, they do not need to be removed but if symptomatic or disfiguring can be removed with shave excision, curettage, and cautery or cryotherapy (Chapters 9 and 10). Histology should be checked for solitary lesions.

Epidermoid Cyst

Cysts are derived from pilar units and often incorrectly called 'sebaceous cysts'. An epidermoid cyst has an epidermal wall surrounding a core of keratin. These cysts are common in young to middle-aged adults and are usually asymptomatic. If they become inflamed and infected then excision may be warranted as they particularly occur on the head, neck, and upper trunk. The lesion is within the dermis with overlying normal epidermis and a punctum (opening on the skin surface) (Figure 38.9a). The pilar type cyst is more common on the scalp (Figure 38.9b) and can be genetically inherited. Contents of pilar cysts are foul smelling and have a cheesy appearance.

Dermatofibroma (Histiocytoma)

This consists of a proliferation of fibroblasts in the dermis. This is thought to be often caused by an insect bite which is usually not noticed in most patients. They are common on the lower limbs of women, presenting as a firm hard nodule which can be itchy (Figure 38.10). Some can be pigmented and cause confusion with benign moles. A useful sign for diagnosis is dimpling on the surface when pressure is exerted laterally on both sides of the dermatofibroma. If the diagnosis is clear then excision should not be undertaken for

cosmetic reasons as healing can be poor, particularly on the lower limbs. If excised, ellipse excision is the best option.

Skin Tag (Fibroepithelial Polyp)

Skin tags are extremely common and present as multiple small, pedunculated, fleshy, skin-coloured lesions, increasing in size and number with age and occurring in the axillae, groins, and neck (Figure 38.11). Snip excision with cautery is the best treatment if requested but not routinely done.

Solar Keratoses (Actinic Keratoses)

These are common pre-malignant lesions occurring on chronic light exposed skin of fair skinned individuals. The risk of malignant transformation to squamous cell carcinoma (SCC) is extremely small. However, these lesions are treated as they are often multiple. They can be asymptomatic or itch and can present as a cutaneous horn (Figure 38.12). Common sites are the backs of hands, face, scalp, and ears and they typically present as multiple pink, rough, scaly, or crusted lesions (Figure 38.13). Any increase in inflammation or size should be biopsied or excised to exclude SCC. General management of solar keratoses involves sun protection with sunscreen and clothing. Individual lesions are treated with liquid nitrogen cryotherapy, curettage and cautery, photodynamic therapy (PDT), topical 5-fluorouracil (Efudix®), 3% diclofenac gel (Solaraze®), and ingenol mebutate gel (Picato®).

Bowen's Disease (Intraepidermal Squamous Cell Carcinoma)

This is a pre-malignant condition that is less common than solar keratosis and can progress to SCC. Sun exposure (and previously arsenic containing tonics) can lead to Bowen's disease which presents as well-defined, persistent, inflamed, scaly patches on the lower limbs of the elderly (Figure 38.14). Differential diagnoses include superficial BCC, psoriasis, discoid eczema, and fungal infections. Surgical excision may be difficult as Bowen's disease occurs commonly on the lower limbs where healing may be slow. Other treatments are liquid nitrogen cryotherapy, topical 5-fluorouracil (Efudix®), and imiquimod (Aldara®).

Key Points

- Reassure the patient that the lesion is benign if you are 100% certain.
- Warn the patient explicitly regarding possible scar and poor cosmesis with any treatment to remove benign lesions.

▶ Warning

- Do not treat a benign lesion unless the patient is 100% sure he or she wants to proceed.
- Removal of benign moles may leave residual pigment and hair growth.

39 Non-Melanoma Skin Cancers

Table 39.1 Risk factors for developing non-melanoma skin cancers (NMSC).

- Skin type – especially Fitzpatrick skin types I and II
- Elderly age
- Long-term sun exposure – outdoors work, holidays abroad, lifestyle, e.g. sunbeds
- Immunosuppression – organ transplant recipients, systemic drugs, e.g. azathioprine, ciclosporin
- Multiple solar keratoses, Bowen's disease

Table 39.2 Poor prognostic indicators in non-melanoma skin cancers.

- Site – face, lips, ear (Figure 39.11)
- Histology – poor differentiation
- Ill-defined tumour
- Previous incomplete treatment
- Recurrent tumour
- Large size

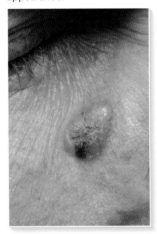

Figure 39.1 Basal cell carcinoma (BCC) – note typical telangiectasia and shiny appearance.

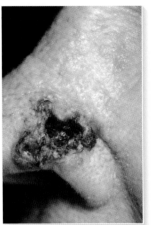

Figure 39.2 Longstanding BCC with ulceration and pigmentation.

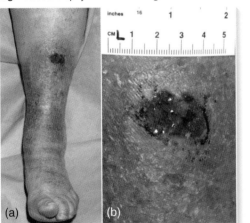

Figure 39.3a and b Superficial BCC on left leg – needs biopsy to confirm diagnosis.

Figure 39.4a and b Ill-defined morphoeic BCCs on nose.

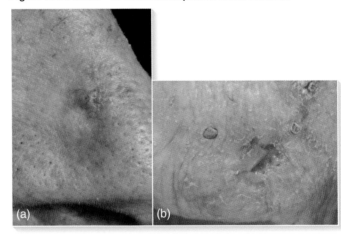

Figure 39.5 BCC histology (H&E ×20).

Peripheral palisading

Artefactual clefting

Central necrosis

Basaloid cells

Dermatology at a Glance, Second Edition. Mahbub M.U. Chowdhury, Ruwani P. Katugampola, and Andrew Y. Finlay.
© 2020 John Wiley & Sons Ltd. Published 2020 by John Wiley & Sons Ltd.
Companion website: www.wiley.com/go/chowdhury/dermatology

Figure 39.6a Multiple squamous cell carcinomas (SCCs) on scalp.

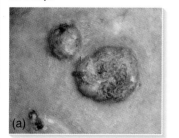

(a)

Figure 39.6b Solitary SCC on nose.

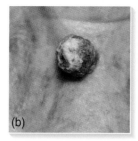

(b)

Figure 39.7 SCC histology (H&E ×10).

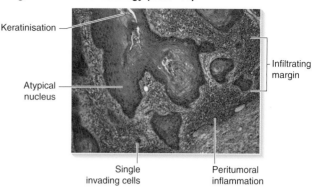

Keratinisation

Atypical nucleus

Infiltrating margin

Single invading cells

Peritumoral inflammation

Figure 39.8 SCC ready for full ellipse excision.

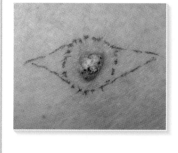

Figure 39.9 Keratoacanthoma (KA) – note central keratin plug and crater.

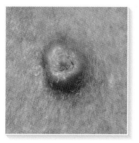

Figure 39.10 Merkel cell carcinoma (MCC).

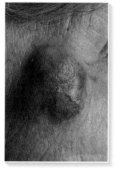

Non-melanoma skin cancers (NMSC) are increasing in number because of the larger elderly population and increased sun exposure. Over 200 000 cases (UK) were recorded in 2015 and this is likely underestimated due to poor data collection. The incidence is at least 250 new cases per 100 000 population. Organ transplant recipients on long-term immuno-suppressive therapy also have high risk for NMSCs (Table 39.1). NMSCs are less likely to metastasise than melanomas.

Basal Cell Carcinoma ('Rodent Ulcer')

Basal cell carcinoma (BCC) is also known as a 'rodent ulcer' as the surface can be damaged and ulcerated. BCC is the most common skin and human malignancy and occurs on sun exposed areas of the head and neck in the elderly. With increasing sun exposure BCCs now affect younger adults in their 30s and 40s. BCCs grow very slowly but can be locally invasive.

Nodulocystic BCC is the most common type. It usually develops on the face as a pearly, skin-coloured, cystic papule or nodule with telangiectasia and a rolled edge. It can ulcerate and there may be a history of bleeding or crusting (Figures 39.1 and 39.2). The lesion can be pigmented causing confusion with a melanoma.

Superficial BCC is the second most common type, usually appearing on the trunk as scaly, pink to red–brown patches or papules and can have a pearly border, more obvious if skin stretched (Figure 39.3). The differential diagnoses include Bowen's disease and inflammatory conditions such as psoriasis and eczema.

Morphoeic (sclerosing) BCC appears as a scar-like, waxy plaque or papule (Figure 39.4). The edges are not well defined, with tumour extension beyond the observed clinical margins. These usually occur on the face and can have ulceration, bleeding, and crusting.

Figure 39.11 Non-melanoma skin cancer common sites.

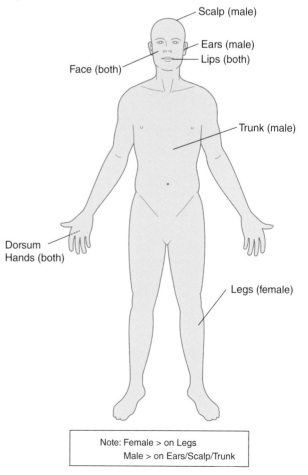

Scalp (male)

Ears (male)

Lips (both)

Face (both)

Trunk (male)

Dorsum Hands (both)

Legs (female)

Note: Female > on Legs
Male > on Ears/Scalp/Trunk

Histology

The histology shows neoplastic basaloid cells occurring in nests that are organised as islands of tumour cells more dense at the periphery (palisading) with a dermal inflammatory infiltrate (Figure 39.5).

Diagnosis

Clinical diagnosis is sufficient for most BCCs; however, if there is clinical doubt a biopsy is required. Superficial shave biopsy is the best diagnostic procedure for this epidermal lesion as punch biopsies risk introducing the tumour deeper into the dermis.

Treatment and Management

• The age, symptoms, patient's general health, risk of the site, and prognostic indicators (Table 39.2) of the tumour need to be assessed before deciding type of treatment.
• Surgical excision is the most appropriate treatment for most BCCs. Larger lesions may require full thickness skin graft or flap repair depending on the site (e.g. face). Mohs' micrographic surgery is indicated in morphoeic BCCs for tumours with ill-defined margins especially if there are recurrent tumours at critical sites (e.g. eyelid or nose) (Chapter 10). BCCs do not always require treatment, especially in the very elderly. Curettage and cautery can be used for tumours located at low risk sites (e.g. trunk and limbs).
• Radiotherapy is useful for large tumours and elderly patients but the skin becomes atrophic and telangiectatic.
• Other treatments include cryotherapy for superficial BCCs (if multiple on the trunk), photodynamic therapy, topical 5-fluorouracil (Efudix®), and imiquimod 5% cream.
• Vismodegib is a tumour growth inhibitor acting on the smoothened (SMO) receptor in the Hedgehog signalling pathway and used in advanced BCCs which are inoperable or where radiotherapy is not possible.

Prognosis

BCCs very rarely metastasise. Sun exposure is the major risk factor and sun protection is essential. There is a risk of recurrence if inadequately treated initially. A second BCC occurs in 20% of patients. Vigilance and early consultation regarding any new lesion is essential.

Squamous Cell Carcinoma

Squamous cell carcinoma (SCC) is the second commonest skin cancer arising from epidermal keratinocytes or appendages. SCCs can be locally invasive and can metastasise. Risk factors include long-term sun exposure, being elderly, having fair skin, and organ transplant recipients (Table 39.1). SCCs occur on the ear, lip, hands, and scalp, as indurated, crusted, or nodular and ulcerated lesions (Figure 39.6). Tumours can arise de novo or within a previous solar keratosis or Bowen's disease.

Histology

Irregular nests of epidermal cells with normal and atypical dysplastic squamous cells are seen. SCCs can be classified as poorly, moderately, or well differentiated tumours (Figure 39.7).

Treatment and Management

• Management needs multi-disciplinary team input by dermatologists, plastic surgeons, and radiotherapists. Full removal with histological confirmation of the primary tumour and any metastasis is needed. The type of SCC, location, and risk of the site involved determine the overall treatment.
• Treatment of choice is surgical with either 3–5 mm margin excision (majority) or up to 1 cm excision margin (larger lesions) (Figure 39.8).

• Small, low risk lesions can be treated with curettage and cautery but radiotherapy and cryotherapy may also be used. Mohs' surgery may be required for ill-defined and high risk lesions (Table 39.1), with radiotherapy after surgery for high risk SCC.
• Regular follow-up is necessary for three to five years after high risk SCC excisions to detect any recurrence at the original site or draining lymph nodes.

Prognosis

Primary cutaneous SCC has a good prognosis. Poorly differentiated tumours are more likely to metastasise. Large size and high risk site (e.g. lip and ear) worsens prognosis.

There is a 30% risk of having a second primary SCC within five years and immunosuppressed patients following organ transplants are more likely to develop multiple and more aggressive tumours. Patients with regional lymphadenopathy have < 20% 10-year survival and those with distant metastases < 10% 10-year survival.

Sun exposure needs to be prevented with sunscreens and protective clothing.

Keratoacanthoma

Keratoacanthoma (KA) is an epithelial tumour of hair follicle similar clinically to SCC. However, KAs grow rapidly over a few weeks and then spontaneously involute or self-heal leaving an ugly 'moon crater' scar. A single nodule with central crater and keratin plug occurs on hair-bearing sun-exposed sites in the elderly (Figure 39.9). Full excision or incisional biopsy is required to exclude invasive SCC. Histology shows well-differentiated squamous epithelium with some cell irregularity with keratin formation centrally. Treatment is usually surgical excision but also curettage and cautery, radiotherapy, and cryotherapy are used.

Merkel Cell Carcinoma

Merkel cell carcinomas (MCC) are believed to arise from Merkel cells (pressure receptors) but recent evidence suggests possible derivation from B lymphocytes in the skin. Polyomavirus has been detected in 80% of MCCs and potentially causes gene mutations in sun-exposed sites, especially if associated immunosuppression. MCCs are relatively rare with incidence of 0.23 per 100 000 population, however, increasing numbers are being diagnosed.

MCCs present as rapidly enlarging, single, red nodules similar in appearance to BCCs but with more rapid growth (Figure 39.10). They can spread as local or distant metastases. Most cases present in men > 50 years of age and on sun-exposed sites, e.g. head and neck, and more commonly in immunosuppressed patients, e.g. HIV, organ transplant recipients, and with drugs such as ciclosporin and azathioprine. Five year survival is around 50% and early aggressive treatment with wide margin surgery and radiotherapy is needed.

Key Points
• NMSC incidence is increasing as a result of the increasing elderly population.
• BCC prognosis is excellent, with metastasis very rare.
• SCC prognosis is variable, depending on the histological differentiation, size and body site affected.

▶ Warnings
• High risk BCCs and SCCs need to be treated urgently.
• Mohs' surgery may be required to ensure complete removal.
• Beware rarer, more aggressive tumours such as MCC presenting clinically as BCCs.

40 Malignant Melanoma

Table 40.1 Malignant Melanoma (MM) diagnostic checklists.

The American A, B, C, D system is:	The Glasgow seven point checklist consists of:

A = Asymmetry
B = Border irregularity
C = Colour variation
D = Diameter > 6 mm
	• **Major features:**
	  – change in size
	  – change in shape
	  – change in colour
	• **Minor features:**
	  – diameter 6 mm or more
	  – inflammation
	  – oozing or bleeding
	  – mild itch or altered sensation
	Note: lesions with any major feature or three minor features are suspicious of melanoma

Table 40.2 Key features of MM on dermoscopy (Figure 40.2 and Chapter 11).

• Asymmetry
• Number of colours
• Structure of the pigment
• Abruptness of the border

Table 40.3 Main types of primary melanoma.

• Superficial spreading melanoma (80%) (Figure 40.6)
• Nodular melanoma (10%) (Figure 40.7)
• Lentigo maligna melanoma (5%)
• Acral lentiginous melanoma (5%) (Figure 40.8)

Figure 40.1 Note moles larger and darker than others.

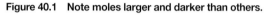

Figure 40.2 Dermatoscope features of MM (Table 40.2).

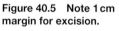

Variable colours — Atypical pigment network — Abruptness of border

Figure 40.3 Breslow thickness determines prognosis by measuring depth from the epidermal granular layer to the deepest melanoma cells.

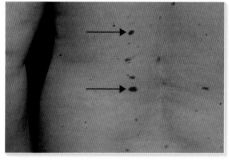

Epidermis — Granular layer
Junction — **Breslow thickness** determines prognosis by measuring depth from the epidermal granular layer to the deepest melanoma cells
Dermis — Melanoma cells

Figure 40.5 Note 1 cm margin for excision.

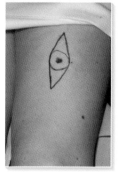

Figure 40.6 Superficial spreading MM – note asymmetry of lesion.

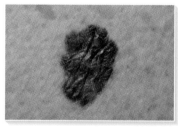

Figure 40.8 Acral MM – note pigment in proximal nail fold.

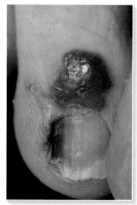

Figure 40.4 MM pathology (H&E ×40).

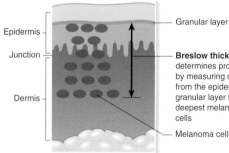

Pagetoid (upward) spread — Mitosis
Melanin pigment — Melanocytes with nuclear atypia

Figure 40.7 Nodular MM – note multiple colours and raised palpable areas.

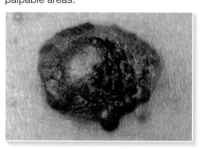

Dermatology at a Glance, Second Edition. Mahbub M.U. Chowdhury, Ruwani P. Katugampola, and Andrew Y. Finlay.
© 2020 John Wiley & Sons Ltd. Published 2020 by John Wiley & Sons Ltd.
Companion website: www.wiley.com/go/chowdhury/dermatology

Malignant melanoma (MM) arises from epidermal melanocytes. These tumours may arise within long-standing or new pigmented lesions. Melanoma occurs at any age in adults and can be unpredictable, with metastasis and death in a significant proportion of patients. Noticing an irregular pigmented lesion is key to early recognition and excision of a melanoma leading to the best opportunity for curative treatment.

Epidemiology

The incidence of melanoma in the UK has quadrupled over the last 40 years and is now around 25 cases per 100 000 population. Incidence rates are predicted to rise by 7% from 2014 to 2035. In 2015, 15 900 new MM cases were diagnosed in the UK with 30% of cases presenting <50 years of age. Melanoma in childhood is extremely rare. Melanoma is the fifth most common cancer in women and the sixth in men. However, it is the second most common cancer presenting in the 20–40 year age group.

Malignant melanoma causes 80% of skin cancer deaths even though <10% of skin cancers are melanoma. More than 2200 deaths were reported in 2016 in the UK, with better survival rates in women because of thinner melanomas.

Risk Factors

Risk factors for MM include exposure to sunlight (especially as a child and teenager) and UV exposure intermittently (holidays and regular sun bed use).
• Moderate risk factors: red hair, freckles, and Celtic Caucasian skin type. Risk is 10–20 times lower in non-whites.
• High risk factors: increasing numbers of melanocytic naevi >6 mm in diameter, dysplastic naevus syndrome (atypical mole syndrome), family history of melanoma, large congenital naevi, and organ transplant recipients on long-term immunosuppression.

Melanoma risk has been linked with major genes including *CDKN2A* gene (chromosome 9), *CDK4* gene (chromosome 12), and melanoma susceptibility gene (chromosome 1).

Diagnosis

Melanoma may arise in new moles, existing melanocytic naevi, or congenital melanocytic naevi. There are a number of simple systems to aid clinical diagnosis of MM by naked eye inspection. The most common systems used are the American A, B, C, D rules and the Glasgow seven point checklist (Table 40.1).

The 'ugly duckling' sign is useful to remember. Any mole that stands out as being irregular compared with other moles present should always be treated with a high degree of suspicion (Figure 40.1).

Clinical examination is aided by a dermatoscope (Chapter 11) which allows closer examination of the surface of pigmented lesions with magnification and oil–glass interface or polarised light to reduce reflection on the surface. A score given can be correlated with the likelihood of malignancy depending on key features seen (Table 40.2; Figure 40.2).

Any suspected MM lesion should be removed fully with primary excision with a 2 mm margin of skin followed by wide local excision, which reduces local recurrence. The local excision margins are determined by the Breslow thickness measuring the histological thickness of the tumour (Figure 40.3). For example, if the Breslow thickness is up to 1 mm then a 1 cm margin is taken. If it is more than 1 mm a 2 cm margin is taken.

An incisional biopsy may occasionally be warranted if a large lentigo maligna on the face or acral melanoma needs to be diagnosed. Shave and punch biopsies should not be used in case they spread the cancer.

Pathology

The essential diagnostic pathological feature of melanoma is the presence of cytologically malignant melanocytes invading the dermis (Figure 40.4). The most common type is the superficial spreading malignant melanoma (SSMM) (Table 40.3).

Additional microscopic features include presence of ulceration, lack of maturation of dermal melanocytic cells, presence of lymphocytic infiltrate, and atypical mitoses with angiogenesis at the base of the lesion.

The Breslow thickness measures the distance of the deepest invasive area of the primary tumour (in millimetres) from the epidermal granular layer. Lesions <1 mm thick are considered lower risk and >4 mm are higher risk. The Clark level, measured on a 1–5 scale, describes the level of anatomical invasion with higher numbers indicating a deeper melanoma. Five-year survival falls with increased thickness of the tumour.

Management

Clinical diagnosis needs to be confirmed with histology and then definitive surgical excision with adequate clear margins (Figure 40.5). Dermatologists follow the 2018 American Joint Committee on Cancer (AJCC) staging system for melanomas. Generally dermatologists tend to manage MM where there is no lymph node or distant metastases involved with multidisciplinary team discussions to guide correct management.

Patients with intermediate, high risk, or recurrent disease can have staging investigations including chest X-ray, liver ultrasound, and CT scan of chest, abdomen, and pelvis. Sentinel node biopsy is recommended by NICE as a staging investigation and is offered for prognostic staging of thicker melanomas but does not have proven benefit in improving clinical outcomes. Lymph node examination and appropriate treatment of draining lymph nodes are essential. Nodal disease and distant metastases may need palliative care.

Ipilimumab, a human anti-CTLA4 monoclonal antibody, has been shown to increase survival in patients with advanced melanoma (Table 14.3, Chapter 14). Targeted therapy with drugs such as vemurafenib may be used for melanomas with BRAF gene mutations which occurs in 50% of melanomas. This treatment inhibits the mutated BRAF protein which usually helps melanomas grow and hence prevents further melanoma growth.

Other treatments include nivolumab (anti-PD1 receptor protein), trametinib (MEK protein inhibitor), and imatinib (c-KIT protein inhibitor). These all act on mutations to proteins in the mitogen activated protein kinase (MAPK) pathway including BRAF, MEK, and c-KIT mutations. Patients should be taught self-examination as early detection of recurrence is important.

Patients with invasive MM should be followed up three monthly for three years and discharged if < 1 mm thickness. Thicker lesions >1 mm should be followed up for a further two years at six-monthly intervals.

Prognosis

• For MMs of Breslow thickness <1 mm the five-year survival is 95–100%.
• For 1–2 mm thick melanomas, five-year survival is 80–96% and for lesions >4 mm thickness this drops to 50%.

Key Points
• MM incidence is increasing.
• MM causes 80% of skin cancer deaths.
• MM with Breslow thickness <1 mm has a better prognosis.
• Always fully surgically excise any suspected melanoma.

▶ Warning
• Beware 'ugly duckling' sign to detect any irregular moles needing removal.
• Do not shave biopsy a mole if any possibility it may be a MM, always excise.

41 Other Malignant Skin Conditions

Figure 41.1a
Plaque and nodular stage cutaneous T cell lymphoma (CTCL) on trunk.

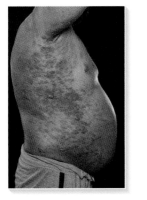

Figure 41.1b   Note atrophy and scaling.

Figure 41.1c and d
Multiple nodules on legs, with closeup.

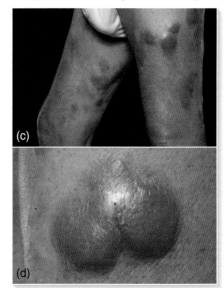
(c)

(d)

Figure 41.1e   Large ulcerating plaque.

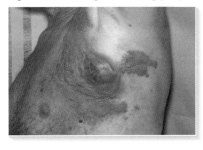

Figure 41.3a, b and c
Kaposi's sarcoma (KS) on feet with closeup.

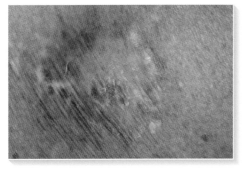
(a)

Figure 41.4a and b
Metastases from malignant melanoma.

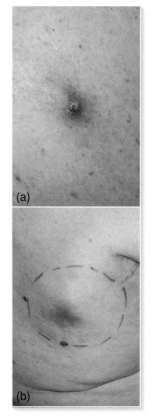
(a)

(b)

Figure 41.2a   Perianal Paget's disease.

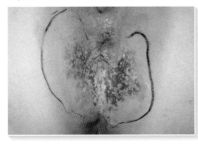

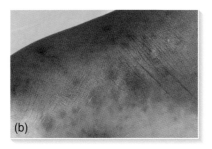
(b)

Figure 41.2b   Scrotal Paget's disease.

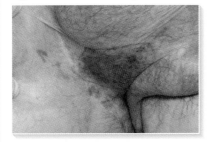

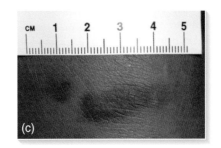
(c)

Dermatology at a Glance, Second Edition. Mahbub M.U. Chowdhury, Ruwani P. Katugampola, and Andrew Y. Finlay.
© 2020 John Wiley & Sons Ltd. Published 2020 by John Wiley & Sons Ltd.
Companion website: www.wiley.com/go/chowdhury/dermatology

Cutaneous T Cell Lymphoma (Mycosis Fungoides)

Mycosis fungoides is the most common variant of primary cutaneous T cell lymphoma (CTCL), a T helper cell lymphoma of the skin. The cause is unknown. It has a male:female ratio of 2:1, with most patients diagnosed in their 50s and 60s.

CTCL can develop from patch stage to limited or extensive plaque stage and then tumour or nodular stage (Figure 41.1). The term parapsoriasis is used to describe a very early pre-diagnostic phase of CTCL. Multiple biopsies may be required over many years prior to definitive diagnosis.

Presentation – patients can present with ill-defined, red to pink, scaly patches with atrophy and telangiectasia. The plaque stage consists of red to brown elevated patches and plaques in the bathing trunk area affecting the buttocks, hip, and upper thighs. Nodules that can ulcerate develop in the tumour stage. The majority of patients have an indolent, slowly evolving disease but any form of CTCL may eventually invade the lymph nodes, peripheral blood, and internal organs with a poor prognosis.

Sézary syndrome is a leukaemic form that can evolve from classic CTCL or develop with erythroderma (generalised scaling and exfoliative dermatitis). Pruritus and lymph node enlargement are common in Sézary syndrome.

Investigations – include physical examination for lymph nodes and hepatosplenomegaly with a peripheral blood smear examination for Sézary cells. T cell receptor gene rearrangement (polymerase chain reaction and/or molecular studies) can be useful to identify monoclonal proliferation of T cell clones in the skin. Renal and liver function, biopsy of enlarged lymph nodes, chest X-ray, CT scan, and bone marrow biopsy may be required.

Histology – typically shows superficial and deep, band-like, perivascular, lymphocytic infiltrate with collections of lymphocytes (Pautrier's micro-abscesses) with thickened epidermis. The infiltrate is mixed with lymphocytes, eosinophils, and plasma cells. Lymphocytes can be atypical with a hyper-convoluted or cerebriform nucleus (Sézary cells).

Differential diagnoses of CTCL include dermatitis, psoriasis, and drug eruption especially in the erythrodermic form. The extent of the body surface area involved is important to document for monitoring any potential progression. In Sézary syndrome >5% of the total lymphocytes are CD4$^+$ Sézary T cells.

Prognosis generally for the patch and plaque stage is good; however, more aggressive disease with spread to lymph nodes and organs, and also Sézary syndrome, have a poor prognosis.

Treatment options – For early stages treatment includes emollients, potent topical corticosteroids, and phototherapy (UVB, topical PUVA). Treatments for later stage disease include topical nitrogen mustard and oral bexarotene (a retinoid). Radiotherapy can be used for localised plaques or tumours. Sézary syndrome may warrant extracorporeal photopheresis. Treatments also include methotrexate, oral prednisolone, and cyclophosphamide; however, chemotherapy is less effective.

Paget's Disease

Paget's disease affecting the breast is a rare intraductal carcinoma presenting in the skin as a well-defined scaly patch or plaque which is eczematous around the nipple areola. This is often unilateral and can be confused with nipple eczema. Biopsy is essential. Extra-mammary Paget's disease is an intraepidermal adenocarcinoma occurring in women >40 years in the vulval area and perineum and in men in the scrotum, penis, anal, and perianal skin (Figure 41.2). This usually develops as a grey, sharply demarcated plaque and may appear eczematous and thickened. Treatment includes local excision and radiotherapy may be needed for recurrences.

Kaposi's Sarcoma

This is a malignancy of lymphatic and epithelial cells caused by human herpes virus 8 (HHV8). There are classic, endemic, transplant, or HIV-associated types.
- Classic Kaposi's sarcoma (KS) is slowly progressive, occurring in 50- to 70-year-olds in the Mediterranean and Eastern Europe (Ashkenazi Jews).
- Endemic forms occur in Africa affecting children and young adults and can be more aggressive affecting the lower limbs.
- KS can occur in immunosuppressed patients, particularly in organ transplant recipients.
- AIDS-related KS affects the trunk, arms, head, and neck and can be more aggressive involving mucosal surfaces. This has now reduced in incidence because of effective HIV treatment.

KS typically presents with small patches on the distal lower extremities which progress proximally (Figure 41.3). Lesions can become thickened and darker and the lower legs can become swollen and ulcerate. Fever, night sweats, and weight loss can occur.

Skin biopsy shows neoplastic spindle cells with clefting and vascular channels. Differential diagnoses include malignant melanoma, pyogenic granuloma, CTCL, or stasis eczema.

Treatment varies with the type of KS. Bigger lesions can be excised surgically. Multiple lesions require radiotherapy with chemotherapy. Immunosuppression-associated KS can improve with reduction in immunosuppression. HIV-associated KS can benefit from radiation, cryosurgery, intralesional vincristine, and topical imiquimod.

Cutaneous Metastases

Metastases present as firm, painless, subcutaneous nodules which can be indistinct. These are uncommon except in terminal malignancy and can be overlooked as a sign of underlying malignancy. Skin biopsy confirms malignant cells of primary tumour origin and specific immunohistochemistry may be required for the final diagnosis. Prognosis is determined by the tumour type, extent of the disease, and treatment options available. The most common causes are breast cancer, gastro-intestinal cancer, melanoma (Figure 41.4) and tumours affecting the lung, kidney, and ovary.

Key Points
- Early CTCL is difficult to diagnose and may require multiple biopsies over many years.
- KS may be an initial sign of HIV or AIDS-related disease.
- Cutaneous metastases are rare but indicate a poor prognosis. The three most common causes are breast cancer, gastro-intestinal cancer, and melanoma.

▶ **Warnings**
- New nodules arising in previous patch stage CTCL suggest transformation to a more severe stage.
- Erythroderma with no previous skin disease should ring alarm bells. Perform a skin biopsy to exclude CTCL.

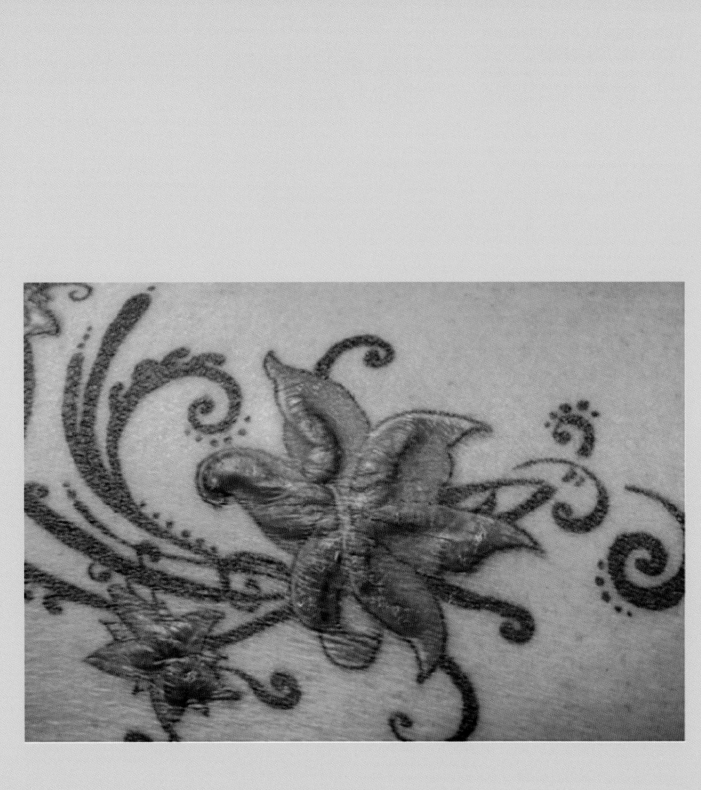

Photodermatology

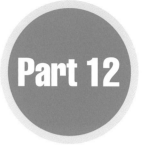

Part 12

Chapters

42 **Pigmentation**

Table 42.1 Tanning.

Protective mechanism against UV damage:

Three phases

1. **Immmediate pigment darkening** – first few minutes after UV exposure, release of preformed melanin from melanocytes, rapidly fades. Induced by UVA
2. **Persistent pigment darkening** – lasts up to 24 hours. Induced by greater exposure to UVA
3. **Delayed tanning** – increased production of melanin first becomes visible after two to three days, lasts up to two weeks. Induced by UVB and UVA

Table 42.2 Tattoos (Figure 42.1).

Common phenomenon from early human history in all cultures, with strong cultural, social, religious, and identity reasons for tattooing. May be accidental e.g. cycle accidents, grit from road

- **Risks of tattooing include** – systemic infection (e.g. hepatitis from amateur tattooing), local infection (e.g. mycobacterium chelonae), hypertrophic scarring or keloids, lichenoid reactions to red pigment, Koebner's phenomenon at site e.g. in psoriasis
- **Treatment** – people change their minds about a tattoo, especially if a person is named or if a visible tattoo later reduces job opportunities. Localised excision is possible for small lesions. Laser therapy is most effective, though the skin does not become totally normal

Table 42.3 Drugs causing pigmentation.

- Amiodarone – grey–blue changes in sun-exposed areas
- Minocycline – dark pigmentation of acne scars or diffuse pigmentation in sun-exposed sites (Figure 42.9)
- Mepacrine – yellow
- Clofazimine – initially red, later blue–brown
- Localised hyperpigmentation in fixed drug eruptions, e.g. co-trimoxazole, naproxen, tetracycline

Figure 42.1 Tattoo with reaction to red pigment.

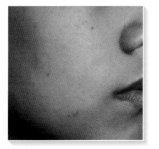

Figure 42.2 Post-inflammatory hypo- and hyper-pigmentation from frequent rubbing.

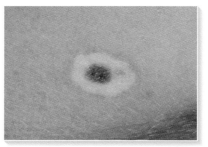

Figure 42.3 Vitiligo of upper eyelid in child.

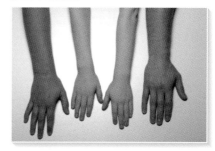

Figure 42.4 Cheek with ill-defined pale areas of pityriasis alba.

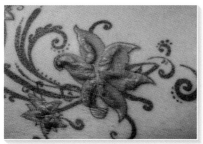

Figure 42.5 Halo naevus – hypopigmentation around a mole.

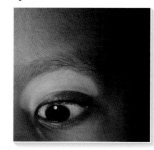

Figure 42.6 Arms of child with oculo-cutaneous albinism between unaffected arms of adults.

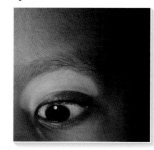

Figure 42.7 Melasma affecting forehead of woman.

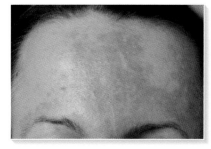

Figure 42.8 Naevus of Ota – pigmentation involving sclera and around eye.

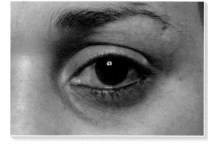

Figure 42.9 Minocycline pigmentation of forehead.

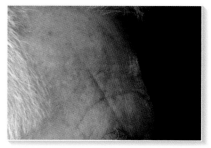

Dermatology at a Glance, Second Edition. Mahbub M.U. Chowdhury, Ruwani P. Katugampola, and Andrew Y. Finlay.
© 2020 John Wiley & Sons Ltd. Published 2020 by John Wiley & Sons Ltd.
Companion website: www.wiley.com/go/chowdhury/dermatology

The visual impact of changes in pigmentation depends on the racial skin type. Vitiligo is more noticeable in people with dark skin and this is complicated by the cultural context: confusion with leprosy gives an extra stigma in some cultures, making it difficult for a woman with vitiligo to marry. Post-inflammatory hyperpigmentation is more obvious in darker skin, so it is even more important to treat inflammatory conditions such as acne effectively.

Effect of Inflammation

Skin inflammation can cause increased (hyper) or decreased (hypo) pigmentation. Psoriasis plaques may leave pale areas after recovery that persist for years. Post-inflammatory hyperpigmentation can be severe if there is deep epidermal disruption (e.g. lichen planus). It follows the pattern of inflammation, which may be diagnostic (e.g. after herpes zoster). Pigmentation may follow trauma (Figure 42.2). Facial acne lesions can leave areas of increased pigmentation.

Skin Lighteners

Lightening of Skin Colour

Reasons for desiring cosmetic skin lightening include cultural attitudes, a view that whiter skin is more attractive, and powerful influences from advertising by cosmetic companies. Medical indications for skin lightening include localised post-inflammatory pigmentation, treatment of solar lentigines, and very widespread vitiligo if the normal darker skin appears abnormal. Reasons not to lighten skin colour include: natural skin colour is normal and attempts at lightening may not produce cosmetic benefit and may result in unnatural pigment variation.

How to Lighten Skin

Topical hydroquinone can be used alone, but it can be irritant and can cause irregular depigmentation. Hydroquinone is banned from cosmetics in Europe. Hydroquinone may be combined with topical tretinoin and/or topical steroids. Azelaic acid may be used. This chemical is produced by *Malassezia furfur* and causes the pigmentary changes in pityriasis versicolor.

Too Little Pigment

Vitiligo

Vitiligo affects 0.4% of the population (Figure 42.3). Flat symmetrical areas of depigmentation develop and enlarge. It is possibly caused by an autoimmune attack on melanocytes: they are absent from affected skin. It causes major psychological/social problems in some cultures or people with dark skin. Vitiligo is associated with pernicious anaemia, thyroid disease, and diabetes.

For treatment narrow-band UVB is more effective than PUVA: other therapies include potent topical steroids or melanocyte transplant from the same person. Melanocytes in hair follicles can multiply and repopulate surrounding skin. However, patchy partial repigmentation may not be of perceived benefit to the patient. Photoprotection and cosmetic camouflage advice should be given.

Pityriasis Alba

Areas of partial depigmentation and fine scaling develop (Figure 42.4) following mild inflammation, typically atopic eczema, on a child's face or limbs. Pityriasis means 'very small bran-like scales' and alba means 'white'. If any eczema persists, treat with topical steroids: normal pigmentation slowly returns.

Halo Naevus

This is a white, flat, circular area around a benign mole, usually in children or teenagers (Figure 42.5). The mole may self-destruct in the autoimmune process that destroyed the surrounding melanocytes. Common and benign in children, so no treatment needed. It is rare in adults, suggesting malignancy: consider biopsy.

Oculocutaneous Albinism

This is an autosomal recessive condition with absence or poor function of tyrosinase enzyme, essential for melanin production. Features include white skin (Figure 42.6), no retinal pigment, photophobia, nystagmus, and squinting. In the most severe type (tyrosinase negative) there is white hair, pink skin, and red eye reflex. If tyrosinase positive there is some pigment. Photoprotection is essential. Squamous cell carcinomas are frequent in tropical areas. In 'ocular albinism' the skin is normal. In some areas of Africa, ignorance and cultural influences lead to albinos becoming social outcasts and poor photoprotection leads to early death from skin cancer.

Piebaldism

This is a rare autosomal dominant condition with white skin patches on the chest, abdomen, and limbs and white hair at the front of the scalp (white forelock). Photoprotection is required.

Too Much Pigment

Melasma (also called Chloasma)

Patchy increased pigmentation, often symmetrical, is seen on the face, especially the forehead (Figure 42.7), cheeks, above the lips, and chin. It mostly occurs in women during pregnancy or on the oral contraceptive pill and gradually fades. Treatment includes sun protection and skin lighteners, such as azelaic acid or the triple combination of hydroquinone, tretinoin, and fluocinolone acetonide. Oral tranexamic acid for three months may be helpful.

Incontinentia Pigmenti

This is an X-linked dominant condition, fatal in males so only seen in females. In infancy recurrent small blisters and papules on trunk and limbs are seen. Blisters settle then hyperkeratotic lesions occur. Later whorled pigmentation persists with atrophic streaks. There may be defects of teeth, eyes, and central nervous system.

Naevus of Ota and Naevus of Ito

- **Ota** – brown–blue hyperpigmentation one side of the face in trigeminal nerve distribution. There is hyperpigmentation of the sclera of the eye (Figure 42.8).
- **Ito** – hyperpigmentation over the shoulder, in posterior supraclavicular and lateral brachial cutaneous nerve distribution.

How not to mix up Ota and Ito: 'A in otA and in fAce, but I not in the eye'.

Argyria

Caused by chronic ingestion of silver, or absorption via lungs or mucosal surfaces, seen in silver mining, and manufacturing. Skin appears blue–grey, especially sun-exposed areas. There is no treatment but the silver is non-toxic.

Key Points
- Skin pigmentation is often altered by skin disease.
- Attempts to alter pigmentation may make matters worse, so first allow natural recovery.

► Warning
- It is essential to ensure good photoprotection in albinism and vitiligo, to try to reduce the risk of skin cancer.

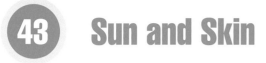

43 Sun and Skin

Table 43.1 **Clinical signs of photoageing.**

- Deep or fine wrinkling
- Coarsening of skin with yellow discolouration
- Skin fragility, scarring
- Deep wrinkles lateral to eye and mouth
- Erythema, pigment changes
- Telangiectasia, atrophy
- Comedones, milia

Table 43.2 **Sun protective measures.**

- Physical and chemical sunscreens
- Clothing
- Hats and sunglasses
- Window protection, e.g. car windows and home windows, glass stops UVB, not UVA
- Stay indoors between 11 a.m.–3 p.m.
- Umbrellas and parasols

Figure 43.1a   Note irregular pigmentation, scaly solar keratoses.

Figure 43.1b   Deep wrinkling.

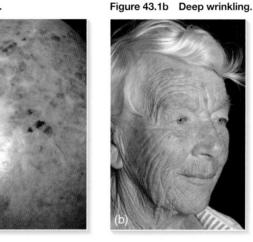

Figure 43.3a and b   Common sunscreens used with ingredients listed.

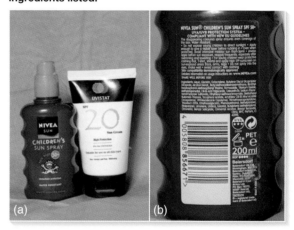

Figure 43.1c   Photoageing comedones.

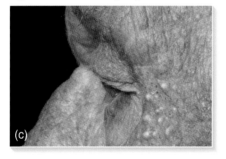

Figure 43.4   Severe sun sensitivity requiring full body cover-up with hat, scarf, and gloves.

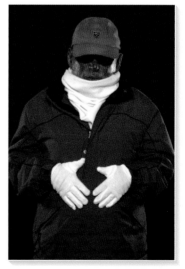

Figure 43.2   Note areas of normal skin tanning with vitiligo spared.

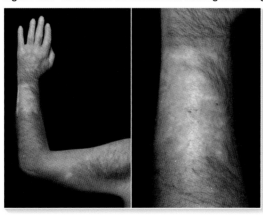

Dermatology at a Glance, Second Edition. Mahbub M.U. Chowdhury, Ruwani P. Katugampola, and Andrew Y. Finlay.
© 2020 John Wiley & Sons Ltd. Published 2020 by John Wiley & Sons Ltd.
Companion website: www.wiley.com/go/chowdhury/dermatology

The sun has many effects on the skin including sunburn, photoageing, and tanning. The various responses to sun exposure depend on skin type and the ultraviolet light wavelength (Chapters 44 and 45). The understanding of normal skin response to ultraviolet light is essential if abnormal responses are to be recognised. Fitzpatrick skin phototyping is most commonly used, from skin type I to skin type VI, based on assessing burning and tanning (Chapter 44, Table 44.1).

Sunburn Reaction

The acute skin response to ultraviolet B (UVB) exposure is termed sunburn reaction and this is an acute inflammatory response.

Sunburn presents with painful erythema on the sites of skin exposure to excess UVB. Onset of sunburn can be delayed for four to six hours after sun exposure and can peak at 16–24 hours. It typically fades over two to three days and can be followed by severe peeling of the skin and tanning.

Sunburn is mediated by an acute inflammatory response that causes damage of the epidermal cells via cytokines and upregulation of inflammatory adhesion molecule expression.

Photoageing

Photoageing or chronic sun damage is brought about by a gradual change in the skin structure and function following long-term, recurrent exposure to sunlight or artificial ultraviolet radiation (UVR) sources. This is due to cumulative DNA damage from recurrent acute DNA injury and from the effects of chronic inflammation. Background intrinsic genetic ageing changes can also occur. The epidermis and dermis are affected mainly by UVB but the dermis is also affected significantly by UVA which can penetrate more deeply.

Clinical signs include fine and deep wrinkling, coarseness, dryness, telangiectasia with pigmentation, increased laxity with loss of skin elasticity and comedones (Table 43.1; Figure 43.1).

Skin types I and II are at greatest risk and photoageing signs may be apparent by the age of 40 years. The distribution is usually the face, neck, and dorsum of the hands. Photodamage can progress even with attempted sun avoidance. It may also present with solar keratoses or skin cancer (Chapters 38 and 39).

Treatment consists of topical retinoids such as tretinoin, alpha hydroxy acid, or tazarotene. Skin peels (e.g. trichloroacetic acid) or phenol and laser resurfacing may be used. The commercial product Boots No. 7 Protect and Perfect® reduces photoageing wrinkles in 20% of subjects after six months.

Tanning

Tanning ability varies with skin phototype: skin type I never tans and skin type IV always tans (Figure 43.2). Tanning can be immediate or delayed and can occur within seconds of exposure to UVA (Table 42.1). Immediate tanning results from photo-oxidative darkening and injury to epidermal melanocytic melanin. Delayed tanning of irradiated skin can persist for weeks to months and can appear over hours to days after exposure to all wavelengths of UVR. There is an increase in melanocyte size mediated by tyrosinase activation and UVR-induced melanocytic DNA damage. This leads to new melanin production. Tanning also varies with differences in UV exposure at different latitudes and heights.

Vitamin D Synthesis and Deficiency

UVB radiation can convert epidermal 7-hydrocholesterol into previtamin D3 which can then be isomerised to vitamin D3 and released into the circulation. Hence, sun exposure is an important step in the manufacture of vitamin D.

Current UK data suggests suboptimal vitamin D levels commonly occur in both adults and children due to limited sun exposure. Sun exposure for 15 minutes two to three times per week should ensure adequate vitamin D levels in fair-skinned individuals. In addition, supplementation recommendations include oral vitamin D at 400 International Units (IU) or 10 micrograms/day.

This may be especially relevant for melanoma patients who are advised to avoid sun exposure. All melanoma patients should have vitamin D levels measured at diagnosis and then should be supplemented if low. There is some evidence linking low serum vitamin D levels and melanoma Breslow thickness at presentation and subsequent survival. Avoidance of sun exposure and subsequent low levels of vitamin D requires careful long-term balance in melanoma patients.

Sunscreens

It is essential to use sunscreens, particularly in photosensitive disorders, to protect the skin from further solar radiation causing damage (Figure 43.3). Sunscreens mainly block UVA, UVB, visible light, or a combination. Sunscreens provide additional protection in combination with other measures such as hats, umbrellas, window protection (stops UVB), and being indoors between 11 a.m. and 3 p.m. (Table 43.2; Figure 43.4).

There are many sunscreens to choose from, which can be confusing. There are physical and chemical sunscreens.
- **Physical sunscreens** are usually opaque, containing titanium dioxide or zinc oxide and reflect UV radiation (UVA, UVB, and visible light). These can look thick and messy on the skin but are more effective and so more protective against skin cancer.
- **Chemical sunscreens** absorb UV radiation, either UVA or UVB. UVB chemical sunscreens protect against UVB-induced sunburn. The sun protection factor (SPF) indicates the UVB photoprotection of the sunscreen. SPF 10 means that after application, the person needs to stay out 10 times as long to reach the same level of tan or sunburn. Usual recommendations have been to use 15–25 SPF sunscreen for most patients but recent evidence suggests SPF 30 or higher is better. Cinnamates and oxybenzone in sunscreens can cause irritation or allergic contact dermatitis. The star rating (up to 5) indicates the UVA protection levels. Broad spectrum blocking sunscreens against UVA and UVB can be used.

Sunscreens need to be used liberally, thickly enough to cover the skin and evenly on all sun-exposed skin areas including the lips, neck, and ears. They need to be reapplied every two to three hours and after activities inducing sweating or swimming. Do not use sunscreens to prolong time spent in the sun.

To detect sunscreen allergy, the specialised test of photopatch testing is required (Chapter 35).

Key Points
- Both UVA and UVB exposure can cause long-term photoageing.
- Sunscreens need to be used regularly and in sufficient amount to have protective effects.
- Sun exposure leads to vitamin D production and avoidance of sun can lead to vitamin D deficiency.

▶ Warning
- Sun exposure leads to photoageing which can be irreversible.

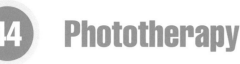

44 Phototherapy

Figure 44.1 The electromagnetic spectrum.

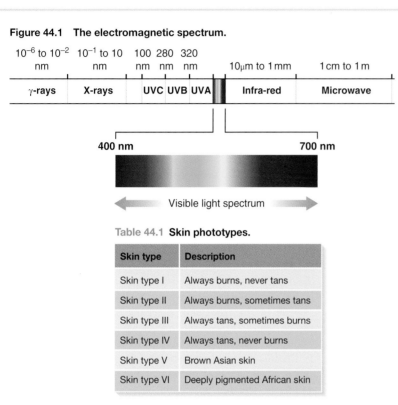

		100	280	320		
10^{-6} to 10^{-2} nm	10^{-1} to 10 nm	nm	nm	nm	10 μm to 1 mm	1 cm to 1 m
γ-rays	X-rays	UVC	UVB	UVA	Infra-red	Microwave

400 nm   700 nm

← Visible light spectrum →

Table 44.1 Skin phototypes.

Skin type	Description
Skin type I	Always burns, never tans
Skin type II	Always burns, sometimes tans
Skin type III	Always tans, sometimes burns
Skin type IV	Always tans, never burns
Skin type V	Brown Asian skin
Skin type VI	Deeply pigmented African skin

Table 44.2 Skin diseases commonly treated with ultraviolet radiation B (UVB).

- Psoriasis (especially widespread plaque psoriasis, guttate psoriasis)
- Widespread atopic eczema
- Nodular prurigo
- Lichen planus
- Cutaneous T cell lymphoma
- Chronic widespread pruritus (especially when secondary to chronic renal failure or liver failure)
- Vitiligo
- Intrahepatic cholestasis of pregnancy

Figure 44.2 UVB cabinet.

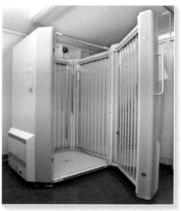

Table 44.3 Skin diseases commonly treated with PUVA photochemotherapy.

- **Systemic (oral) PUVA**
  - widespread plaque psoriasis
  - cutaneous T cell lymphoma
  - palmoplantar pustulosis
- **Bath PUVA**
  - widespread plaque psoriasis
  - vitiligo
- **Topical (gel) PUVA**
  - granuloma annulare
  - necrobiosis lipoidica

Figure 44.3 A patient receiving PUVA to their feet.
(a) The patient soaks their feet in psoralen solution diluted in water for 10 minutes and then (b) exposes the feet to UVA.

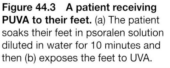

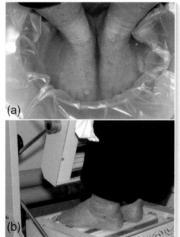

(a)

(b)

Figure 44.4 A patient receiving photodynamic therapy (PDT).

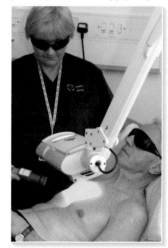

Table 44.4 Potential side effects of phototherapy.

- Short-term side effects
  - sunburn-like reaction with redness and burning sensation of the skin (Chapter 43)
  - dry skin
  - reactivation of cold sores
- Long-term side effects
  - skin ageing (Chapter 43)
  - freckles and lentigos (Chapter 38)
  - pre-malignant skin lesions such as actinic keratoses and Bowen's disease (Chapter 38)
  - non-melanoma skin cancer (Chapter 39)

Dermatology at a Glance, Second Edition. Mahbub M.U. Chowdhury, Ruwani P. Katugampola, and Andrew Y. Finlay.
© 2020 John Wiley & Sons Ltd. Published 2020 by John Wiley & Sons Ltd.
Companion website: www.wiley.com/go/chowdhury/dermatology

Some skin diseases improve following sunlight exposure. Phototherapy is the use of ultraviolet radiation A or ultraviolet radiation B (UVA 320–400 nm or UVB 280–320 nm) as a treatment (Figure 44.1).

Phototherapy: General Principles

The skin response following exposure to UVA or UVB ranges from mild erythema or burning to blistering. 'Skin types' describe the tanning and burning response of individuals to natural sunlight as well as to phototherapy (Table 44.1). During lifelong exposure to sunlight, UVA is responsible for skin ageing whereas UVB is responsible for sunburn. Prolonged exposure to natural or other UV radiation (sunbeds, repeated phototherapy) can increase the risk of pre-malignant skin lesions and non-melanoma skin cancers. Patients who have received repeated courses of phototherapy should be educated and followed up to identify potential pre-malignant and malignant skin lesions.

Treatment is commenced with a dose of UVA or UVB that causes just visible erythema on that particular individual's skin (minimal erythema dose [MED]). The dose of UVA or UVB is then gradually increased depending on the clinical response. It is important to know what other treatment patients are taking during the course of phototherapy, as some drugs can make patients more photosensitive (e.g. tetracycline, amiodarone).

Phototherapy is considered as a second-line treatment option when topical treatments have failed, when a large body surface area is affected, or where treating the individual lesions of the rash with active topical treatment is difficult as the lesions are small and widespread (e.g. guttate psoriasis).

UVB Phototherapy

This is administered within a cabinet containing tubes emitting UVB at a predetermined dose set by the operator (Figure 44.2). Narrowband UVB (311 nm) has replaced the previous use of broadband UVB phototherapy in many dermatology units.
- Skin diseases treated with UVB are listed in Table 44.2.
- Treatment is usually given three times a week up to a maximum of 20–24 treatments per course, depending on disease response. Some patients require repeated courses of UVB treatment during flare-ups of their disease (e.g. psoriasis); other conditions may require a longer course of treatment (e.g. cutaneous T cell lymphoma, vitiligo).

UVA Phototherapy

- UVA is given with psoralen, a photosensitising agent (PUVA). Skin diseases treated with PUVA are listed in Table 44.3.
- Psoralen can be given orally (in the form of 8-methoxypsoralen or 5-methoxypsoralen), or as 8-methoxypsoralen solution diluted in water for the patient to soak in for about 10 minutes (bath PUVA) or applied as a gel, prior to exposure to UVA.
- UVA is given in a phototherapy cabinet when a large body surface area is being treated, or in hand and foot PUVA units (e.g. for palmoplantar pustulosis, Figure 44.3).
- PUVA can be administered with an oral retinoid (Re-PUVA) for the treatment of plaque psoriasis and palmoplantar pustulosis.

Important Safety Issues Related to Phototherapy

Before starting phototherapy (UVA or UVB), patients are counselled regarding the treatment-related risks and side effects (Table 44.4). The long-term side effects of phototherapy are related to the lifetime cumulative dose of UV exposure in addition to factors such as skin type and photoprotective behaviour. The following safety precautions are recommended to patients during phototherapy:
- Wear UV-protective goggles within the UV cabinet to minimise the risk of cataract. Patients having systemic psoralen should continue to wear UV-protective sunglasses for up to 24 hours post-treatment.
- Protection of genital area of men with appropriate clothing.
- Protection of non-treatment areas (e.g. use of visor for face).
- Photoprotection of skin on a long-term basis (Chapter 43).
- Monitor for abnormal skin lesions by regular self-examination.

Phototherapy in Special Circumstances

- **Pregnancy and breast feeding** – UVB phototherapy is considered relatively safe in treating skin diseases during pregnancy and breast-feeding (e.g. psoriasis, widespread atopic eczema). UVB phototherapy should be considered where topical treatments alone fail to improve the skin disease and systemic treatment is contraindicated because of pregnancy or breast-feeding.
- **Children** – the age at which a child is considered suitable for phototherapy depends on their ability to comply with the safety precautions within the phototherapy cabinet.

Photodynamic Therapy

Photodynamic therapy (PDT) is a form of phototherapy that utilises high-intensity visible light as opposed to ultraviolet light. PDT is used for the treatment of pre-malignant skin lesions (solar keratoses, Bowen's disease) and superficial basal cell carcinomas.

During PDT, methyl aminolevulinate cream, a photosensitiser, is applied to the lesion being treated and kept under occlusion for three hours. Selective uptake of the porphyrin precursor in this cream by the abnormal cells localises the treatment to the target area. After three hours, the cream is wiped away and the lesion(s) exposed to visible red light (570–670 nm) (Figure 44.4). This wavelength corresponds to the absorption peak of protoporphyrin IX, resulting in formation of highly reactive oxygen singlet species leading to localised destruction of the abnormal cells.

Daylight PDT is an alternative form of PDT where natural daylight is used instead of the artificial red light mentioned above. During daylight PDT, total sun block is applied to the treatment area including the pre-malignant lesion. Methyl aminolevulinate cream is then applied to the lesion being treated and kept under occlusion. After 30 minutes, the cream is wiped away and the lesion exposed to natural daylight for two hours, which can be in the patient's own home, making this treatment more patient-friendly.

The common side effects of PDT include pain during treatment and localised swelling, erythema, scabbing, and, rarely, ulceration of the treatment area post-treatment.

Key Point
- UVA or UVB phototherapy is a suitable second-line treatment option for certain skin diseases where topical treatment has failed or when the disease affects a large body surface area.

► Warning
- Long-term risk of repeated phototherapy includes the risk of skin cancers. Patients receiving phototherapy should be counselled about this risk and educated to self-examine their skin to identify suspicious skin lesions.

Photodermatoses

Table 45.1 Classification of photodermatoses.

	Immediate photosensitivity (trigger: visible light)	Delayed photosensitivity (trigger: visible light and/or UV)
Idiopathic photodermatoses	• Solar urticaria	• Polymorphic light eruption (PLE) • Chronic actinic dermatitis (CAD) • Actinic prurigo (AP)
Inherited	• Erythropoietic protoporphyria (EPP)	• Congenital erythropoietic porphyria (CEP) • Xeroderma pigmentosa (XP) • Porphyria cutanea tarda (PCT)
Secondary causes		• Plants (phytophotodermatitis, Figure 45.1), e.g. contact with psoralen containing plants: rue, giant hogweed, celery • Drugs, e.g. tetracyclines, amiodarone, thiazide diuretics • Metabolic, e.g. PCT secondary to haemochromatosis or alcoholic liver disease

Table 45.2 Approach to a patient with a suspected photodermatosis.

Clinical history
- Age of onset
- Seasonal variation in rash (worse in spring/summer, improves in autumn/winter)
- Time interval between sunlight exposure and onset of symptoms and signs of skin disease
- Symptoms, e.g. skin burning/pain (EPP), itching (solar urticaria, PLE)
- Signs, e.g. no signs (EPP), urticaria (solar urticaria), papules and plaques (PLE), blisters (CEP, PCT)
- Family history, e.g. XP, porphyrias
- Impact on daily activities and quality of life, e.g. restricted indoors, unable to do outdoor work and leisure activities
- Photo-protection measures
- Drug history, contact with plants, alcohol intake

Clinical examination
- Distribution of the rash: photodermatoses generally affect skin on exposed sites and spare covered sites
- Skin manifestations: e.g. scars and milia (EPP), blisters, photomutilation, hypertrichosis (PCT and CEP), marked freckling (XP)
- Morphology of lesions: e.g. phytophotodermatitis presents with linear erythema/blisters at the site of contact between the plant and skin (Figure 45.1)
- Nails: photo-onycholysis (lifting of nail plate due to subungual blisters) noted mostly on fingernails
- Scalp: scarring alopecia due to recurrent blistering, e.g. CEP

Investigations
- Serum autoantibodies: antinuclear antibodies, extractable nuclear antigens, Ro and La antibodies, anti-double-stranded DNA antibodies
- Urine, blood, and faecal samples for porphyria screen (samples need to be covered to protect from direct light)
- Monochromator light test
- Photopatch testing when a chemical or plant contact allergy exacerbated by sunlight exposure is suspected

Table 45.3 Classification of porphyrias.

Main category of porphyria	Characteristic features	Examples
1. Cutaneous porphyrias: (a) Bullous (b) Non-bullous	**Photosensitivity to visible light with:** (a) Blisters hours to days after light exposure, milia, skin fragility, scarring, hypertrichosis (b) Skin oedema immediately following light exposure	(a) Porphyria cutanea tarda (PCT) Congenital erythropoietic porphyria (CEP, extremely rare) (b) Erythropoietic protoporphyria (EPP)
2. Acute porphyrias	Neurological and visceral features, e.g. peripheral neuropathy, abdominal pain, vomiting	Acute intermittent porphyria (AIP)
3. Cutaneous and acute porphyrias	Combination of the features of cutaneous bullous and acute porphyrias	Variegate porphyria (VP)

Dermatology at a Glance, Second Edition. Mahbub M.U. Chowdhury, Ruwani P. Katugampola, and Andrew Y. Finlay.
© 2020 John Wiley & Sons Ltd. Published 2020 by John Wiley & Sons Ltd.
Companion website: www.wiley.com/go/chowdhury/dermatology

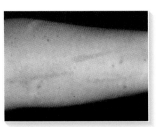

Figure 45.1 Phytophotodermatitis – note the linear erythema/ blisters at the site of contact between the plant and the skin.

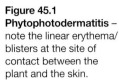

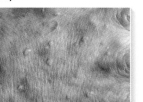

Figure 45.5 Milia and subtle scars on the hand of a patient with porphyria cutanea tarda (PCT).

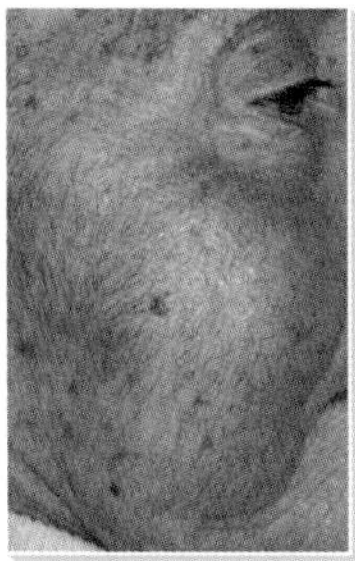

Figure 45.6 Hypertrichosis on the face of a female patient with PCT.

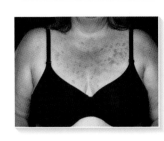

Figure 45.2 Polymorphic light eruption (PLE) – note the distribution of the rash to the light-exposed skin on the upper anterior chest wall.

Figure 45.7 Blistering due to PCT.

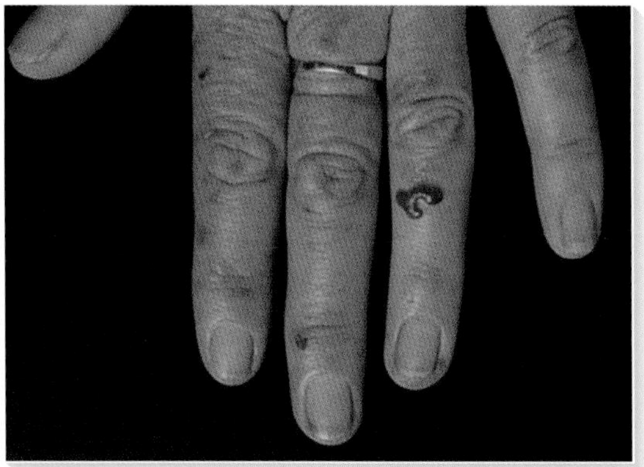

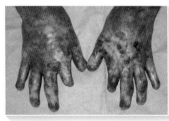

Figure 45.3a and b Chronic actinic dermatitis (CAD) – note the eczematous rash on photo-exposed skin and sparing of the photo-protected skin.

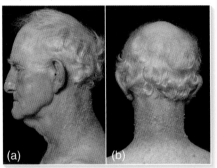

Figure 45.9 The back of a patient 24 hours following monochromator light testing – the dark circles mark the sites of the different wavelengths that were shone on the patient's back. The erythema within some of the circles identifies the wavelength(s) that precipitated the patient's photodermatosis and helps confirm the diagnosis based on the history and clinical examination.

Figure 45.8 Hands of a patient with congenital erythropoietic porphyria (CEP) – note the blisters on the dorsum of the left hand, superficial ulcers due to burst blisters, severe scarring resulting in loss of fingernails, shortening of fingers, and deformity of hands.

Figure 45.4a and b Actinic prurigo (AP) – note the eczematous rash with papules and nodules on photo-exposed skin.

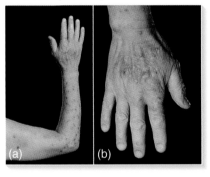

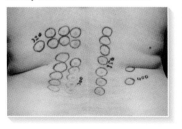

Photodermatoses are skin diseases that are precipitated or aggravated by exposure to sunlight. They may be precipitated by one or a combination of different wavelengths of light: ultraviolet A (UVA 320–400 nm), ultraviolet B (UVB 290–320 nm), and visible light (400–750 nm) (Chapter 44, Figure 44.1). Photodermatoses can be idiopathic, inherited, or secondary to other causes (Table 45.1). They affect exposed skin such as the face, anterior neck, upper chest wall, and dorsum of the hands; photoprotected skin including behind the ears is usually spared (Table 45.2).

The onset of the rash following light exposure can be immediate or delayed. Patients with immediate photosensitivity usually present with an urticarial rash. Patients with delayed photosensitivity present with blistering, papules, increased freckling, and/or eczematous rash.

Certain inflammatory skin diseases can be exacerbated by sunlight (e.g. rosacea, cutaneous discoid lupus erythematosus [DLE]) or improved with sunlight (e.g. psoriasis).

Individuals with severe photodermatoses may develop vitamin D insufficiency or deficiency as a result of decreased sunlight exposure (Chapter 43).

Polymorphic Light Eruption

Polymorphic light eruption (PLE) is one of the most common photodermatoses, usually occurring at the beginning of spring and resolving by autumn. Itchy erythematous papules, plaques, and vesicles on exposed skin appear about one day following exposure to bright sunlight (Figure 45.2).

Treatment includes sun protection (clothing, broad spectrum sunscreen) and moderately potent topical corticosteroids. Severe cases benefit from a one week course of oral prednisolone 20 mg/day at the onset of the rash. Narrowband UVB or psoralen plus UVA (PUVA) treatment at the beginning of spring can desensitise and 'harden' the skin to decrease the severity of PLE.

Chronic Actinic Dermatitis

Chronic actinic dermatitis (CAD) is caused by photosensitivity mainly to UVB but also extending to UVA and visible wavelengths. CAD usually affects men over the age of 50 years, usually worse during summer months. It is characterised by an eczematous rash in photo-exposed skin up to a few days after exposure; with time, the affected skin becomes lichenified with post-inflammatory pigmentary changes (Figure 45.3a and b). Some patients may have coexisting atopic dermatitis or allergic contact dermatitis affecting other parts of the body thus confusing the clinical presentation and delaying the diagnosis of CAD.

A clinical diagnosis of CAD can be confirmed by phototesting. Patch testing (Chapter 35) should be considered to exclude coexistent allergic contact dermatitis.

Treatment includes sun protection as for PLE, topical emollients, moderate to potent topical corticosteroids, or topical calcineurin inhibitors (pimecrolimus or tacrolimus ointment). Severe disease requires short courses of oral steroids and long-term systemic immunosuppressant therapy such as azathioprine or ciclosporin (Chapter 14). PUVA treatment to 'harden' the skin can be used with caution not to precipitate an acute flare of CAD.

Actinic Prurigo

Actinic prurigo (AP) is caused by photosensitivity to UVA and UVB radiation with the symptoms being worse during spring and summer months. It presents with itchy papules, nodules, vesicles, and eczematous patches on photo-exposed skin up to a few days after light exposure, resulting in scarring (Figure 45.4a and b). Cheilitis and conjunctivitis also occur. Onset of disease can be in childhood or early adulthood, affecting females twice as commonly than males. About 70% of individuals with AP have the specific HLA type HLA-DRB1*0407.

A clinical diagnosis of AP can be confirmed by HLA typing and phototesting. Treatment is as for CAD. Narrowband UVB or PUVA treatment can be used with caution, in conjunction with topical corticosteroids to avoid precipitating a flare of AP.

Solar Urticaria

Itchy urticarial wheals develop on sun-exposed body sites within minutes of sunlight exposure. Lesions resolve within 24 hours. Solar urticaria is often precipitated by visible light, but UVA and/or UVB may also precipitate the rash. It may occur in association with PLE. Rarely, anaphylaxis may occur with bronchospasm.

Treatment includes sun protection (clothing, broad spectrum sunscreen) and antihistamines. Gradual, cautious exposure to UVA phototherapy has been beneficial to 'harden' the skin.

Porphyrias

Porphyrias are a group of inherited metabolic disorders (Figures 45.5–45.8). The individual porphyrias are caused by deficiency of the different enzymes involved in the haem biosynthetic pathway. The metabolites that accumulate upstream of the deficient enzyme lead to the manifestations of the individual porphyrias. The measurements of these metabolites in the patient's blood, urine and faeces aids in the diagnosis of the type of porphyria.

Based on the clinical manifestations, porphyrias are broadly divided into three categories (Table 45.3).

Treatment of all the cutaneous porphyrias is photoprotection from visible light with appropriate clothing and reflectant physical sunscreens that provide protection from both visible light and ultraviolet radiation (as opposed to chemical sunscreens that only protect from UV radiation).

Porphyria Cutanea Tarda

Porphyria cutanea tarda (PCT) is the most common cutaneous porphyria. It may develop from secondary causes such as alcoholic liver disease or haemochromatosis.

Treatment – regular venesection or oral hydroxychloroquine.

Erythropoietic Protoporphyria

Patients require monitoring of liver function as they may develop liver failure necessitating a liver transplant. Patients with erythropoietic protoporphyria may benefit from oral beta-carotene to improve their tolerance to sunlight.

Xeroderma Pigmentosa

This is a group of autosomal recessive diseases caused by defective DNA repair mechanisms.

Xeroderma pigmentosa (XP) is characterised by marked photosensitivity to sunlight, freckling, and increased risk of multiple premalignant and malignant lesions of the skin (basal cell and squamous cell carcinomas, melanoma) and eyes from childhood.

Some 20–30% of cases may also develop neurological manifestations ranging from hyporeflexia to ataxia and quadriparesis.

XP is also associated with an increased risk of malignancies of the brain, lungs, kidneys, oral cavity, and gastro-intestinal tract.

Management includes diligent photoprotection, regular surveillance, and treatment of pre-malignant and malignant lesions by a multi-disciplinary team. Oral retinoids have been used to decrease frequency of skin malignancies in XP.

Phototesting

Phototesting is used to detect the wavelength(s) of light that may provoke a particular photodermatosis. In monochromator light testing, light at different known wavelengths, which correspond to UVA, UVB, and visible light, are shone on the patient's back. Evidence of localised visible erythema and/or skin oedema is checked immediately after and 24-hours post-irradiation (Figure 45.9).

Key Points

- A rash in light exposed sites should raise the possibility of a photodermatosis.
- Photoprotection is essential in the management of all photodermatoses.

▶ **Warning**

- Phototherapy should be commenced cautiously in solar urticaria, as it may precipitate the rash and/or anaphylaxis.
- Patients with severe photodermatoses may require supplementation to avoid vitamin D deficiency resulting from decreased sunlight exposure.
- Numerous drugs can precipitate an acute attack of porphyria. The following website provides information on the safe use of drugs in acute forms of porphyria: https://www.wmic.wales.nhs.uk/specialist-services/drugs-in-porphyria/

Systemic Diseases

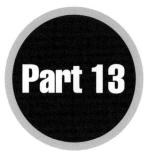

Part 13

Chapters

46 Skin Signs of Systemic Disease

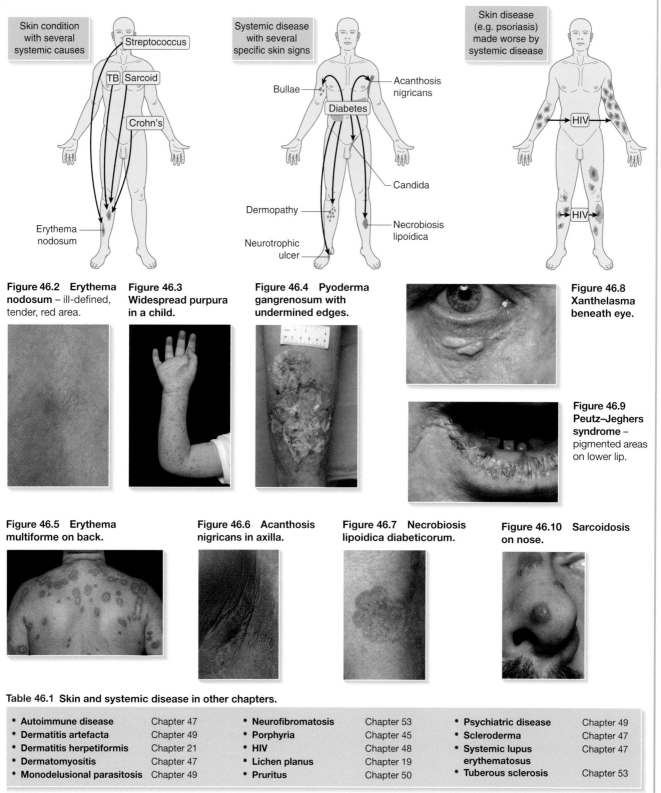

Figure 46.1 How the skin and systemic disease interact.

Skin condition with several systemic causes
Streptococcus
TB | Sarcoid
Crohn's
Erythema nodosum

Systemic disease with several specific skin signs
Bullae
Diabetes
Acanthosis nigricans
Candida
Dermopathy
Neurotrophic ulcer
Necrobiosis lipoidica

Skin disease (e.g. psoriasis) made worse by systemic disease
HIV
HIV

Figure 46.2 Erythema nodosum – ill-defined, tender, red area.

Figure 46.3 Widespread purpura in a child.

Figure 46.4 Pyoderma gangrenosum with undermined edges.

Figure 46.8 Xanthelasma beneath eye.

Figure 46.9 Peutz–Jeghers syndrome – pigmented areas on lower lip.

Figure 46.5 Erythema multiforme on back.

Figure 46.6 Acanthosis nigricans in axilla.

Figure 46.7 Necrobiosis lipoidica diabeticorum.

Figure 46.10 Sarcoidosis on nose.

Table 46.1 Skin and systemic disease in other chapters.

• Autoimmune disease	Chapter 47	• Neurofibromatosis	Chapter 53	• Psychiatric disease	Chapter 49
• Dermatitis artefacta	Chapter 49	• Porphyria	Chapter 45	• Scleroderma	Chapter 47
• Dermatitis herpetiformis	Chapter 21	• HIV	Chapter 48	• Systemic lupus	Chapter 47
• Dermatomyositis	Chapter 47	• Lichen planus	Chapter 19	erythematosus	
• Monodelusional parasitosis	Chapter 49	• Pruritus	Chapter 50	• Tuberous sclerosis	Chapter 53

Dermatology at a Glance, Second Edition. Mahbub M.U. Chowdhury, Ruwani P. Katugampola, and Andrew Y. Finlay.
© 2020 John Wiley & Sons Ltd. Published 2020 by John Wiley & Sons Ltd.
Companion website: www.wiley.com/go/chowdhury/dermatology

It is not surprising that the skin is involved in many systemic diseases – it would be odd if it wasn't. Knowing about these clues to systemic disease is satisfying and gives you ('Sherlock Holmes') the chance of astonishing your colleagues with an accurate diagnosis on apparently little information (Figure 46.1).

Conditions with Several Causes

Erythema Nodosum
Ill-defined, tender, raised, red lesions, several centimetres across, on the shins (Figure 46.2).
- Tuberculosis
- Sarcoidosis
- Beta-haemolytic *Streptococcus* – upper respiratory tract infection
- Drugs (e.g. oral contraceptive pill, sulphonamides)
- Autoimmune disease (e.g. systemic lupus erythematosus)
- Inflammatory bowel disease, especially Crohn's disease.

Pruritus (Note Correct Spelling) (Chapter 50)
Generalised itchiness. First rule out skin causes of pruritus such as early pemphigoid, dermatitis herpetiformis, or scabies.
- Hyperthyroidism
- Lymphoma (e.g. Hodgkin's disease)
- Renal failure
- Hepatobiliary disease, including cholestasis, primary biliary cirrhosis
- Iron deficiency
- Polycythaemia rubra vera. Pruritus provoked by water contact (e.g. having a shower)
- HIV infection.

Purpura
Red or dark blue areas, usually flat. Does not blanche on pressure because the red blood cells have come out of the blood vessels and are in the dermis (Figure 46.3).
- Low platelets (thrombocytopenia)
- Drugs (e.g. warfarin)
- Scurvy (vitamin C deficiency)
- Amyloidosis
- Henoch–Schönlein purpura
- Infections (e.g. meningococcal meningitis).

Pyoderma Gangrenosum
Persistent ulceration with purple undermined edge (Figure 46.4).
- Ulcerative colitis, Crohn's disease
- Rheumatoid arthritis
- Myeloproliferative disease (e.g. acute lymphoblastic leukaemia, chronic myeloid leukaemia, myelodysplasia, paraproteinaemia)
- Systemic malignancy.

Erythema Multiforme
Many red ('erythema') lesions over body and limbs (Figure 46.5). May be target-like but can be many shapes ('multiforme').
- Viral disease, especially herpes simplex
- Mycoplasma infection
- Drugs (e.g. sulphonamides), but many implicated
- Depending on the cause, withdraw drug or treat infection and provide urgent inpatient supportive therapy.

Acanthosis Nigricans
Dark velvety thickening in flexures, especially axillae, groin (Figure 46.6).
- Diabetes
- Insulin resistance and obesity
- Gastric adenocarcinoma.

Systemic Diseases with Specific Signs
Endocrine Disease
Diabetes
- Diabetic dermopathy. Atrophic brown scars on shins, thighs
- *Candida* infection
- Acanthosis nigricans (Figure 46.6)
- Diabetic bullae
- Neurotrophic ulceration
- Necrobiosis lipoidica diabeticorum (Figure 46.7).

This has a waxy, yellow, shiny appearance centrally and is typically on the shins. It indicates either the presence of diabetes or a strong risk of developing it. There is little evidence of effective therapy.

Addison's Disease (Adrenal Insufficiency)
- Hyperpigmentation

Thyroid Disease
Hyperthyroidism is associated with pruritus, pre-tibial myxoedema, and protruding eyes. In hypothyroidism there is dry skin with an ivory-yellow colour, coarse scanty scalp hair, and enlarged tongue.

Metabolic Disease
Hyperlipidaemia
Xanthelasma (around the eyes) may occur with normal lipid levels but indicate increased risk of heart disease (Figure 46.8). Tendon xanthomas suggest familial hypercholesterolaemia and tuberous xanthomas (elbows and knees) suggest type III hyperlipoproteinaemia. Eruptive xanthomas (buttocks, back, limbs) indicate severe hypertriglyceridaemia.

Systemic Cancer
Skin signs of systemic cancer:
- Cutaneous metastases (Chapter 41)
- Tylosis (palmar keratoderma)
  - oesophageal cancer
- Acanthosis nigricans (Figure 46.6)
  - gastric adenocarcinoma
- Acquired ichthyosis (generalised stratum corneum thickening)
  - Hodgkin's disease
- Dermatomyositis (proximal muscle weakness and mauve facial rash) (Chapter 47)
  - common systemic malignancies
- Erythema gyratum repens (extremely rare, waves of erythema reminiscent of the grain of cut wood)
  - lung cancer
- Necrolytic migratory erythema (itchy red rash groin, lower abdomen, buttocks)
  - glucagonoma (alpha cell tumour of pancreas)
- Migratory thrombophlebitis (Trousseau's sign: in 1867 he self-diagnosed the sign and died)
  - pancreatic carcinoma
- Acquired hypertrichosis lanuginosa (widespread excessive hair growth)
  - lung, colorectal carcinoma.

Genetic diseases with skin signs and risk of systemic malignancy:
- Neurofibromatosis types 1 and 2 (Chapter 53)
  - Malignant neurofibrosarcoma
  - Astrocytoma.

- Peutz–Jeghers syndrome (pigmented mucosal and skin macules and gastro-intestinal polyps) (Figure 46.9)
  ○ Pancreas, breast cancer.
- Gardner's syndrome (subcutaneous fibromas, benign cysts, gastro-intestinal polyposis)
  ○ Colonic cancer.
- Gorlin's syndrome (naevoid basal cell carcinoma syndrome)
  ○ Medulloblastoma.
- Tuberous sclerosis (epilepsy, mental retardation) (Chapter 53)
  ○ Malignant sarcoma
  ○ Renal cell carcinoma.
- Muir–Torre syndrome (sebaceous tumours)
  ○ Colonic adenocarcinoma (50%)
  ○ Urogenital malignancies (25%).

Systemic Infection
Meningococcal meningitis: purpura.

Gastro-intestinal Disease
- Dermatitis herpetiformis (intensely itchy, small blisters). There is gluten sensitive enteropathy associated with villous atrophy of small bowel and IgA anti-endomysial antibodies (Chapter 21).
- Acrodermatitis enteropathica (blisters and scaling: perioral and acral [i.e. at end of limbs or fingers/toes]). Deficient zinc absorption leads to zinc deficiency.
- Liver cirrhosis. Signs include jaundice, pruritus, spider angiomas, and body hair loss.
- Primary biliary cirrhosis. Associated with lichen planus (Chapter 19) and hepatitis C infection.

Cardiology
LEOPARD Syndrome
Lentigines widespread (brown flat areas), Electrocardiographic abnormalities, Ocular hypertelorism, Pulmonary stenosis, Abnormal genitalia, Retardation of growth, Deafness.

LAMB and NAME Syndromes (Carney Complex)
LAMB: Lentigines, Atrial Myxoma, mucocutaneous myxomas, Blue naevi.
NAME: Naevi, Atrial Myxoma, myxoid neurofibromas, Ephelides (freckles).

Important because identifies atrial myxoma which must be removed.

Sarcoidosis
Sarcoidosis (Figure 46.10) can be either primarily systemic or primarily cutaneous. Systemic sarcoidosis, typically with hilar lymphadenopathy, may present with erythema nodosum. Cutaneous sarcoidosis occurs as plaques, nodules, or papules. Specific features include occurrence in scars (Koebner's phenomenon), red–blue swellings on ears or tip of nose (lupus pernio), and annular lesions especially on the face. There may be nail destruction with resorption of terminal phalanges. Diagnosis is based on skin biopsy, raised serum angiotensin-converting enzyme, chest X-ray, and lung function tests. Therapy is with topical, intralesional, or oral corticosteroids, or with chloroquine or hydroxychloroquine.

Key Points
- Skin changes are often critical clues to systemic disease.
- The same pattern of disease can have several causes (e.g. erythema nodosum).

▶ Warning
- Skin diseases may be altered by systemic disease. Pityriasis versicolor and psoriasis may become worse in HIV infection and viral warts may become worse on immunosuppressive drugs.

47 Autoimmune Disease and Vasculitis

Table 47.1 Classification of vasculitis.

- **Large vessel vasculitis** – giant cell temporal arteritis, Takayasu's arteritis
- **Small/medium vessel vasculitis** – Wegener's granulomatosis, Churg–Strauss syndrome, polyarteritis nodosa, Kawasaki disease
- **Small vessel vasculitis** – Leukocytoclastic vasculitis, Henoch–Schönlein syndrome, cryoglobulinaemia and drug induced vasculitis, rheumatoid arthritis, systemic lupus erythematosus (SLE), Sjögren's syndrome

Table 47.2 Causes of small vessel vasculitis.

- **Bacterial infections** – *Streptococcus* group A, *Staphylococcus aureus*
- **Other infections** – Hepatitis, herpes simplex, fungal, and parasitic infections
- **Drugs** – Penicillin, thiazides, quinine, oral contraceptives
- **Diseases** – Systemic lupus erythematosus (SLE), rheumatoid arthritis, malignancies, capillary disorders, cutaneous T cell lymphoma (mycosis fungoides), multiple myeloma, lung cancer, renal cancer, cryoglobulinaemia, ulcerative colitis, HIV infection

Table 47.3 Tests to investigate vasculitis.

- Autoantibody screen (ANA, ANCA)
- Full blood count (normochromic anaemia, neutrophilia, eosinophilia)
- ESR, CRP
- Urea and electrolytes, liver function tests
- Chest X-ray
- Skin biopsy to show leukocytoclastic vasculitis

Note: Churg–Strauss syndrome is c-ANCA (cytoplasmic staining) positive and Wegener's granulomatosis is p-ANCA (perinuclear staining) positive

Figure 47.1a and b Discoid lupus erythematosus (DLE) with scaly plaques and scarring alopecia on scalp.

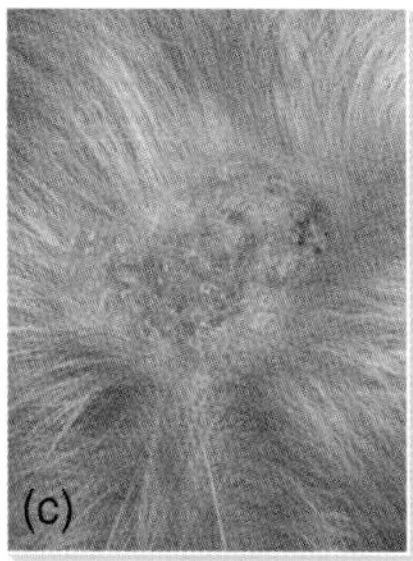

Figure 47.1c Note follicular plugging.

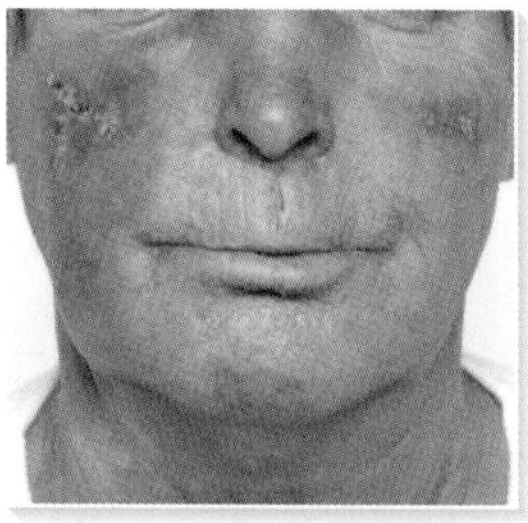

Figure 47.2a DLE.

Figure 47.2b DLE on cheek with atrophy and scaling (closeup).

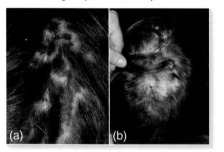

Figure 47.3a and b Subacute LE with annular patches on chest/arms.

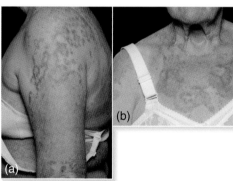

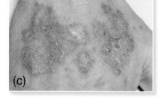

Figure 47.3c Subacute LE on dorsum of hand.

Figure 47.4a and b Nail fold capillary loops/telangiectasia.

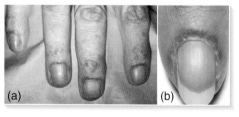

Figure 47.5a and b Sclerodactyly and calcinosis with closeup.

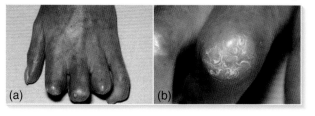

Figure 47.6a and b Heliotrope rash in dermatomyositis with closeup.

Dermatology at a Glance, Second Edition. Mahbub M.U. Chowdhury, Ruwani P. Katugampola, and Andrew Y. Finlay.

Companion website: www.wiley.com/go/chowdhury/dermatology

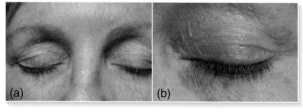

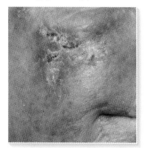

Figure 47.6c and d Rash in dermatomyositis on photoexposed areas, e.g. chest/arms.

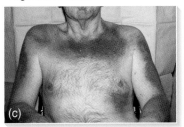

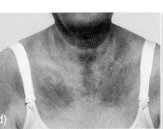

Figure 47.6e Gottron's papules on knuckles.

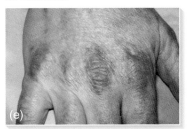

Figure 47.6f Gottron's sign on elbow.

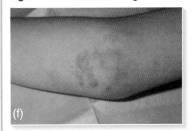

Figure 47.6g Gottron's sign on knees.

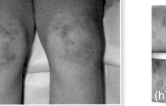

Figure 47.6h Nail fold changes and ragged cuticles with Gottron's papules.

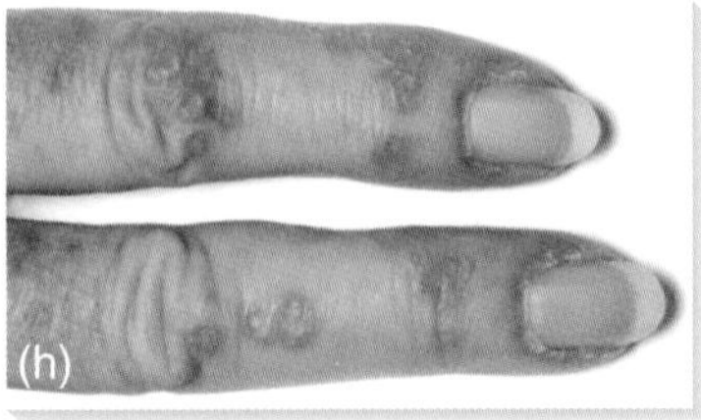

Figure 47.7a Vasculitis with palpable purpura on legs.

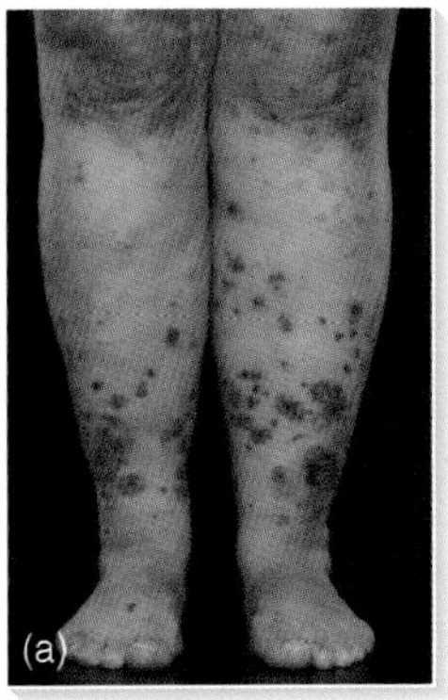

Figure 47.7b and c Vasculitis on feet with closeup.

Figure 47.7d Extensive vasculitis on buttocks and thighs.

Figure 47.7e Severe ulceration post-vasculitis.

Figure 47.7f Urticarial vasculitis lasts > 24 hours confirmed with skin biopsy.

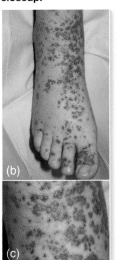

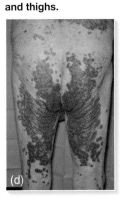

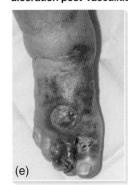

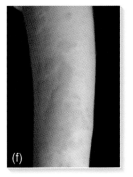

This chapter covers a broad range of diseases including lupus erythematosus (LE), scleroderma, dermatomyositis, and vasculitis.

Lupus Erythematosus

There are many forms of lupus erythematosus with a wide range of manifestations ranging from localised chronic skin disease in discoid lupus erythematosus (DLE) to subacute cutaneous or systemic lupus erythematosus (SLE) with multiple organ disease. These diseases are thought to be caused by a variety of autoantibodies against cellular antigens including DNA, RNA, and other proteins.

Treatment options include oral, intralesional, and topical corticosteroids (potent to very potent), antimalarials (e.g. hydroxychloroquine), and dapsone.

Sunscreens are essential, with strict sun avoidance (Chapter 43).

Discoid Lupus Erythematosus

This is the most common form with localised or widespread, scaly, red papules and plaques with central atrophy and scarring. DLE is more common in women with peak incidence in the forties.

Photosensitivity is present in 50% with 1–5% of cases progressing to SLE. The main sites affected are scalp, face, and ears (Figures 47.1 and 47.2). Scarring alopecia can occur.

Clinical features include follicular plugging and adherent scaling with wrinkled epidermal atrophy. Lesions can be hypertrophic (thickened) leading to white or hyperpigmented depressed scars with telangiectasia.

Subacute Cutaneous Lupus Erythematosus

This subtype has non-scarring red annular patches (Figure 47.3) or plaques in sun-exposed areas on the upper trunk, neck, face, and dorsum of hands. Photosensitivity is present in 70–90%.

Blood tests show positive ANA (anti-nuclear), anti-Ro (anti-SSA) and anti-La (anti-SSB) antibodies. Systemic involvement with kidney disease and leukopenia can occur.

Children of affected women may develop neonatal lupus erythematosus following transplacental transmission of antibodies (Chapter 31).

Systemic Lupus Erythematosus

This is a multi-system disease affecting mainly women (8 : 1 ratio) aged 30–40 years.

Butterfly rash can occur (in 50% of patients) on malar areas of the cheeks and nose with red, violaceous plaques or patches on the chest, shoulders, and hands with scaling and follicular plugging: there is no atrophy. Alopecia occurs in 20% of cases.

Skin biopsy is needed for histology and immunofluorescence with autoantibody screen of blood to confirm positive ANA and anti-double-stranded DNA.

Other manifestations include fever, arthritis, vasculitis, Raynaud's phenomenon, oral mucosal ulceration, and nail fold capillary changes with prominent capillary loops (Figure 47.4), and renal, cardiac, lung, and nervous system abnormalities.

Scleroderma (Systemic Sclerosus)

This is an idiopathic condition causing diffuse or localised fibrosis. The diffuse form can have internal organ fibrosis and vascular abnormalities.

CREST syndrome is a localised form with **C**alcinosis, **R**aynaud's disease, o**E**sophageal dysmotility, **S**clerodactyly, and **T**elangiectasia. This most commonly involves the hands (Figure 47.5) and face. This occurs mainly in women (3:1 ratio) with peak onset at 30–50 years.

Skin changes include smooth, shiny, pigmented, indurated skin with restricted mouth opening, perioral puckering, Raynaud's phenomenon, facial telangiectasia, sclerodactyly, dilated nail fold capillaries with ragged cuticles, calcinosis cutis (Figure 47.5b), and livedo reticularis. Fingertip ulceration and gangrene is common and diffuse calcification of the skin may occur.

Tests to confirm diagnosis include positive ANA (90%) with nucleolar pattern staining, antibodies to Scl-70 and anti-centromere antibodies (highly specific for CREST syndrome).

There is no treatment that reverses skin fibrosis. Raynaud's phenomenon is treated with calcium channel blockers. Cessation of smoking can improve digital ulceration and resistance to trauma.

Dermatomyositis

This is an idiopathic inflammatory myopathy which may be linked with underlying malignancy (paraneoplastic) especially in the elderly. Fatigue, proximal symmetrical muscle weakness, and dysphagia can occur.

Skin features include a peri-orbital heliotrope (blue–purple colour) rash (Figure 47.6a and b), Gottron's papules (red plaques on extensor finger joints) (Figure 47.6e), erythema over knees and elbows (Gottron's sign) (Figure 47.6f and g), dilated nail fold capillaries, and ragged cuticles (Figure 47.6h). Ten per cent of patients have skin findings without muscle disease (amyopathic dermatomyositis).

Serum creatinine kinase is usually raised and a muscle biopsy may be required. Anti-Jo-1 antibody positive (20%) is associated with interstitial lung disease and arthritis.

The disease course may progress or remit spontaneously.

Treatments include sun protection, systemic corticosteroids, hydroxychloroquine, and steroid-sparing agents (e.g. methotrexate, azathioprine).

Screening tests for underlying malignancy should be carried out.

Small Vessel Vasculitis

Vasculitis can be classified depending on the type of inflammation in specific blood vessel walls (Table 47.1). In 60% of patients no cause is found, in others there is deposition of IgG or IgM immune complexes in post-capillary venules.

The principal skin sign is palpable purpura which can be painful. Skin signs include livedo reticularis (a blotchy, net-like pattern), purpura, erythema multiforme, and urticaria. These signs occur on the lowermost areas of the back, buttocks, and lower legs (Figure 47.7).

Vasculitis can be caused by infection, drugs, food allergy, connective tissue diseases, and malignancy (Table 47.2). A full vasculitis screen (Table 47.3) includes full blood count, renal and liver function, autoantibody screen (ANA, anti-neutrophil cytoplasmic antibody [ANCA]), ESR, chest X-ray, and skin biopsy to show leukocytoclastic vasculitis.

Patients with systemic vasculitis can present with malaise, fever, weight loss, and glomerulonephritis, sensory neuropathy, abdominal pain and haemorrhage, angina, and stroke.

Prognosis is dependent on factors such as renal involvement. The condition resolves within a few weeks if precipitating factors can be removed. NSAIDs can be used for general symptoms and systemic steroids (60–80 mg/day) with other immunosuppressive agents can help (e.g. cyclophosphamide, methotrexate, azathioprine, or ciclosporin).

Key Points
- All forms of lupus erythematosus need strict sun avoidance.
- Think widely for causes of vasculitis including drugs, infections, and systemic diseases.

▶ Warning
- Suspected vasculitis should be urgently investigated and treated.

48 The Immunosuppressed Patient

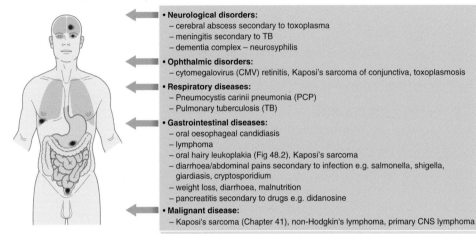

Figure 48.1 Systemic manifestations of HIV.

- **Neurological disorders:**
  - cerebral abscess secondary to toxoplasma
  - meningitis secondary to TB
  - dementia complex – neurosyphilis
- **Ophthalmic disorders:**
  - cytomegalovirus (CMV) retinitis, Kaposi's sarcoma of conjunctiva, toxoplasmosis
- **Respiratory diseases:**
  - Pneumocystis carinii pneumonia (PCP)
  - Pulmonary tuberculosis (TB)
- **Gastrointestinal diseases:**
  - oral oesophageal candidiasis
  - lymphoma
  - oral hairy leukoplakia (Fig 48.2), Kaposi's sarcoma
  - diarrhoea/abdominal pains secondary to infection e.g. salmonella, shigella, giardiasis, cryptosporidium
  - weight loss, diarrhoea, malnutrition
  - pancreatitis secondary to drugs e.g. didanosine
- **Malignant disease:**
  - Kaposi's sarcoma (Chapter 41), non-Hodgkin's lymphoma, primary CNS lymphoma

Table 48.1 Common skin manifestations of HIV/AIDS.

- **Inflammatory skin diseases:**
  - Psoriasis, eczema, seborrhoeic dermatitis (Figure 48.3), folliculitis
- **Infections:**
  - Viral – herpes zoster/herpes simplex, CMV, molluscum contagiosum (Figure 48.5), human papilloma virus (HPV)
  - Fungal – *Malassezia, Cryptococcus, Histoplasma, Candida*
  - Bacterial – *TB, syphilis, bacillary angiomatosis*
- **Problems due to drugs:**
  - Stevens–Johnson syndrome – cotrimoxazole, nevirapine, efavirenz
  - Nail pigmentation – indinavir, zidovudine, ritonavir
  - Lipodystrophy – indinavir, ritonavir
  - Hair loss – lamivudine, indinavir
- **Malignancy:**
  - Kaposi's sarcoma (Figure 48.4), lymphoma

Table 48.2 Skin conditions associated with immunosuppression.

- HIV-related skin conditions (Table 48.1)
- Skin cancer in transplant recipients (Chapter 39)
- Molluscum contagiosum
- Melanoma/SCC/BCC (Chapters 39 and 40)
- Skin lymphoma (Chapter 41)
- Varicella zoster, herpes simplex infections (Chapter 24)
- Warts, e.g. common viral wart, HPV (Chapter 24)

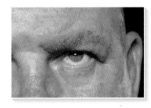

Figure 48.3 Seborrhoeic dermatitis affecting eyebrows.

Figure 48.2a and b Oral hairy leukoplakia on lateral tongue border.

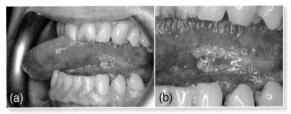

(a)   (b)

Figure 48.4a and b Kaposi's sarcoma on sole showing patch and nodule, with closeup.

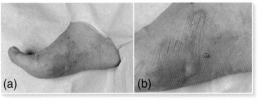

(a)   (b)

Figure 48.5a Typical molluscum.

Figure 48.5b Widespread molluscum in HIV.

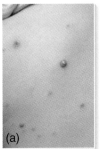

(a)

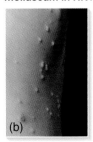

(b)

Figure 48.5c Note central dimples in molluscum papules.

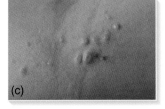

(c)

Figure 48.5d Molluscum on upper eyelid after topical steroid use.

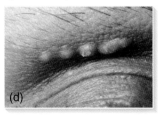

(d)

Dermatology at a Glance, Second Edition. Mahbub M.U. Chowdhury, Ruwani P. Katugampola, and Andrew Y. Finlay.
© 2020 John Wiley & Sons Ltd. Published 2020 by John Wiley & Sons Ltd.
Companion website: www.wiley.com/go/chowdhury/dermatology

Immunosuppressed patients are prone to infections and skin cancers. This chapter covers HIV infection and skin conditions seen in immunocompromised patients.

Human Immunodeficiency Virus Infection

Over 36 million people are infected with HIV and 70% of these are in sub-Saharan Africa. In the UK around 100 000 individuals are affected. There are around 4000 new cases per year with 10% presenting with advanced HIV disease or AIDS (acquired immunodeficiency syndrome). In 2017, there were 400 AIDS-related deaths in the UK.

The HIV virus is transmitted by sexual intercourse, contaminated injections used by drug abusers, blood products, breast milk, and by perinatal transmission. This can coexist with other sexually transmitted infections such as hepatitis C.

HIV is a human retrovirus containing RNA which transcribes DNA via a reverse transcriptase enzyme. HIV infection leads to CD4 cell depletion starting as a primary cell immunity defect progressing to general immune dysfunction. A CD4 count of $< 200\,mm^2$ (normal $> 500\,mm^2$) is regarded as diagnostic of AIDS. Markers of disease progression include high HIV viral load measured by polymerase chain reaction (PCR) assay. These markers can also be used to monitor response to treatment.

HIV seroconversion (HIV p24 antigen detectable) can occur up to three months after infection. Twenty-five per cent develop clinical seroconversion illness consisting of fever, malaise, rash, sore throat, lymphadenopathy, and arthralgia. HIV PCR and p24 antigen confirm the diagnosis of HIV and an antibody test (Western blot or immunofluorescence assay) can also be carried out, but 75% seroconvert without symptoms.

The Centers for Disease Control and Prevention (CDC) classification stages the disease from primary seroconversion illness through to AIDS-related complex (advanced HIV disease with opportunistic infection or tumours) (Figure 48.1).

Skin manifestations of HIV/AIDS can affect up to 75% of HIV patients (Table 48.1). The acute HIV illness can present with an asymptomatic macular or papular rash affecting the face and trunk and also seborrhoeic dermatitis (Figure 48.3).

All skin diseases and other infections can be atypical and more persistent and severe than usual, often responding poorly to standard treatment. If this occurs with any common conditions such as psoriasis or seborrhoeic dermatitis, HIV screening should be considered at an early stage.

Active retroviral therapy (ART) involves three drug combinations to suppress viral replication and to reduce the risk of viral resistance. Prognosis is predicted by viral resistance as well as factors such as drug tolerance, side effects, and adherence (i.e. compliance). Drugs used include nucleoside reverse transcriptase inhibitors (abacavir, lamivudine, zidovudine, didanosine), protease inhibitors (atazanavir, darunavir, ritonavir, indinavir, saquinavir), or non-nucleoside reverse transcriptase inhibitors (efavirenz, nevirapine, rilpivirine). Twenty-five per cent of hospital admissions with HIV are a result of drug side effects (Table 48.1).

Generalised macular and papular rashes are common with co-trimoxazole and nevirapine. Nevirapine and efavirenz can cause Stevens–Johnson syndrome or toxic epidermal necrolysis. Eight per cent of abacavir treated patients develop hypersensitivity within two weeks with fever, rash, and flu-like symptoms but this can be avoided with gene screening for HLA-B*5701 which indicates patient predisposition to hypersensitivity reactions.

Prognosis was markedly improved with the introduction of ART therapy in 1997 and death rates have reduced for those aged 25–40 years. In the UK, 98% of HIV infected people are now on treatment. Opportunistic infections have reduced but lymphoma is increasing in incidence.

Immune reconstitution inflammatory syndrome (IRIS) may be triggered by ART therapy and skin conditions can develop when CD4 and CD8 counts increase (e.g. herpes and viral wart infections, Kaposi's sarcoma (Figure 48.4) and eosinophilic folliculitis).

Immunocompromised Patients and Skin Conditions

Any immunocompromised patient can be more prone to skin problems. Therapies such as oral tacrolimus, azathioprine, ciclosporin, and mycophenolate mofetil may predispose to skin tumours and skin infections. The commonly associated conditions are listed in Table 48.2.

Skin cancer in immunosuppressed transplant recipients can be more aggressive with early recurrences and metastases. Therapy to ensure full surgical removal is needed.

In some centres regular monitoring of transplant patients for skin cancers may be undertaken ensuring increased vigilance at follow-up.

Squamous cell carcinoma, melanoma, and basal cell carcinoma are all more common in immunocompromised patients (Chapters 39 and 40).

Key Points

- Always consider HIV infection if skin conditions are severe, atypical, and less responsive to standard treatments.
- Drug therapy for HIV infection may cause skin problems including dermatological emergencies such as Stevens–Johnson syndrome or toxic epidermal necrolysis.
- Immunosuppressed patients present with a wide range of common skin conditions which may be more severe and persistent (e.g. viral warts).

▶ Warning

- Skin cancers in immunosuppressed transplant patients may be more aggressive and metastasise early. Full surgical clearance of the tumour and close monitoring is required.

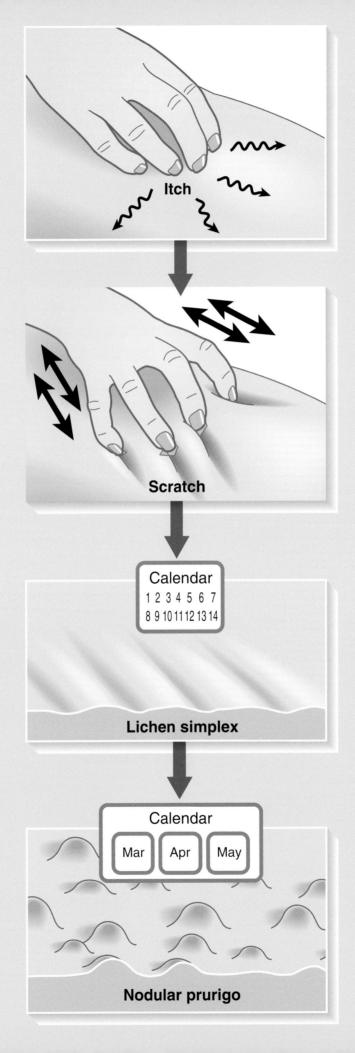

Miscellaneous Conditions

49 Psychodermatology

Table 49.1 Skin disease aggravated/provoked by psychological problems.

- **Alopecia areata**
  Severe stress can result in hair loss (alopecia areata). Before the Battle of Corruna (1809) General Sir John Moore's hair turned white: typically in alopecia areata the dark hairs are shed more easily

- **Psoriasis**
  Many patients feel that their psoriasis started or became worse after stressful events such as a family death or financial problems. Stress may affect cortisol levels and provoke increased psoriasis severity

- **Atopic eczema**
  Adult atopic eczema is associated with depression, stress-related and behavioural disorders. It is difficult to separate out which aspects of behaviour are caused by the disease, and which by personality

Figure 49.1   Mind–skin–interpersonal interaction.

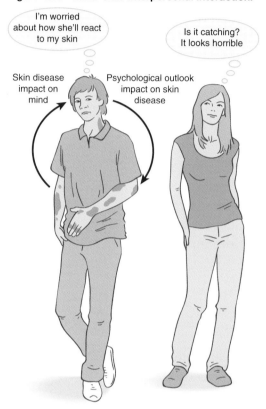

I'm worried about how she'll react to my skin

Is it catching? It looks horrible

Skin disease impact on mind

Psychological outlook impact on skin disease

Figure 49.2   Dermatitis artefacta – ulcers.

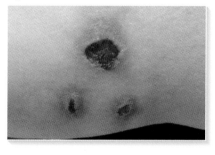

Figure 49.3   Factitial purpura, caused by sucking on a glass.

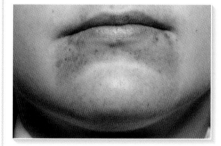

Figure 49.4   Dermatitis artefacta – odd shaped ulcerated areas left thigh.

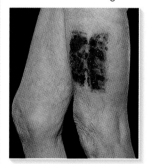

Figure 49.5   How itch leads to nodular prurigo.

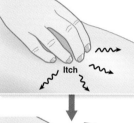

Itch

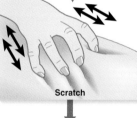

Scratch

Calendar
1 2 3 4 5 6 7
8 9 10 11 12 13 14

Lichen simplex

Calendar
Mar Apr May

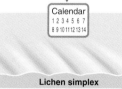

Nodular prurigo

Figure 49.6   Lichen simplex on elbow – thickening after frequent rubbing.

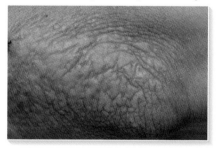

Figure 49.7   Nodular prurigo with excoriations.

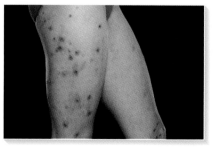

Dermatology at a Glance, Second Edition. Mahbub M.U. Chowdhury, Ruwani P. Katugampola, and Andrew Y. Finlay.
© 2020 John Wiley & Sons Ltd. Published 2020 by John Wiley & Sons Ltd.
Companion website: www.wiley.com/go/chowdhury/dermatology

Skin disease often results in psychological problems. As the skin is so visible and because it has such a major role in formal and intimate communication, relationships may be impaired and self-esteem lowered, resulting in distress that may be hard to resolve (Figure 49.1). The prevalence of depression is high in people with widespread skin disease; this is often unrecognised by their carers. Therefore, it is important in all patients to consider their psychological state, especially in chronic widespread inflammatory skin disease (Table 49.1). There are a few skin diseases in which psychological influences or mental illness have a major causative role.

Psychiatric and Skin Co-morbidity

- **Depression** – high prevalence in severe psoriasis.
- **Obsessive–compulsive disorder** (OCD) – may cause excessive scratching in atopic dermatitis. Hand dermatitis occurs with frequent hand washing.
- **Social phobia** – anxious avoidance of social situations where previously their skin condition resulted in problems.
- **Body dysmorphic disorder** – distorted self-image.

Skin Diseases Primarily Caused by Psychological and Psychiatric Problems

Factitious Dermatitis

Rarely, people deliberately damage their skin, sometimes repeatedly over many months or years. They draw attention to the damaged skin and seek treatment, but deny any knowledge of how it was caused: both lesions and history are false. They may cause non-healing ulcers by constantly picking at the skin (Figure 49.2), by injecting toxic matter, or by cigarette burns. Lesions may be odd shapes (Figures 49.3 and 49.4). Patients may gain by taking on a sickness role.

Management is very difficult. Clearly, the patient needs psychological help. It is debatable whether it is helpful to confront a patient with the diagnosis. A face-saving strategy is to allow the patient to retreat from the self-harming procedure without having to admit their responsibility for it.

Delusional Infestation (Parasitosis)

This is a monodelusion, a psychiatric disorder with a single focus in a person who otherwise functions normally. Patients become unshakeably convinced that they are infested by an insect or parasite, or have fibres in the skin. They convince friends and family of this and their partners may become convinced that they are also infested (folie à deux). 'Morgellons syndrome' is a descriptor now adopted by many patients whom most dermatologists and psychiatrists consider have delusional infestation.

Typically, patients bring in a small piece of matter that they claim is a parasite that they have squeezed out of their skin: invariably under the microscope there is no evidence of any parasite. Patients 'doctor shop', and often complain about their care, as they are convinced that they are 'infected' and do not accept that they have a psychiatric problem. Often homes have been fumigated after others have taken the patient's complaint at face value.

First examine the patient to make sure there is no infestation. Management then involves reaching an agreement with the patient that they have a problem (unspecified) that needs solving and prescribing anti-psychotics, e.g. amisulpride, olanzapine, or risperidone.

Dysmorphic Disorder

Most people have an inaccurate self-perception of how they look to others: for example, medical students when watching a video recording of themselves in a clinic may be surprised at how they appear. However, some people's self-perception is so widely distorted that their behaviour is inappropriately affected.

Body dysmorphic disorder may focus on different body aspects, such as weight or skin. A very small amount of physiological acne, barely visible to even a close observer, may be perceived as of huge significance and be blamed by the patient for problems in their life. The doctor's difficulty in not being able to see what the patient is concerned about resulted in the term 'dermatological non-disease'.

Patients may insist on powerful systemic therapy or on cosmetic procedures that do not appear to be indicated. Often, any procedure carried out does not satisfy the patient, with risks of complaints and litigation. There may be an association with OCD and there is a risk of suicide.

Management requires reaching agreement with the patient that there is distress and disability, and considering cognitive behaviour therapy or use of specific serotonin reuptake inhibitors.

Damaging Habits

Trichotillomania

There is shortening or baldness of scalp hair caused by the patient deliberately pulling individual hairs out. Children often deny doing this. A major clue is that the hairs in the affected area are usually of different lengths. In a child this is a sign of psychological distress but in an adult it may be a more serious sign of psychiatric disease.

Neurodermatitis

If you have itchy skin it is very difficult not to scratch (Figure 49.5) and current therapies for itch are not very effective. Repeated scratching results in damage to the skin, 'neurodermatitis'. To begin with there is superficial damage to the skin, 'excoriations' (scratches). Repeated trauma induces the skin protective mechanism of thickening, resulting in 'lichen simplex' (Figure 49.6). This is itchy itself, so the scratching and rubbing continue, eventually resulting in a lumpy or cobblestone appearance, 'nodular prurigo' (Figure 49.7).

The underlying skin disease is treated and topical steroids applied to the inflammatory changes, along with antibiotics if there are signs of secondary bacterial infection. Protection of the skin with occlusive bandages (where possible) is the single most useful technique, in order to break the vicious itch–scratch cycle.

Key Points

- Educational and psychological training programmes can improve the quality of life of patients with chronic skin disease.
- Psychodermatology conditions are ideally managed in joint dermatology/psychiatry clinics.

▶ Warning

- There is a suicide risk in body dysmorphic disorder: don't dismiss it.

50 Pruritus

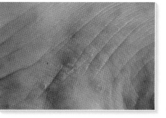

Figure 50.1 **The four types of itch.**

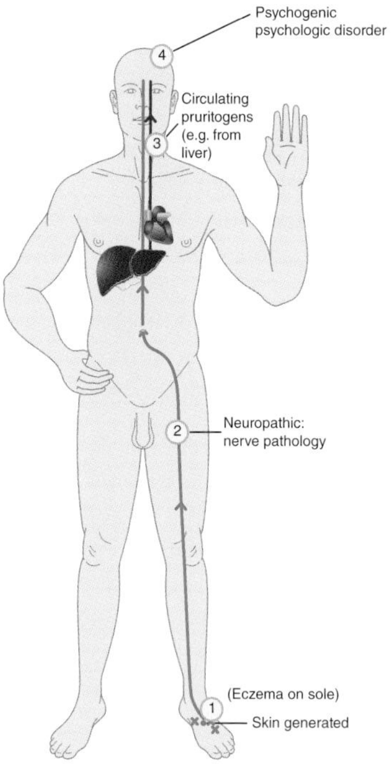

- 4 — Psychogenic psychologic disorder
- 3 — Circulating pruritogens (e.g. from liver)
- 2 — Neuropathic: nerve pathology
- 1 — (Eczema on sole) Skin generated

Figure 50.4 **Scabies** – on the palm.

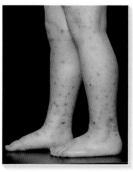

Figure 50.5 **Insect bites** – lower leg.

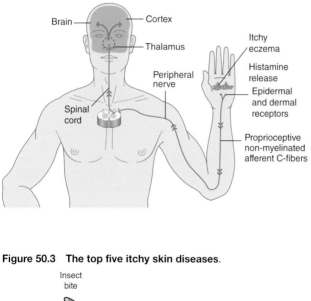

Figure 50.6 **Dermatitis herpetiformis** – sacral area.

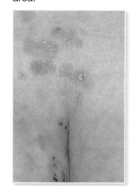

Figure 50.7 **Eczema.**

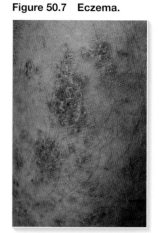

Figure 50.8 **Urticaria.**

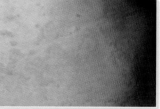

Figure 50.2 **The itch pathway** – skin generated itch.

- Brain
- Cortex
- Thalamus
- Itchy eczema
- Histamine release
- Epidermal and dermal receptors
- Peripheral nerve
- Spinal cord
- Proprioceptive non-myelinated afferent C-fibers

Figure 50.9 **Systemic (non-skin) causes of itch.**

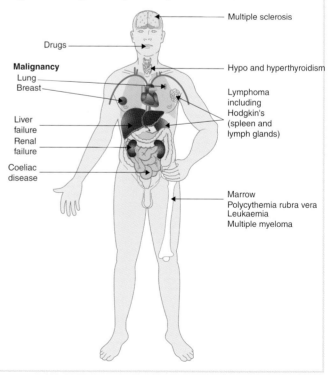

- Multiple sclerosis
- Drugs
- **Malignancy**
  - Lung
  - Breast
  - Liver failure
  - Renal failure
- Coeliac disease
- Hypo and hyperthyroidism
- Lymphoma including Hodgkin's (spleen and lymph glands)
- Marrow Polycythemia rubra vera Leukaemia Multiple myeloma

Figure 50.3 **The top five itchy skin diseases.**

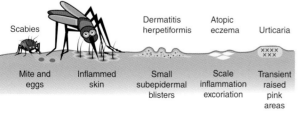

- Insect bite
- Scabies
- Dermatitis herpetiformis
- Atopic eczema
- Urticaria
- Mite and eggs
- Inflammed skin
- Small subepidermal blisters
- Scale inflammation excoriation
- Transient raised pink areas

Dermatology at a Glance, Second Edition. Mahbub M.U. Chowdhury, Ruwani P. Katugampola, and Andrew Y. Finlay.
© 2020 John Wiley & Sons Ltd. Published 2020 by John Wiley & Sons Ltd.
Companion website: www.wiley.com/go/chowdhury/dermatology

Introduction

Itch presumably evolved by conferring some survival benefit. Maybe scratching reduced the health impairment caused by being bitten by insects or other disease carrying predators. Or maybe itch allowed an animal to learn to avoid being bitten. Whatever its origin, itch is now experienced by people with inflammatory skin disease, and with systemic diseases. Although very distressing and common, itch treatment is still unsatisfactory. Itch is often more severe in the evening and during the night.

What Causes the Sensation of Itch?

The itch sensation is of course actually experienced in the cortex, fooling us into thinking that we feel it on (say) the hand. Itch may originate in four different ways (Figure 50.1):

1 **Skin generated** – usually by inflammation or other visible pathological processes involving the skin.
2 **Neuropathic** – caused by neuronal pathology along the afferent pathways.
3 **Neurogenic and systemic** – generated in the central nervous system in response to circulating chemicals that promote itch (pruritogens), but with no evidence of neural pathology.
4 **Psychogenic** – itching caused by a psychological disorder.

Histamine is the main chemical involved in the sensation of itch, but other neurotransmitters may also be involved. The itch sensation is transmitted from epidermal and dermal receptors to non-myelinated afferent C-fibres (I'm itching to C you). The impulses continue from the peripheral nervous system through to the thalamus and primary somatosensory cortex (Figure 50.2)

Itch in the Elderly

Itch in the elderly can be caused by any or all of the causes seen in adults, but is often multifactorial. 'Dry skin' (xerosis) is very common in the elderly by itself or along with other causes of pruritus.

Itch in Pregnancy

Pruritus of pregnancy affects 20% of pregnant women. Common causes include intrahepatic cholestasis, polymorphic eruption of pregnancy, and dry skin. Rare causes include pemphigoid gestationalis.

Intrahepatic cholestasis (pruritus gravidarum) is hormonally triggered (Chapter 33). A defect in bile acid secretion leads to raised serum bile acids. Severe pruritus starts on the palms and soles, in the second or third trimester. Treatment is with ursodeoxycholic acid. Although prognosis is generally good, severe intrahepatic cholestasis is associated with adverse foetal outcomes including premature labour or stillbirth.

Impact of Itch

Itch, the skin equivalent of pain, can have a major impact on quality of life, preventing sleep, and causing problems with social life, personal relationships, work, and study. The natural reaction is to scratch, but scratching damages the skin and can result in nodular prurigo (Chapter 49).

What Diseases Cause Itch?

Skin Diseases Causing Itch

Most inflammatory skin diseases cause some itch. However, some skin diseases cause especially intense severe itch (Figure 50.3), including scabies, insect bites, dermatitis herpetiformis, atopic eczema, and urticaria (Figures 50.4–50.8). Don't get caught out, early pemphigoid, before the blistering, is very itchy.

Systemic Diseases Causing Itch

Itch: the dashboard warning light (Go to the nearest garage! Or at least think and investigate).

Itch can be the presenting symptom of many systemic, non-dermatological diseases, including lymphoma, hypo- and hyperthyroidism, and liver and renal failure (Figure 50.9).

Management of Itch
Clinical Approach

1 Examine skin for primary skin lesions.
2 Systemic examination – check lymph nodes, liver, spleen, kidneys.
3 Only diagnose a psychological cause on the basis of a diagnostic psychological history, not on the absence of finding a physical cause (Chapter 49).

Treatments for Itch

The key to itch management is to make the correct diagnosis and to treat whatever disease is causing the itch. The evidence base for itch therapy is generally very poor: despite the high prevalence of pruritus there are few properly controlled trials.

Antihistamines

Antihistamines are only of benefit if the itch is caused by the release of histamine. 'Non-sedative' (or more accurately 'low-sedative') antihistamines such as cetirizine or loratadine are therefore effective in urticaria, but not in atopic eczema. Confusingly, 'sedative' antihistamines such as piriton cause drowsiness and so may appear to give some benefit in atopic eczema.

Corticosteroids

Topical or systemic corticosteroids may rapidly reduce pruritus in severe inflammatory skin disease such as atopic eczema. This is because they rapidly settle the inflammation, not by any direct anti-itch effect.

Menthol and Calamine

This 'old-fashioned' topical application is cooling and may provide some symptomatic relief.

How can you Measure Itch?

As for pain, it is not possible to directly measure itch sensation, but objective measurement of scratch is used as a surrogate. Wristwatch monitors can measure frequency of scratching, and for research purposes patients can be video-monitored during sleep.

More simply, itch can be measured with standardised patient completed questionnaires: there are many described, including ItchyQuant, 5-D Itch Scale, and the Itch Numeric Scale. Not all itch is the same: itch can vary in intensity, position, and course and have associated sensations such as pain, stinging, or burning. These distinctions can be recorded using questionnaires.

The impact of itch on life quality can be measured with a questionnaire specific for itch (e.g. ItchyQoL), or with a generic measure such as the DLQI.

Key Points
- Itch can be extremely distressing, it's the dermatology 'pain'.
- Itch may be the first clue to a systemic disease.

► Warning
- Never assume that itch is 'psychological'. Always examine carefully for skin or systemic disease.

Cosmetic Dermatology

Dr Maria Gonzalez

Table 51.1 **Glogau photoageing classification.** (This classification refers to patients with Fitzpatrick skin types I and II only.)

Severity	Age	Pigmentation	Wrinkles	Actinic keratoses
Type 1 = Mild	This is typical of someone who is usually aged between **28 and 35**	Minimal pigment change	There are few if any wrinkles or scars present	Keratosis is not yet visible
Type 2 = Moderate	Typically aged between **35 and 50**	The colour of the skin is sallow	Smile lines may start to become visible. Early signs of lines and wrinkles will be seen in motion, such as smile lines	Keratosis is palpable but not easily visible
Type 3 = Advanced	Typically aged between **50 and 65**	Obvious discolouration of the skin is evident. Telangiectasias often referred to as 'broken capillaries' are now very visible	Wrinkles are now apparent, even when not smiling	Keratosis present and visible
Type 4 = Severe	Aged between **60 and 75**	Sallow-yellow, greyish skin colour	Severe wrinkling throughout	Actinic keratosis, with or without skin cancer

Table 51.2 **Commonest cosmetic dermatology conditions, treatments and indications.**

Skin condition	Treatment and mechanism of action	Clinical indications	Precautions
Excess hair growth	Long pulsed lasers 1064 nm, 755 nm, 800 nm. Target pigment cells of hair follicles. Results in long-term reduction of facial and body hair	1064 nm – hair removal in Fitzpatrick (FP) skin types V/VI skin, 755 nm – types I–IV skin, 800 nm – types I–V skin	Wavelength of treatment must match the skin type to avoid complications including blister formation, pigmentary problems such as post-inflammatory hyper or hypopigmentation. Avoid treatment if patient's skin is tanned. Cooling of the skin essential during treatment
Pigmentation	Q-switched lasers (nanosecond pulses) 532 nm/1064 nm. Targets pigment cells (melanosomes) or tattoo ink breaking up the pigment into smaller fragments which are slowly scavenged by the body's immune system	Birthmarks (café au lait spots), freckles, photodamage (solar lentigos), tattoos (all colours but best results with black and red inks)	Caution in pigmented skin where complications more likely. 1064 nm safer in FP skin types V/VI
Facial redness	595 nm pulse dye laser. Target haemoglobin which heats up the vessels causing thrombosis and damage. Damaged vessel slowly scavenged by the immune system	Telangiectasia due to photodamage and rosacea. Red lesions such as port wine stains, spider naevi	Comparatively safe laser but often unsightly bruising required to obtain the best results in port wine stains (PWS) and other vascular lesions
Leg and facial veins	532 nm, 595 nm, 800 nm, 1064 nm lasers all used in the treatment of vessels. Target chromophore is haemoglobin	Superficial facial vessels respond better to shorter wavelengths such as 532 nm. Deeper vessels such as leg veins treated with longer wavelengths such as 1064 nm	Treatment not recommended in darker skin types such as FP skin types V/VI. However telangiectasia/leg veins not visible in darker skin so often not a cosmetic problem
Acne	Lasers have a limited effect on acne. Possible mechanisms of action include targeting of *P. acnes* or heating and damage to sebaceous glands. Conventional dermatological treatments remain the mainstay of treatment	Because of inconsistent results lasers best reserved for patients in whom conventional treatments are contraindicated. Mild inflammatory acne may improve for short periods with laser treatment	Treatment is safe but not very effective
Acne scarring	Treatments which cause limited wounding of the skin triggering a wound healing response with an increase in collagen production are most effective in treating acne scarring. CO_2 laser resurfacing most effective treatment for acne scarring. Microneedling and other devices such as radiofrequency devices also moderately effective	All forms of acne scarring suitable for these treatments but laser treatment of ice pick and rolling scars produce poor results. Surgical intervention with subcision or excision may be necessary	CO_2 laser resurfacing can cause hypopigmentation in darker skin types (FP skin types IV–VI). Alternatives such as microneedling or radiofrequency more appropriate. Fillers may be used for deeper scars

Dermatology at a Glance, Second Edition. Mahbub M.U. Chowdhury, Ruwani P. Katugampola, and Andrew Y. Finlay.
© 2020 John Wiley & Sons Ltd. Published 2020 by John Wiley & Sons Ltd.
Companion website: www.wiley.com/go/chowdhury/dermatology

145

Chapter 51 Cosmetic Dermatology

Table 51.3 Common treatments for facial rejuvenation.

Treatment	Mechanism of action	Clinical indications	Precautions
Botulinum toxin	Temporary weakening of muscle action by disrupting the release of acetylcholine at the neuromuscular junction. Duration of action is three months	Reduction of hyperdynamic lines of the face caused by muscle movement including frown lines (glabella lines), crows-feet lines, horizontal forehead lines. Indicated in patients with Glogau photodamage types 2–3	Not suitable in patients with myasthenia gravis. Caution in older patients in whom brow ptosis more likely if too much toxin injected into horizontal forehead rhytides
Dermal fillers	Hyaluronic acid injected into dermis and subdermal areas of the skin to volumise the skin	Patients in whom photodamage or intrinsic ageing have resulted in volume loss of the face usually due to atrophy of soft tissues such as skin, fat, and bone. Suitable for patients with Glogau photodamage types 2–4	Caution in patients with lupus or sarcoidosis because of risk of granuloma formation. Risk of blindness if injected into facial vessels which anastomose with ophthalmic arteries. Risk of skin necrosis if injected into facial vessels
Chemical peels	Epidermolysis/dermolysis induced by application of acidic chemical to the skin	Signs of photodamage including pigmentation (dyschromia) or roughness of the skin secondary to collagen damage. Results last for weeks to years depending on the depth and aggressiveness of the peel. Results can be prolonged by lifestyle changes which minimise sun exposure. Suitable for patients with Glogau photodamage types 1–4	Cannot be used in patients on oral isotretinoin as may cause scarring
Laser treatment	All available lasers may have a rejuvenating effect. The most commonly used lasers are those which target pigmentation e.g. non-ablative lasers (where the epidermis remains intact) and ablative lasers (where the epidermis is disrupted) which stimulate collagen production	Signs of photodamage including pigmentation (dyschromia) or roughness of the skin secondary to collagen damage. Results last for weeks to years depending on laser used. Results can be prolonged by lifestyle changes which minimise sun exposure. Suitable for patients with Glogau photodamage types 1–4	Caution necessary in pigmented skin as ablative lasers can cause prolonged pigmentation. Non-ablative lasers more suitable

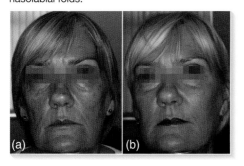

Figure 51.1 (a) A 60-year-old patient with features of photodamage including dyschromia, malar fat atrophy, and increased skin laxity. (b) Post treatment with a Q-switched 532 nm laser for treatment of epidermal hyperpigmentation and dermal fillers injected into the cheeks and nasolabial folds.

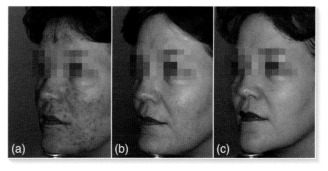

Figure 51.2 (a) A 45-year-old patient with multiple inflamed papules and pustules on extensive areas of the face supporting a diagnosis of rosacea. (b) Twelve weeks after successful treatment with lymecycline and ivermectin cream. (c) Marked improvement in skin texture and resolution of erythema following five treatments with the pulsed dye laser at intervals of six weeks.

Cosmetic dermatology is cosmetic enhancement of patients using cosmetic procedures such as botulinum toxin, dermal fillers, laser treatments, and cosmetic or cosmeceutical products. There is a blurring between clinical and cosmetic dermatology as conditions such as rosacea, acne, and photodamage merge into the practice of cosmetic dermatology. There is no consensus on what is truly a cosmetic treatment. In the UK the definition is also influenced by the limits of the health service where 'cosmetic' conditions may be denied treatment due to cost implications.

Motivation to Seek Cosmetic Treatment

Multiple factors will influence whether a patient seeks cosmetic treatments:

- Patient perception of own appearance
- Failure of make-up cover (e.g. large birthmarks, scars)
- Comments on appearance from colleagues, partner, peers
- Major life changes (e.g. divorce, new partner)

Medical Assessment and Contraindications

All patients requesting cosmetic treatment should have a thorough medical assessment.

The following cautions and contraindications need to be considered:

- **Skin cancer** – ensure no current malignancy before cosmetic procedures.
- **Multiple allergies or eczema** – sensitivity to cosmetic products, e.g. glycolic acid.
- **Herpes infection** – chemical peel may provoke permanent scarring, consider prophylactic aciclovir.
- **Recent oral isotretinoin** – unusual scarring may occur with chemical peels or laser therapy.

- **Psoriasis** – Koebnerisation at site of skin trauma caused by chemical peel or lasers.
- **Keloid scar history** – risk of inducing more scarring with chemical peel or lasers.
- **Lupus erythematosus** – dermal fillers may provoke delayed granuloma formation.

Skin 'Ageing' (Table 51.1)

Intrinsic ageing is the normal deterioration and atrophy of components of skin, bones, and cartilage occurring regardless of lifestyle. Extrinsic ageing is caused by patient lifestyle, such as excessive sun exposure, impacting on cosmetic appearance. Activities that increase oxidative stress in the skin increase cellular skin damage, with a reduction in collagen and elastin. This results in cosmetic changes including coarse and fine rhytides (wrinkles), multiple small vessels visible on the skin, dilatation of follicular ostia, loss of skin elasticity, or abnormal uneven pigmentation (dyschromia). Excessive sun exposure is the key cause of oxidative damage to the skin. However, smoking, excessive alcohol intake, high personal stress, and irregular sleep patterns may also contribute to oxidative damage.

Skin Type

Cosmetic concerns are influenced by the patient's skin type. The Fitzpatrick (FP) classification (Chapter 44 Phototherapy) categorises different skin types based largely on the skin's reaction to sunlight. People with the fairest skin (skin types I and II) are highly susceptible to the effects of sunlight and often seek cosmetic treatments for signs of photodamage including wrinkles, telangiectasia, and pigmentation. Darker skinned patients (skin types V–VI) are less affected by photodamage and tend to focus on signs of intrinsic ageing and pigmentary issues such as melasma.

Aims of Treatment

Most cosmetic dermatology treatments aim to produce greater facial symmetry, smooth convex facial contours, and homogenous skin tone and texture. This usually requires a combination of treatments. Dermal fillers and botulinum toxin are used to achieve facial symmetry and smooth contours. Chemical peels and laser treatments are focused on homogenous skin tone.

Commonest Cosmetic Dermatology Treatments (Tables 51.2 and 51.3)

Laser Treatment

Lasers use a specific wavelength of light to target appropriate chromophores in the skin depending on the aim of the treatment. The commonest target chromophores are melanin in pigmentary disorders, haemoglobin in vascular or red face problems, and collagen for targeting wrinkles and scars (Figures 51.1 and 51.2). Once these chromophores are targeted light energy is converted to heat energy resulting in damage to or stimulation of the target organelles.

Chemical and Physical Abrasion

Before the advent of lasers, skin rejuvenation techniques included the use of physical and chemical techniques to abrade or exfoliate the skin. These continue to be popular techniques largely because of the sometimes prohibitive cost of lasers and also because of the specialised training required for the use of lasers. Chemical peels are carried out using chemicals such as trichloroacetic acid, glycolic acid, and salicylic acid. These acids are used to lyse or destroy the bonds between the cells of the stratum corneum, epidermis, or dermis, depending on the strength of the peel. Once this occurs this section of the skin is lysed and 'peels' away over several days. The new skin which regenerates in its place is smoother with less defined wrinkles and improved pigmentation.

For physical abrasion a range of different types of equipment are used to remove the superficial layers of skin. The most popular technique for achieving this is microdermabrasion. This procedure utilises abrasive crystals or devices with metallic tips which abrade the skin. Their usage is more widespread among non-medical practitioners.

Injection of Dermal Fillers

The commonest dermal filler is made from hyaluronic acid, which is found normally throughout the skin. Hyaluronic acid is injected as a clear gel into the dermis, subdermis, and just above the bone (pre-periosteal area) to provide a lifting effect. This results in an improvement of skin contours and reduction in the appearance of rhytides (wrinkles). Most fillers persist in the skin for 6–12 months.

Injection of Botulinum Toxin

Botulinum toxin acts by blocking the release of acetylcholine at the neuromuscular junction. This results in partial paralysis of the muscle in which it is injected. This has the effect of smoothing the wrinkles caused by dynamic movement of the face. The most commonly treated areas are the forehead, glabella, and the crow's feet area around the outer corners of the eyes. The duration of action is three months.

Ethical Issues

Ethical considerations should play a role in all patient cosmetic consultations, as in other fields of medicine. Cosmetic dermatology clinics attract many patients with unrealistic expectations of what treatment can achieve. It is important to recognise that there are vulnerable patients that seek aesthetic treatments, including those with body dysmorphic disorder (Chapter 49) and also young patients easily influenced by celebrity media endorsements. Proper medical assessment must be carried out to ensure appropriate treatment is offered: the patient should understand the therapy being offered and be made aware of likely outcomes and risks.

Key Points

- A thorough medical assessment is essential for all patients considering cosmetic procedures.
- Avoid chemical peels and laser treatment after recent isotretinoin treatment.
- Provide honest and realistic options for all cosmetic treatments.

▶ Warning

- Beware unrealistic expectations of patients requesting cosmetic treatments especially those with body dysmorphic disorder.

52 Skin Breakdown

Table 52.1 Causes of leg ulceration.

- Venous disease 80%
- Arterial disease
- Vasculitis
- Trauma
- Burns
- Pressure sore
- Obesity
- Immobility
- Diabetes
- Peripheral neuropathy
- Cancer – basal or squamous cell cancer
- Pyoderma gangrenosum

Table 52.2 How to use Doppler to measure Ankle Brachial Pressure Index (ABPI).

1. Wrap blood pressure cuff around upper arm
2. Place Doppler probe over brachial artery in antecubital fossa (same site where stethoscope normally placed)
3. Inflate then slowly release pressure until Doppler detects return of pulse
4. Repeat on leg, with cuff around lower thigh and Doppler probe over artery behind medial ankle
5. If (ankle pressure)÷(arm pressure) > 0.9: no arterial disease

Table 52.3 The four phases of wound healing (Orstead et al. 2011).

Immediate	Haemostasis
Days 1–4	Inflammation
Days 4–21	Granulation and contraction
Day 21–2 years	Remodelling

Figure 52.1 Venous eczema with ill-defined erythema and crusting.

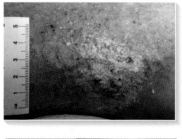

Figure 52.2 Atrophie blanche at ankle.

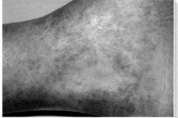

Table 52.4 Features to distinguish arterial ulcers from venous ulcers (Newton, 2011).

Arterial ulcers	Venous ulcers
History	**History**
Diabetes	Previous DVT
Hypertension	Recurrent phlebitis
Smoking	Varicose veins
Inability to elevate limb	Reduced mobility
Vascular disease	
Position	**Position**
Lateral malleolus	Gaiter area lower leg
Tibial area	Medial side
Pressure points	
Pain	**Pain**
Intermittent claudication	Throbbing, aching, heavy feeling legs
Worse at night and at rest	Improves with elevation, rest
Improves with dependency	
Ulcer characteristics	**Ulcer characteristics**
Punched out, occasionally deep	Shallow, flat margins
Irregular	Moderate exudate
Low exudate	
Lower leg	**Lower leg**
Thin shiny dry skin	Haemosiderin staining
Reduced hair	Thickening, fibrosis
Skin cool	Dilated veins
Pallor on elevation	Crusty dry eczematous skin
Weak/absent pedal pulses	Pedal pulses present
Delayed (>3 s) capillary refill	Normal rapid capillary refill
Development of gangrene	Limb oedema

Table 52.5 Burns assessment.

- **Burn Area assessment**
  - assess roughly using 'Rule of Nines' (Figure 52.9)
  - assess more accurately using Handprint concept
  - one Handprint area = approx. 1% body surface area (Chapter 12)
- **Burn Depth assessment**
  - *superficial partial* — epidermis lost
  - *deep partial* — epidermis and dermis lost
  - *full thickness* — epidermis, dermis, and subcutaneous fat lost

Assess clinically two days after burn. If no capillary refill after pressure or stretching, suggests deep partial or full thickness

Figure 52.3 Bilateral lipodermatosclerosis – firm woody feel.

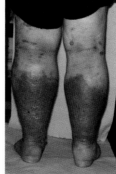

Figure 52.4 Venous ulcer at ankle with surrounding haemosiderin.

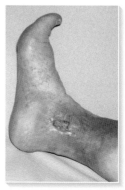

Dermatology at a Glance, Second Edition. Mahbub M.U. Chowdhury, Ruwani P. Katugampola, and Andrew Y. Finlay.
© 2020 John Wiley & Sons Ltd. Published 2020 by John Wiley & Sons Ltd.
Companion website: www.wiley.com/go/chowdhury/dermatology

Figure 52.5   Arterial ulcer on dorsum of foot with surrounding cellulitis.

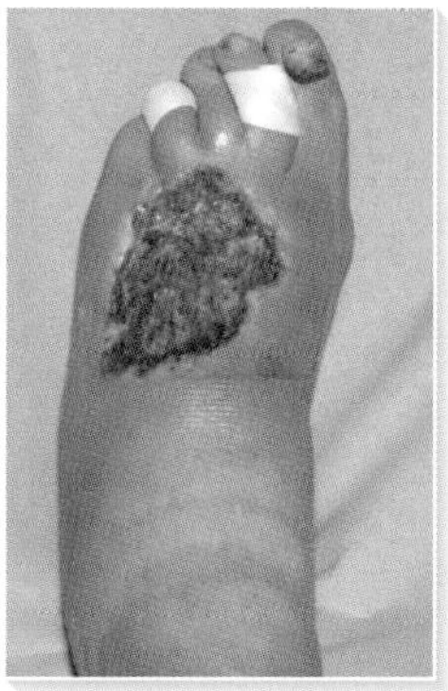

Figure 52.6   Neurotrophic ulcer, distal sole.

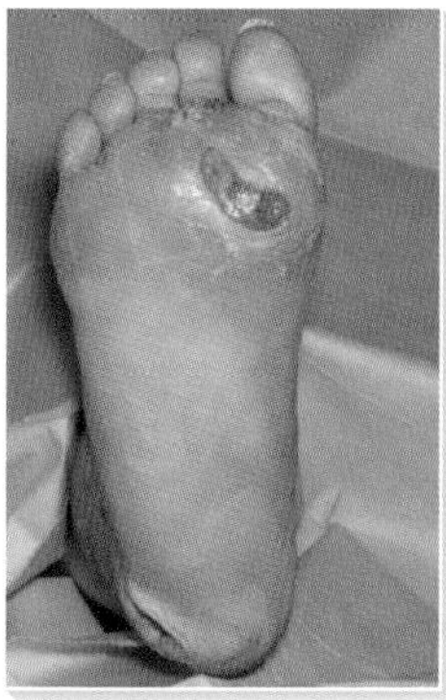

Figure 52.7   Burn of palm.

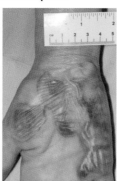

Figure 52.9   Rule of Nines, rough percentages to assess area of burns.

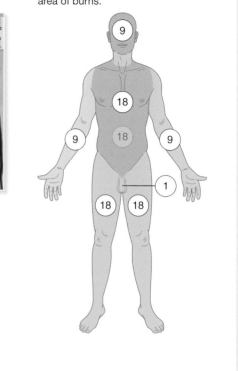

Figure 52.8   Burn reaction to cryotherapy.

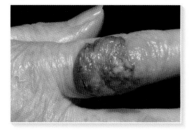

Leg Ulcers

An ulcer is defined as a break in the skin with loss of epidermis or also dermis. Leg ulcers have a major impact on quality of life causing social restriction and pain, costing a total of £940 million each year in the UK. There are many causes of leg ulcers (Table 52.1).

Venous Hypertension and Pathogenesis of Venous Ulcers

The pressure in the veins in the lower leg depends on the height of blood directly above pressing down: this is usually 0–20 mmHg. Disease of the veins, immobility, and obesity results in the valves in the large veins in the leg not working properly (incompetent) and so the pressure rises above 20 mmHg (venous hypertension). This high pressure results in leakage of fluid (oedema) and fibrin from the veins into the dermis. Fibrin cuffs form around the small veins in the dermis, causing venous insufficiency and ulceration.

Venous Eczema (Stasis Dermatitis, Gravitational Eczema, Varicose Eczema)

Occurs on the lower legs and is itchy. There is mild scaling with redness and oozing (Figure 52.1). The hyperpigmentation looks like melanin but is caused by dermal haemosiderin from red blood cells.

Treatment – emollients and low potency topical steroids.

Atrophie Blanche

Small white atrophic lesions typically near a painful lower leg ulcer, with red dots (large capillaries) visible. May suggest other systemic inflammatory disease (e.g. SLE) (Figure 52.2).

Lipodermatosclerosis

A hard painful 'wooden feeling' area around the lower leg, with overlying redness and palpable edge (Figure 52.3). The leg shape may look like an upside down cola or wine bottle. It is caused by long-standing venous hypertension, chronic inflammation, and fibrin in dermis and underlying fat. Often confused with cellulitis, but this is inflammation without infection. There is a high risk of ulceration. Compression may help long-term but is 'too late'.

Examination of Leg Ulcers

Ninety-five per cent of venous leg ulcers are near the ankles (Figure 52.4). Examine the nearby skin for atrophy, hair follicle loss, pitting oedema, pigmentation, or sign of other disease such as malignancy.

Management of Leg Ulcers

Investigations

* Measure ankle brachial pressure index (ABPI) (Table 52.2).
* Check haemoglobin, white cell count, or CRP (to detect infection), serum glucose, and sickle-cell test if at risk.
* Biopsy if malignancy suspected.

Venous Leg Ulcer Treatment: Compression Bandaging

Sustained compression is much more important to the outcome than the type of dressing. Only use if a Doppler study (Table 52.2) confirms no arterial disease. Evidence-based benefit with optimum healing taking four months if compression pressure is 40 mmHg at the ankle. Use four- or three-layer compression bandaging and elevate the leg when sitting or lying down. Obese or oedematous ankles need more bandages to maintain pressure. Encourage weight loss and increased mobility. Maintain treatment as 25% risk of recurrence after one year.

Antibiotics and Ulcers

All wounds have surface bacteria. Only treat pathogenic organisms if there is clinical evidence of bacteria doing harm. Give systemic antibiotics if surrounding cellulitis, redness, tenderness, or exudate of pus. Avoid topical antibiotics as they encourage growth of resistant organisms, do not reach the bacteria that cause cellulitis deep within the skin, and may cause contact dermatitis.

Risk of Allergic Contact Dermatitis

Multiple topical preparations may be used for chronic ulcers. The skin barrier is already broken so it is easy for allergens to get in (e.g. antibiotics, preservatives, lanolin, rubber in elastic bandages).

How an Ulcer Heals

There are four phases of wound healing (Table 52.3). Granulation tissue forms as an early response to injury. Re-epithelialisation starts from the edge and from any persisting appendages such as hair follicles within the ulcer. Newly formed keratinocytes migrate across the wound beneath the scab.

Other Ulcers

(Figures 52.5 and 52.6)

Pressure Sores

Normally people turn over during sleep, but they cannot turn if immobile (e.g. after a stroke). If over many days the pressure of the weight of the body goes through one area such as a bony prominence, the skin will become relatively ischaemic and may ulcerate. Pressure sores must be prevented by regular turning of immobile patients and by using special weight distributing mattresses. Pressure sores take months to heal and can be disastrous, complicating rehabilitation after illness. Bed sore frequency is an indicator of the quality of nursing care.

Arterial Ulcers

Occur on toes, feet, shins, with well-defined edges and severe pain (Figure 52.5). Most common cause atheroma: essential to stop smoking. It is important to distinguish between venous and arterial ulcers (Table 52.4).

Treatment – if ABPI very low, surgery to restore blood flow.

Pyoderma Gangrenosum

Ulcers occur at odd sites, with undermined purple edges. Associated with rheumatoid arthritis, inflammatory bowel disease, leukaemia, and IgA monoclonal gammopathy. High dose systemic steroids are indicated.

Burns (Table 52.5; Figures 52.7–52.9)

Burns may be from fire, electricity, or chemicals and cause permanent scarring, major disability, or death. Common in mobile infants (e.g. cooker, hot water): there is a need for prevention strategies.

Emergency treatment – put out the flames (e.g. by rolling the person in a blanket), and cool the injured site with cold water. Maintain airway and get to hospital fast.

Management – fluid replacement; careful estimation as over-hydration can be dangerous. Control pain and maintain body core temperature. Consider transfer to specialised burns unit.

Long-term management – management of scarring and risk of squamous cell carcinoma in scars (Marjolin ulcers).

Key Points
- Compression bandaging is critical for venous leg ulcers.
- Do not confuse lipodermatosclerosis with cellulitis.

▶ Warning
- In venous eczema there is a risk of cellulitis or ulceration, consider pressure stockings.

53 Hereditary Skin Diseases

Table 53.1 Examples of hereditary skin disease and their mode of inheritance.

- **Autosomal recessive (AR)** – xeroderma pigmentosa (XP) (Chapter 45), recessive dystrophic epidermolysis bullosa (EB)
- **Autosomal dominant (AD)** – ichthyosis vulgaris, Darier's disease, epidermolysis bullosa simplex, bullous ichthyosiform erythroderma, neurofibromatosis 1, tuberous sclerosis (TS)
- **X-linked recessive (XLR)** – X-linked recessive ichthyosis
- **X-linked dominant (XLD)** – incontinentia pigmenti (IP)

Table 53.2 What to do when a hereditary skin disease is suspected.

- Detailed clinical history, including detailed family history of the suspected disease manifestations
- Thorough clinical examination of the affected individual and, when possible, other affected relatives
- Blood from index case and, when possible, relatives for DNA analysis to identify disease-causing mutation(s)
- Skin biopsies may be required for histological examination for characteristic features of the disease
- Refer patient and relatives for genetic counselling, prenatal and/or antenatal counselling and testing

Table 53.3 Characteristics of some inherited ichthyoses.

Disease	Inheritance	Pathogenesis	Clinical features
Ichthyosis vulgaris (Figure 53.1)	AD	Filaggrin gene mutations	Fine scales on trunk, large scales on legs, spares flexures
X-linked recessive ichthyosis (Figure 53.2)	XLR	Reduced steroid sulphatase	Affects males, females are carriers. Fine to large dark scales on trunk, limbs, and sides of face. Female carriers: delayed labour with male infants
Bullous ichthyosiform erythroderma (Figure 53.3)	AD	Keratin 1 or Keratin 10 mutations	Erythroderma and blistering at birth and neonatal period followed by marked hyperkeratosis on trunk and limbs, with a velvety appearance, prominent on flexures
Netherton syndrome	AR	SPINK5 gene mutations	Erythroderma, double-edged scale, bamboo appearance of hair-shafts, high serum IgE
Harlequin ichthyosis	AR	ABCA12 gene mutations	Thick, large plates of scale encase the neonate at birth. Most die within few weeks

Table 53.4 The main types of epidermolysis bullosa (EB).

Disease	Inheritance	Pathogenesis	Clinical features	Level of blister formation in the skin (Figure 21.1)
EB simplex	AD	Abnormal keratin 5 or 14	Blistering mainly of the palms and soles	Epidermis (intraepidermal)
Junctional EB	AR	Abnormal laminin or type XVII collagen	Skin fragility with denuded skin, often on axillae and groins, may be more widespread	Lamina lucida and lamina lucida-densa interface of the basement membrane
Dystrophic EB	AD or AR	Type VII collagen	Hands and feet with marked scarring and deformities	Sublamina densa of the basement membrane

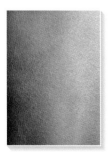

Figure 53.1 Ichthyosis vulgaris – note the fine scaling on the trunk.

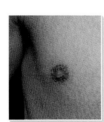

Figure 53.2 X-linked recessive ichthyosis – note the dark scales on the chest wall.

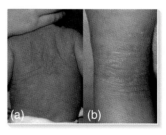

(a)   (b)

Figure 53.3 Bullous ichthyosiform erythroderma. (a) Note the generalised erythroderma and scaling of the trunk. (b) Note the marked hyperkeratosis with a velvety appearance on flexures.

Dermatology at a Glance, Second Edition. Mahbub M.U. Chowdhury, Ruwani P. Katugampola, and Andrew Y. Finlay.
© 2020 John Wiley & Sons Ltd. Published 2020 by John Wiley & Sons Ltd.
Companion website: www.wiley.com/go/chowdhury/dermatology

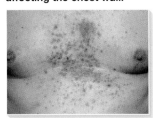

Figure 53.4   Darier's disease affecting the chest wall.

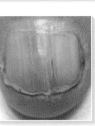

Figure 53.5 Notching of the distal nail plate in Darier's disease.

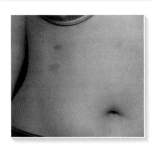

Figure 53.6 Café-au-lait macules in neurofibromatosis 1 (NF1).

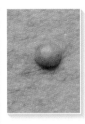

Figure 53.7 Neurofibroma in neurofibromatosis (NF1).

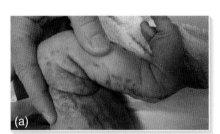

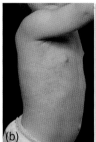

(a)   (b)

Figure 53.8   Incontinentia pigmenti (IP). (a) Note the blisters on an erythematous background in a linear distribution on the limbs during the neonatal period. (b) Note the streaks and whorls of macular hyperpigmentation from about six months onwards.

The human genome, which compromises over three billion DNA base pairs, was first mapped in 2003 through an international collaborative project, the Human Genome Project. Advanced technology has led to the ability to sequence the genome to aid research, diagnosis, and impact on clinical management in a vast number of diseases including rare genetic diseases, polygenic common diseases, and cancers. These new sequencing techniques include whole genome sequencing, whole exome sequencing, and targeted sequencing where a specific group of predetermined genes known to cause a specific phenotype are sequenced. Identification and understanding of the genetic basis of diseases has led to research into potential gene therapy for rare, severe hereditary skin diseases such as epidermolysis bullosa (EB). Gene therapy aims to correct the disease-causing genetic abnormality or defect via viral mediated ex-vivo DNA or RNA transfer into patient's skin cells in culture, as in EB. The use of viral vectors is however, associated with the risk of insertional mutagenesis, and therefore these techniques will need further refining prior to use in routine clinical practice.

There are a vast number of hereditary skin diseases. Examples of hereditary skin diseases and the clinical approach are summarised in Tables 53.1 and 53.2.

Ichthyoses

These are a group of inherited disorders resulting in abnormal keratinisation, differentiation, and desquamation of the epidermis (Table 53.3). They are characterised by generalised scaling of the skin to varying degrees from mild (ichthyosis vulgaris) to severe life-threatening (harlequin ichthyosis). Ichthyoses usually present at birth, in the neonatal period, or early infancy. Presence or absence of erythroderma or blistering, distribution, and features of the scale help to differentiate between the ichthyoses.

Diagnosis can often be made clinically and confirmed by the characteristic histological features on skin biopsy ± DNA analysis to identify disease causing mutation(s) ± biochemical analysis for defect in disease-causing molecules.

Treatment is symptomatic, aimed at decreasing the hyperkeratosis: topical emollients, keratolytics (10% urea or 5% salicylic acid), retinoids. Oral retinoids (acitretin) may dramatically improve some forms of ichthyosis. However, the benefits of lifelong use need to be weighed against its potential side effects and the risk of its use in women of childbearing age (teratogenic).

Epidermolysis Bullosa

A group of inherited disorders where different disease-causing mutations result in defects in the structural proteins of the basement membrane (Chapter 21, Figure 21.1). Characterised by skin fragility and blistering following minor trauma, ulceration, and infection of wounds followed by scarring.

Mucosal surfaces may be affected: eyes, gastro-intestinal tract (e.g. dysphagia due to oesophageal strictures may lead to nutritional deficiencies and complications such as iron-deficiency anaemia).

There are three main types, with many subtypes of varying severity according to the level of blister formation in the skin (Table 53.4).

Diagnosis is made clinically and confirmed by the characteristic electron microscopic features on skin biopsy and DNA analysis.

Treatment is supportive and aimed at:
- **Avoiding or minimising skin trauma** – use of foam pads to pressure points, elbows, and knees; non-adherent dressing for wounds.
- **Avoiding or managing infected wounds** with antibiotics.
- **Nutritional support** – multivitamin and iron supplementation.
- **Monitoring** chronic non-healing wounds for evidence of malignant transformation to squamous cell carcinoma (SCC), and its prompt treatment, in the dystrophic forms of EB.

Darier's Disease

An autosomal dominant disease: mutations in the *ATP2A2* gene on chromosome 12 interfere with intracellular Ca^{2+} signalling. Characterised by red–brown, keratotic, crusted papules on the trunk and face which are often prone to secondary bacterial infection (Figure 53.4), palmar pits, and notching of distal nail plate (Figure 53.5).

Treatment – antimicrobial washes, keratolytic emollients (with 10% urea), topical retinoids or corticosteroids, oral retinoids (acitretin).

Neurofibromatosis 1 (NF1)

An autosomal dominant neurocutaneous disease: mutations in the neurofibromin gene on chromosome 17 result in loss of its tumour suppressor effect and uncontrolled cell growth.

Cutaneous manifestations – café-au-lait macules (Figure 53.6). These are light brown macules up to several centimetres in diameter that develop in childhood, ≥ 6 macules is one of the diagnostic features of NF1. Neurofibromas are derived from peripheral nerves and their surrounding tissue (Figure 53.7). These are multiple soft, pedunculated, skin-coloured nodules that develop in older children and young adults. Large, painful, plexiform neurofibromas and axillary freckling may also develop.

Extracutaneous manifestations – ocular (Lisch nodules on iris, optic nerve glioma), neurological (involvement of the spinal cord or brain with neurofibromas), malignant change (sarcomas).

Diagnosis is made clinically; can be confirmed on DNA analysis. MRI of brain and spinal cord is required for symptomatic patients. No specific treatment is available except surgical excision of troublesome or disfiguring neurofibromas.

Tuberous Sclerosis (TS)

This is an autosomal dominant neurocutaneous disease caused by mutations in genes encoding tumour suppressor proteins harmartin (chromosome 9) and tuberin (chromosome 16).

Cutaneous manifestations – ash-leaf macules (oval, hypopigmented macule(s) appear in infancy), adenoma sebaceum (firm, skin-coloured/erythematous papules of the face, especially on the nasolabial region, appear in childhood), shagreen patches (skin-coloured patch with papular surface, usually seen on the lower back), periungual fibromas (firm, skin-coloured papules).

Extra-cutaneous manifestations – neurological (seizures, learning disabilities), ocular (retinal phacomas: grey–yellow plaques near the optic disc), tumours (cardiac rhabdomyomas, angiomyolipomas, astrocytomas).

Diagnosis is made clinically; can be confirmed on DNA analysis. MRI is helpful in identifying tumours. There is no specific cure for TS. Surgical or laser treatment can be useful for disfiguring or troublesome adenoma sebaceum and periungual fibromas, and adenoma sebaceum responds to topical rapamycin.

Incontinentia Pigmenti (IP)

This is an X-linked dominant disease that affects the skin, hair, nails, teeth, eye, and central nervous system. It is caused by mutations in the inhibitor of nuclear factor kappa-B kinase subunit gamma (*IKBKG*) gene on chromosome X, a gene involved in cell survival, immunity, and inflammation. IP is seen mainly in females, as it is lethal in male foetuses due to the single affected X chromosome; surviving males have been found to be 47XXY.

Cutaneous manifestations – the skin involvement often corresponds to Blaschko lines. Blaschko lines are invisible lines that correspond to epidermal cell migration during embryogenesis. These are linear on the limbs and circumferential on the trunk. Unlike dermatomes, they do not correspond to spinal cord levels or innervations. The four stages in IP are characteristic, and include: (i) blisters on an erythematous background usually noted in the neonatal period to about four months of age, on the trunk and in a linear distribution on the limbs, usually sparing the face (Figure 53.8a), followed by (ii) a warty rash for the next few months, (iii) streaks and whorls of macular hyperpigmentation from about six months onwards (Figure 53.8b), (iv) linear atrophic hypopigmentation. Other features include alopecia and pitting, ridging, or hypertrophy of nails.

Extracutaneous manifestations – dental (hypodontia, complete absence of teeth, conical teeth), eyes (retinal neovascularisation, increased risk of retinal detachment in infancy and early childhood), central nervous system (seizures, learning disabilities).

Diagnosis is made clinically; can be confirmed on DNA analysis. Regular ophthalmological surveillance is essential for early detection of retinal detachment. Management of the skin includes trying to keep the skin clean and blisters intact to reduce the risk of superadded infection.

Xeroderma Pigmentosa

See Chapter 45.

Key Points

- A detailed family history is essential in inherited skin diseases.
- Genetic counselling should be offered to those with inherited skin diseases.
- The mainstay of management of ichthyosis is emollients and/or keratolytics and acitretin for severe cases.
- For EB, try to prevent skin trauma and wound infections.
- Inherited skin diseases may be associated with extracutaneous complications.

▶ Warning

- Some inherited skin diseases are complicated by malignant transformation of skin or extracutaneous tissue.
- Oral retinoids (acitretin) can be beneficial in the ichthyoses. However, acitretin is teratogenic so use it with extreme caution in women of childbearing age.

Clinical Picture Quiz

Answer True or False to the following questions.

Case 1

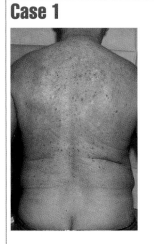
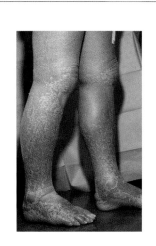

This man presented with a widespread, red, scaly rash affecting most of his face, body, arms, and legs. He had a previous history of well-defined scaly plaques on his knees and elbows.
1 *This patient has erythroderma.*
2 *The most likely underlying cause for this patient's current skin status is psoriasis.*
3 *This patient is at risk of hyperthermia.*
4 *This patient is at risk of cardiac failure.*
5 *All patients with this skin manifestation should be treated with systemic steroids.*

Case 2

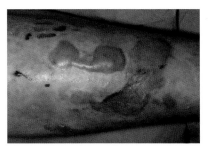

An elderly patient presented with tense, itchy blisters on his legs and trunk.
1 *The most likely diagnosis is bullous pemphigoid.*
2 *The oral mucosa is never affected in this skin disease.*
3 *Direct immunofluorescence is used to confirm the diagnosis.*
4 *This patient's skin blistering may be associated with coeliac disease.*
5 *Localised areas of this condition can be treated with topical steroids.*

Case 3

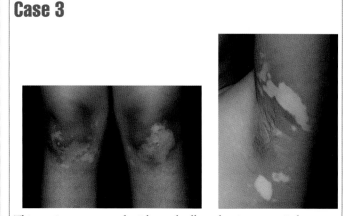

This patient presented with gradually enlarging, non-itchy, non-scaly white patches on both knees and axillae.
1 *The most likely diagnosis is vitiligo.*
2 *May be associated with thyroid disease.*
3 *Topical corticosteroids should not be used for treating this condition.*
4 *UVB or UVA phototherapy can be used to treat this condition.*
5 *Repigmentation following treatment may be patchy.*

Case 4

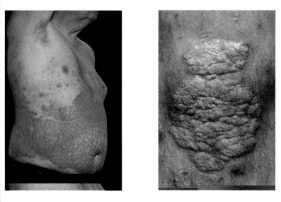

This patient presented with a several year history of thick, scaly, erythematous plaques on his trunk, elbows, and knees.
1 *The most likely diagnosis is psoriasis.*
2 *This rash typically occurs in an asymmetrical distribution.*
3 *The scalp, nails, and joints may be affected in this condition.*
4 *This disease does not demonstrate Koebner's phenomenon.*
5 *Widespread disease can be treated with UVB phototherapy.*

Dermatology at a Glance, Second Edition. Mahbub M.U. Chowdhury, Ruwani P. Katugampola, and Andrew Y. Finlay.
© 2020 John Wiley & Sons Ltd. Published 2020 by John Wiley & Sons Ltd.
Companion website: www.wiley.com/go/chowdhury/dermatology

Case 5

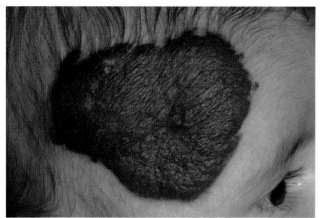

This rapidly growing red lesion appeared within the first few weeks of life of this otherwise well infant.
1 *The most likely diagnosis is a vascular malformation.*
2 *These lesions usually regress spontaneously over years.*
3 *These lesions may bleed and/or ulcerate.*
4 *These lesions should always be treated with systemic steroids.*
5 *Oral propranolol is used to treat these lesions if they interfere with function or rapidly enlarge.*

Case 6

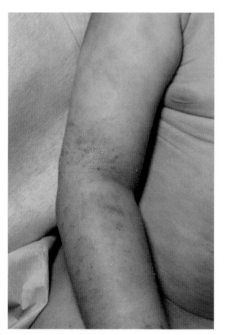

This child gave a history of an itchy, dry rash since the age of three months. The rash affected the face, body, and limbs, and was worse on the skin creases of limbs.
1 *The most likely diagnosis is atopic dermatitis.*
2 *Epidermal barrier function is usually defective in this condition.*
3 *Pitting of nails is a common finding in these patients.*
4 *This rash may be complicated by herpes simplex virus infection.*
5 *Topical corticosteroids are the treatment of choice in this condition.*

Case 7

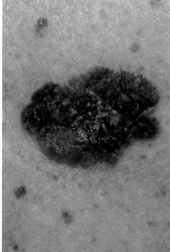

What is the diagnosis for this presentation and what other lesions could this be confused with?
1 *The incidence of this type of skin growth is reducing.*
2 *These cause 80% of skin cancer deaths.*
3 *Red hair increases the risk of developing melanoma.*
4 *Change in shape of a mole suggests possibility of melanoma.*
5 *A partial skin biopsy is ideal for diagnosis.*

Case 8

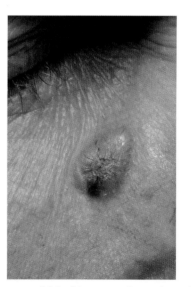

What different types of this skin cancer do you know?
1 *This is the most common type of human malignancy.*
2 *These tumours are aggressive and grow rapidly.*
3 *A biopsy is always needed to confirm the diagnosis.*
4 *Mohs' surgery is indicated for treatment of ill-defined skin cancers.*
5 *These occur in sun-exposed sites.*

Case 9

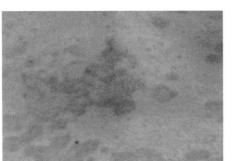

What is the diagnosis of this presentation and what history would you need to take?

1 *This condition is usually non-itchy.*
2 *The chronic form lasts more than six weeks.*
3 *Bizarre shapes can occur.*
4 *Angioedema of the face is rare.*
5 *The mainstay of treatment is antihistamines.*

Case 10

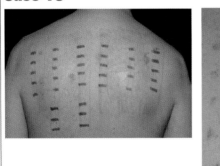 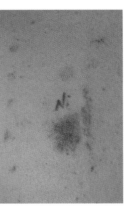

What test is shown here and what are the indications?

1 *This test detects type I allergy.*
2 *This test detects type IV allergy.*
3 *This test can diagnose irritant contact dermatitis.*
4 *Allergic contact dermatitis caused by nickel is common.*
5 *Allergic contact dermatitis can coexist with atopic eczema.*

Case 11

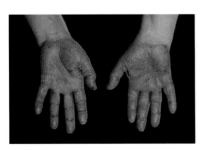

What is the most likely diagnosis for this presentation?

1 *This condition is usually itchy.*
2 *Psoriasis of the hands can be made worse with friction.*
3 *Tinea usually affects both hands.*
4 *Hairdressers are at increased risk of this condition.*
5 *Potent topical steroids are indicated.*

Case 12

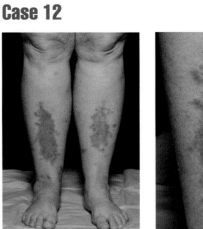 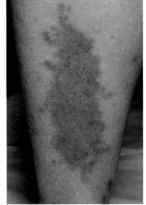

What is this condition?

1 *This occurs in diabetics.*
2 *This usually occurs on the legs.*
3 *This can be treated with topical steroids.*
4 *This can be treated with phototherapy.*
5 *This improves with better diabetic control.*

Case 13

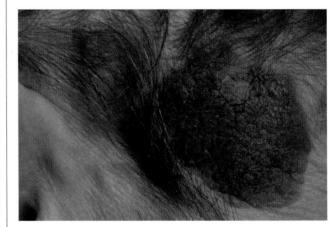

What is the most likely diagnosis for this presentation?

1 *These lesions are benign.*
2 *These commonly occur on the trunk of the elderly.*
3 *These can be of variable pigmentation.*
4 *These always need to be removed.*
5 *These have no malignant potential.*

Case 14

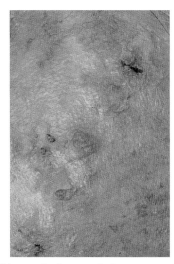

This 87-year-old man had noticed these non-itchy, scaly, rough patches on his scalp for many years. He was an ex-builder and had worked outdoors for most of his life.
1 *The most likely diagnosis is solar keratosis.*
2 *These are related to his previous occupation.*
3 *There is a risk of basal cell carcinoma.*
4 *The scalp is a commonly affected site.*
5 *Biopsy is not essential.*

Case 15

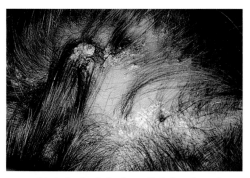

This 45-year-old lady had had well-defined, itchy, thickened plaques on her scalp for six months. She noticed they got worse with sun exposure. On examination, there were signs of follicular plugging, scarring, and some telangiectasia.
1 *This condition can cause severe scarring.*
2 *There is a risk of systemic disease.*
3 *Potent topical steroid can be used for facial disease.*
4 *Raised white cell count can occur.*
5 *Hydroxychloroquine can be very effective treatment.*

Case 16

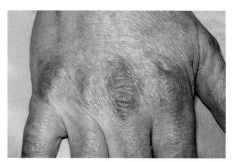

This 76-year-old gentleman presented with this rash on his hands and a periorbital blue–purple rash. He had noticed difficulty brushing his hair and walking up stairs in the last three months.
1 *The diagnosis is a connective tissue disease.*
2 *This disease can be linked with underlying malignancy.*
3 *Nail fold changes are uncommon.*
4 *Serum creatinine kinase is usually low.*
5 *Systemic steroids are used commonly as treatment.*

Case 17

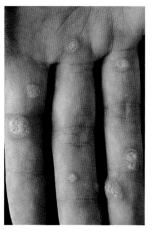

This 13-year-old child presented with unsightly, non-itchy lumps on the fingers. His older brother also had similar lesions.
1 *These lesions are contagious.*
2 *These are caused by a bacterial infection.*
3 *Treatment with cryotherapy is essential.*
4 *Salicylic acid-based preparations can be used.*
5 *Immunosuppressed adults are prone to these.*

Case 18

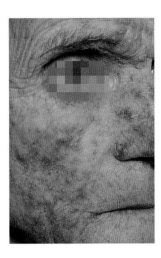

This 55-year-old gentleman had facial flushing and redness with occasional pustules. He liked eating spicy food with a few beers on a frequent basis.

1 *The most likely diagnosis is acne.*
2 *Scaling is unlikely to be seen.*
3 *There may be signs of eye disease.*
4 *Oral tetracyclines are not indicated.*
5 *Pulse dye laser may be helpful.*

Case 20

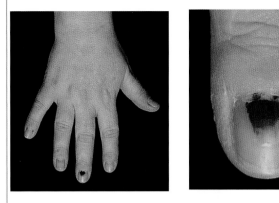

This 25-year-old woman presented with a few weeks' history of pigmentation of her right middle finger nail. She gave a history of having caught her finger in a door a few weeks previously. She was otherwise well and not on any medication.

1 *The most likely diagnosis is a subungual melanoma.*
2 *Pigmentation of the posterior nail fold is highly suggestive of a subungual melanoma.*
3 *A longitudinal nail biopsy should be undertaken on any suspicious pigmented subungual lesions to exclude or confirm a diagnosis of melanoma.*
4 *Longitudinal melanonychia is a normal finding in racially pigmented individuals.*
5 *Nail discolouration is an uncommon feature of fungal nail infections.*

Case 19

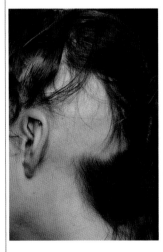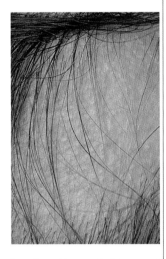

This 25-year-old woman presented with a 12-month history of patchy hair loss. Some patches of hair loss spontaneously regrew. She was otherwise well, apart from a history of vitamin B12 deficiency for which she was on replacement therapy.

1 *The most likely diagnosis is alopecia areata.*
2 *The vitamin B12 deficiency may be relevant to her hair loss.*
3 *The scalp is not the only affected part of the body in this type of hair loss.*
4 *Scalp biopsy is essential to confirm the diagnosis.*
5 *Topical steroids are a treatment option for this condition.*

Case 21

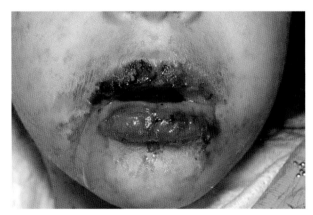

This 7-year-old girl complained of a sore mouth and eyes with peeling and crusting of the lips a day after commencing antibiotics for a chest infection.

1 *The most likely diagnosis is herpes simplex (cold sore).*
2 *Immediate management includes stopping the antibiotic.*
3 *Systemic steroids are curative.*
4 *The child needs to be managed in a high dependency unit with supportive care.*
5 *Ophthalmology input is essential in the management of this child.*

Case 22

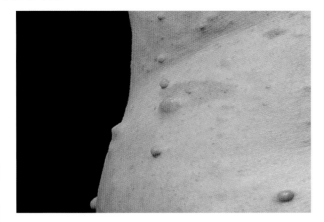

This 30-year-old woman requested removal of some of the soft, skin-coloured nodules on her skin which were getting irritated when rubbing on her clothing. She gave a history of multiple brown patches (at least 15 lesions) on her skin at different body sites since early childhood. Since her mid-teens, she recalls developing these multiple skin coloured nodules. On examination, she was also noted to have freckling in both axillae. She was otherwise well.

1 *The most likely diagnosis is neurofibromatosis 1.*
2 *The multiple brown patches on her skin are not diagnostic of this condition.*
3 *A detailed family history is relevant in this patient.*
4 *The patient has a 50% chance of passing on this condition to her children.*
5 *This patient should also be seen by an ophthalmologist.*

Case 23

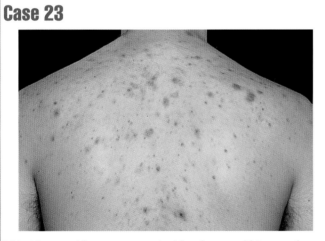

This 18-year-old man presented with a few years' history of worsening 'spots' on his face, neck, chest, and back that were starting to leave unsightly scars. He had tried numerous over the counter skin creams with no improvement. He was requesting some treatment as the appearance of his skin was now starting to affect him socially, especially preventing him going swimming.

1 *The most likely diagnosis is acne.*
2 *Acne is a disease of the pilosebaceous units of the skin.*
3 *Comedones are a common feature of acne and rosacea.*
4 *Scarring is a potential complication of acne.*
5 *Female patients of childbearing age treated with isotretinoin should be counselled about its teratogenic effects.*

Case 24

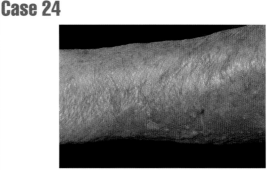

This 51-year-old patient had developed tenderness, redness, and swelling on the right forearm over the last week. The patient had well-controlled diabetes. On examination, there was scaling and fissuring on the right palm.

1 *This patient has cellulitis.*
2 *The palmar rash may have facilitated infection getting into the skin.*
3 *Antibiotics should not be given as they may lead to resistance.*
4 *Long-term prophylaxis antibiotics may reduce the likelihood of recurrence.*
5 *When affecting the lower leg, cellulitis can be confused with lipodermatosclerosis.*

Case 25

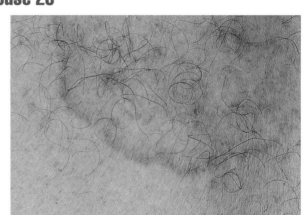

This 35-year-old patient has noticed itchiness on the chest over the last two weeks. On examination there is a well-defined, red rash with minimal visible scale.

1 *The most likely diagnosis is erythrasma.*
2 *The toe webs should be examined as 'athlete's foot' can lead to fungal infection elsewhere.*
3 *As there is little scale, this rash is probably not fungal.*
4 *Scrapings should be taken from the edge of the rash for mycology.*
5 *The treatment of choice for localised dermatophyte infection is topical terbinafine.*

Case 26

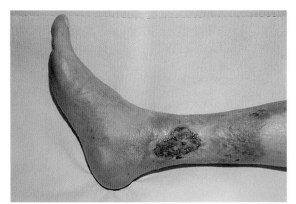

This 60-year-old, non-smoking patient presented with an ulcerated area near the left lateral malleolus. There was a history of a DVT in this leg 15 years previously. On examination the patient was in pain.
1 *The most likely diagnosis is venous ulcer.*
2 *The Ankle Brachial Pressure Index should be measured.*
3 *Compression bandaging should be avoided as it may increase the pain.*
4 *Any bacteria isolated from wound swab culture should be treated with antibiotics.*
5 *Treatment of venous ulcers may cause allergic contact dermatitis.*

Case 27

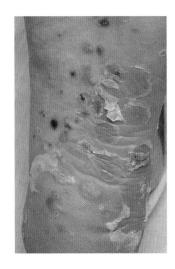

This 35-year-old man has had a persisting problem of recurrent pustules on his palms and soles over the last eight years. He is otherwise well.
1 *This is probably a type of localised psoriasis.*
2 *Swabs from the pustules grow streptococci.*
3 *Antibiotics are the treatment of choice.*
4 *Oral retinoids are effective, but value limited by side effects.*
5 *Palmoplantar pustulosis is an autosomal dominant condition.*

Case 28

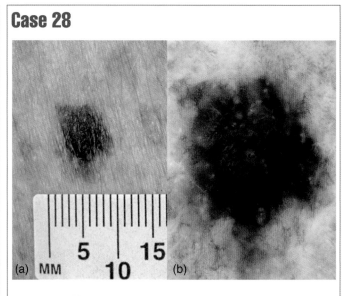

A 52-year-old man presented with a non-symptomatic, growing mole on his back. Figure A shows the clinical appearance and Figure B shows the dermoscopy image.
1 *This is a benign seborrhoeic keratosis and no treatment is required.*
2 *It is a benign dermatofibroma and no treatment is required.*
3 *It is suspected melanoma and urgent excision is needed.*
4 *It is a benign reticular naevus and the patient can be reassured.*
5 *It is a basal cell carcinoma and excision is needed.*

Case 29

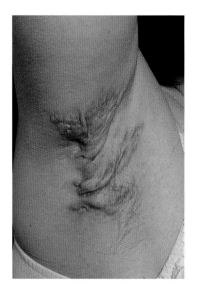

This lady presented with a several year history of inflammatory nodules and abscesses affecting both axillae, resulting in rope-like scars.
1 *This patient has hidradenitis suppurativa.*
2 *A skin biopsy is required to confirm the diagnosis.*
3 *Smoking is a risk factor for the condition.*
4 *Long-term penicillin-based antibiotics help to prevent flares.*
5 *Management of acute flares includes pain relief.*

Case 30

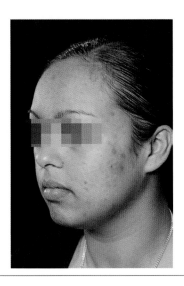

This 26-year-old female patient with scarring acne has been on a six-month course of oral isotretinoin which she completed one week ago. Today she requested treatment for the post-inflammatory hyperpigmentation (PIH) that has occurred as a result of her acne. She is also keen to have treatment to improve the scars on her cheeks.

1 CO_2 laser resurfacing should be started immediately.

2 Microneedling treatment will eradicate a significant number of ice pick scars.

3 Pulsed dye laser treatment may be useful for improving pigmentation secondary to post-inflammatory hyperpigmentation.

4 Q-switched Nd:YAG 1064 nm laser treatment is the safest laser for treating PIH in this patient.

5 Q-switched Nd:YAG 532 nm laser treatments would provide excellent results for PIH treatment in this patient.

Clinical Picture Quiz Answers

Case 1

1 True (for further details on erythroderma see Chapter 20).
2 True. The clinical description of the patient's previous rash is suggestive of psoriasis (for further details on psoriasis see Chapter 15).
3 False. Patients with erythroderma are at risk of hypothermia.
4 True
5 False

Case 2

1 True (for further details on bullous pemphigoid see Chapter 21).
2 False
3 True (for further details on immunofluorescence see Chapter 21).
4 False. Dermatitis herpetiformis (not pemphigoid) can be associated with coeliac disease (for further details on dermatitis herpetiformis see Chapter 21).
5 True

Case 3

1 True (for further details on vitiligo see Chapter 42).
2 True
3 False
4 True
5 True

Case 4

1 True (for further details on psoriasis see Chapter 15).
2 False
3 True
4 False. Koebner's phenomenon is the appearance of skin lesions on sites of trauma, often in a linear distribution. The following skin diseases demonstrate this phenomenon: psoriasis, lichen planus, vitiligo, viral warts, molluscum contagiosum.
5 True (for further details on phototherapy see Chapter 44).

Case 5

1 False. This is an infantile haemangioma (for further details on haemangiomas and differentiating features between vascular malformation and infantile haemangiomas see Chapter 31).
2 True
3 True
4 False
5 True

Case 6

1 True (for further details on atopic dermatitis see Chapter 16).
2 True
3 False (for further details on nail pitting see Chapter 30).
4 True
5 True (for further details on topical corticosteroids see Chapter 12).

Case 7

1 False
2 True
3 True
4 True
5 False

Discussion

This is a malignant melanoma (for diagnostic criteria and types of melanoma see Chapter 40).
• Other pigmented lesions that most commonly cause confusion with malignant melanoma include moles, pigmented basal cell carcinomas, and seborrhoeic keratoses.
• Malignant melanoma incidence has increased steadily over the last 40 years. A full excision with a 2 mm margin is ideal for initial diagnosis. A partial biopsy can be difficult to interpret histologically (e.g. depth: Breslow thickness) to determine prognosis.

Case 8

1 True
2 False
3 False
4 True
5 True

Discussion

This is a basal cell carcinoma (BCC) (Chapter 39 for types of BCC).
• BCCs are slow growing and usually only locally invasive, metastasis is very rare.
• Initial clinical diagnosis can be sufficient for most BCCs with histological confirmation after removal. However, a biopsy is required if there is any doubt.
• Sun exposure is an important risk factor for BCC.

Dermatology at a Glance, Second Edition. Mahbub M.U. Chowdhury, Ruwani P. Katugampola, and Andrew Y. Finlay.
© 2020 John Wiley & Sons Ltd. Published 2020 by John Wiley & Sons Ltd.
Companion website: www.wiley.com/go/chowdhury/dermatology

Case 9

1 False
2 True
3 True
4 False
5 True

Discussion

This is urticaria (for history points see Chapter 37 and Table 37.2).
- Urticaria is usually very itchy and this can be the main problem in some patients.
- Chronic urticaria lasts longer than six weeks with no cause found in 80%.
- Bizarre shapes such as annular patterns can be seen.
- Angioedema of the face including lips and eyelids can occur in up to 50% of patients.
- Antihistamines are the main treatment used (Table 37.4).

Case 10

1 False
1 True
2 False
3 True
4 True

Discussion

This shows the back four days after the patch tests were applied. A nickel allergy reaction is seen (Chapter 35).
- Patch testing is a specialised technique applying allergens to the back to detect delayed type IV hypersensitivity. This does not diagnose irritant contact dermatitis but excludes allergic contact dermatitis if negative.
- Nickel is the most common metal allergen detected. Exposure is common in many metal objects such as jewellery.
- Any patient with treatment resistant atopic or endogenous eczema should have patch testing to exclude allergic contact dermatitis.

Case 11

1 True
2 True
3 False
4 True
5 True

Discussion

This picture shows hand eczema (Chapter 36).
- This is usually itchy and 5–10% of the population are affected during their life. Other differential diagnoses include psoriasis and tinea (Table 36.1).
- Psoriasis can be worsened with friction and tinea manuum is usually unilateral.
- Certain occupations (e.g. hairdressing) are more prone to hand eczema including irritation and allergy.
- Potent topical steroids can be used for short periods (e.g. six weeks).

Case 12

1 True
2 True

3 True
4 True
5 False

Discussion

This is necrobiosis lipoidica (Chapter 46).
- Necrobiosis lipoidica occurs in diabetics and usually affects the shins. Better diabetic control does not lead to improvement.
- Topical steroids and PUVA phototherapy can be used but both may be unsatisfactory.

Case 13

1 True
2 True
3 True
4 False
5 True

Discussion

This shows a seborrhoeic keratosis (Chapter 38).
- Seborrhoeic keratoses are benign and very common on the trunk of elderly patients.
- Variable pigmentation of seborrhoeic keratoses can cause diagnostic confusion with malignant melanoma. However, they have no malignant potential and do not need to be removed if clinical diagnosis is confident.

Case 14

1 True
2 True
3 False
4 True
5 True

Discussion

These are solar keratoses commonly seen on the scalp and other sun-exposed sites (Chapter 38).
- Outdoor occupations will increase the risk of developing solar keratosis especially in fair-skinned individuals.
- Biopsy is not essential unless changes such as tenderness, increase in size, and inflammation occur which may indicate transformation to squamous cell carcinoma.

Case 15

1 True
2 True
3 True
4 False
5 True

Discussion

This shows discoid lupus erythematosus (Chapters 28 and 47).
- Progression to systemic lupus erythematosus (SLE) occurs in 1–5% of cases. Low white cell count can be a sign of SLE.
- Very potent and potent topical steroids can be used on the face for this condition to prevent permanent facial scarring.
- Hydroxychloroquine (anti-malarial drug) can be an effective treatment.

Case 16

1 True
2 True
3 False
4 False
5 True

Discussion

This is dermatomyositis which is an idiopathic inflammatory myopathy (Chapter 47).
• This can be linked with underlying malignancy (paraneoplastic) especially in elderly patients.
• Proximal muscle weakness is a classical sign which should be enquired about. Nail fold changes such as dilated capillaries are common. Serum creatinine kinase is usually raised.
• Systemic steroids are the mainstay of treatment with steroid-sparing agents such as methotrexate.

Case 17

1 True
2 False
3 False
4 True
5 True

Discussion

These are viral warts seen in a child (Chapter 24).
• They are caused by human papilloma virus and can be contagious especially in young children.
• Treatment is not essential and cryotherapy can be painful in young children. Salicylic acid-based preparations can be used but not on the face.
• Immunosuppressed adults are more prone to multiple viral warts e.g. HIV infection, transplant patients on long-term ciclosporin.

Case 18

1 False
2 True
3 True
4 False
5 True

Discussion

This is rosacea (see Chapter 28 on how to differentiate from other facial rashes).
• Acne usually affects teenagers and younger adults and comedones are a common feature.
• Rosacea is not scaly and can present with eye diseases such as keratitis and iritis.
• Oral tetracyclines are the mainstay of treatment if papules and pustules are present. Pulse dye laser can be effective treatment for telangiectasia.

Case 19

1 True
2 True
3 True
4 False
5 True

Discussion

This is alopecia areata, which can affect the scalp, and other hair-bearing sites (Chapter 30). There may be a personal or family history of other autoimmune diseases. The diagnosis can be made clinically without the need for a scalp biopsy. Diagnostic features are patchy, non-scarring alopecia on normal scalp skin with or without presence of exclamation mark hairs.

Case 20

1 False
2 True
3 True
4 True
5 False

Discussion

This is a subungual haematoma supported by the history of preceding trauma. However, if a subungual melanoma is suspected, a nail biopsy will help with the diagnosis (Chapter 30). Yellow–brown, crumbly, thickened nails are a common feature of fungal nail infections or 'onychomycosis' (Chapter 25).

Case 21

1 False
2 True
3 False
4 True
5 True

Discussion

This is Stevens–Johnson syndrome (SJS; Chapter 20). In this child, the most likely cause is the antibiotic. Use of systemic steroids to manage SJS is controversial due to increased risk of sepsis. Management includes identifying and withdrawing the underlying cause and supportive care to prevent complications.

Case 22

1 True
2 False
3 True
4 True
5 True

Discussion

This is neurofibromatosis 1 (NF1; Chapter 53). NF1 is inherited in an autosomal dominant manner, and therefore 50% of an affected individual's children are likely to inherit the disease. In some affected individuals there may be a family history of NF1, whereas in others, the disease may develop due to a new mutation in the neurofibromin gene. Having ≥6 café au lait macules is one of the diagnostic features of NF1. Individuals with NF1 need an ophthalmology review in view of its ocular manifestations including Lisch nodules of the iris and optic nerve gliomas.

Case 23

1 True
2 True
3 False
4 True
5 True

Discussion

This is acne, a disease of the pilosebaceous units of the skin, the pathogenesis which is multifactorial (Chapter 17). Comedones are a feature of acne, but not of rosacea (Chapter 28). Scarring from acne can range from subtle pitted to keloid scars. The aim of treatment is to control the disease and prevent scarring.

Case 24

1 True
2 True
3 False
4 True
5 True

Discussion

Cellulitis (Chapter 23) is often 'caused' by bacteria gaining entry via the disordered barrier function of skin. Systemic antibiotics are needed to treat bacterial cellulitis. There is evidence that long-term, low dose, prophylactic antibiotics may reduce the likelihood of recurrence. Lipodermatosclerosis of the leg at first glance may look very similar to cellulitis. However, lipodermatosclerosis has a very "woody", tough feel and the patient has no systemic signs of infection.

Case 25

1 False
2 True
3 False
4 True
5 True

Discussion

An itchy rash with a well-defined edge is most likely a fungal dermatophyte infection (Chapter 25). Erythrasma is a possible cause of a rash in the flexures, but is less likely. Toe web dermatophyte infection may be the source. A fungal rash may not be scaly either because topical creams may have been applied or because the rash is in the flexures.

Case 26

1 True
2 True
3 False
4 False
5 True

Discussion

This is most likely a venous ulcer (Chapter 52). Ankle brachial pressure index (ABPI) should be measured to confirm that there is not also an arterial problem. Compression bandaging is the treatment of choice: patients should be warned that it may be uncomfortable. The many different components of topical applications may lead to allergic contact dermatitis (Chapter 35).

Case 27

1 True
2 False
3 False
4 True
5 False

Discussion

There is some controversy over whether palmoplantar pustulosis is a subtype of psoriasis (Chapter 15). It has a very distinctive presentation. The pustules are sterile and antibiotics are not indicated.

Case 28

1 False
2 False
3 True
4 False
5 False

Discussion

Dermoscopy (Chapter 11) does not show features of seborrhoeic keratosis (comedo-like openings, milia-like cysts), basal cell carcinoma (arborizing vessels), or dermatofibroma (structureless centre with a delicate peripheral network). The presence of network and globules indicate a melanocytic lesion. However, the pigment network is asymmetrical in colour and structure, and there are scattered globules indicating growth. Hence this is suspicious of a malignant melanoma which requires urgent excision (Chapter 40).

Case 29

1 True
2 False
3 True
4 False
5 True

Discussion

For further details on hidradenitis suppurativa see Chapter 18. The diagnosis is primarily clinical. Long-term tetracyclines can be beneficial or the combination of clindamycin and rifampicin for 10–12 weeks.

Case 30

1 False
2 False
3 False
4 True
5 False

Discussion

This patient has darker Fitzpatrick skin type (IV–VI). These patients often develop prolonged pigmentation in the site of previous lesions following inflammatory conditions such as acne (Chapter 51).

• Treatments such as CO_2 laser resurfacing, microneedling, and chemical peels are all contraindicated in patients who are having treatment with oral isotretinoin or within six months of completing the course of treatment due to a high risk of irregular scarring.

• Pulsed dye laser treatment is effective in treating erythema of the skin as seen in rosacea and vascular problems such as port wine stains. It has no impact on pigmentary problems such as post-inflammatory hyperpigmentation (PIH).

• The safest and most effective treatment for PIH in this patient would be treatment with a Q-switched Nd:YAG 1064 nm laser.

• Q-switched Nd:YAG 532 nm lasers treat epidermal pigmentation and are not suitable for patients with darker Fitzpatrick skin types (IV–VI). As PIH is a dermal condition 532 nm lasers are unlikely to have any impact on this condition and may actually burn pigmented skin and worsen PIH.

References

Feldman, S.R. (2010). The prime directive for enhancing patients' medical experience. *Journal of Dermatological Treatment* 21 (4): 217.

Finlay, A.Y. and Chowdhury, M.M.U. (eds.) (2007). *Specialist Training in Dermatology*. Edinburgh: Elsevier.

Meulenberg, F. (1997). The hidden delight of psoriasis. *British Medical Journal* 315: 1709.

Newton, H. (2011). Wound essentials 6: leg ulcers: differences between venous and arterial. *Wound Essentials* 6: 26.

Orstead, H.L., Keast, D., Forest-Lalande, L. et al. (2011). Basic principles of wound healing. *Wound Care Canada* 9 (2): 4–12.

Companion website: www.wiley.com/go/chowdhury/dermatology

Index

Page locators in *italics* indicate figures/tables/boxes. This index uses letter-by-letter alphabetization.